MEDICINE RESEARCH SUMMARIES

MEDICINE RESEARCH SUMMARIES

VOLUME 17

(WITH BIOGRAPHICAL SKETCHES)

MEDICINE RESEARCH SUMMARIES

Additional books in this series can be found on Nova's website
under the Series tab.

Additional e-books in this series can be found on Nova's website
under the eBooks tab.

MEDICINE RESEARCH SUMMARIES

VOLUME 17

(WITH BIOGRAPHICAL SKETCHES)

ZHONGWEN LIÁNG
AND
BIBAO ZHANG
EDITORS

nova biomedical
New York

NOTICE TO THE READER

The Publisher has taken reasonable care in the preparation of this book, but makes no expressed or implied warranty of any kind and assumes no responsibility for any errors or omissions. No liability is assumed for incidental or consequential damages in connection with or arising out of information contained in this book. The Publisher shall not be liable for any special, consequential, or exemplary damages resulting, in whole or in part, from the readers' use of, or reliance upon, this material. Any parts of this book based on government reports are so indicated and copyright is claimed for those parts to the extent applicable to compilations of such works.

Independent verification should be sought for any data, advice or recommendations contained in this book. In addition, no responsibility is assumed by the publisher for any injury and/or damage to persons or property arising from any methods, products, instructions, ideas or otherwise contained in this publication.

This publication is designed to provide accurate and authoritative information with regard to the subject matter covered herein. It is sold with the clear understanding that the Publisher is not engaged in rendering legal or any other professional services. If legal or any other expert assistance is required, the services of a competent person should be sought. FROM A DECLARATION OF PARTICIPANTS JOINTLY ADOPTED BY A COMMITTEE OF THE AMERICAN BAR ASSOCIATION AND A COMMITTEE OF PUBLISHERS.

Additional color graphics may be available in the e-book version of this book.

Library of Congress Cataloging-in-Publication Data

ISBN: 978-1-53612-751-5
ISSN: 2168-6467

Published by Nova Science Publishers, Inc. † New York

CONTENTS

PREFACE

This new book compiles biographical sketches of top professionals in the field of medicine as well as research summaries from a number of different focuses in this important field.

Part I

Researcher Biographical Sketches

In: Medicine Research Summaries. Volume 17
Editors: Zhongwen Liáng and Bibao Zhang
ISBN: 978-1-53612-751-5

Chapter 1

Yangzom Doma Bhutia

Affiliation:
Texas Tech Univ. Health Science Center

Address:
3601 4th St Stop 6540
Lubbock TX, 79430, US
Phone: 806-743-1282
E-mail: yangzom.d.bhutia@ttuhsc.edu

Education:

2004- 2008	Ph.D. Veterinary Medicine, Indian Veterinary Research Institute, Izatnagar, Uttar Pradesh, India
2001- 2004	M.V.Sc. Clinical Veterinary Medicine, Acharya N.G. Ranga Agricultural University, Andhra Pradesh, India
1996- 2001	B.V.Sc. & A.H. (DVM), Marathwada Agricultural University, Parbhani, Maharashtra, India

Research and Professional Experience:

2014- Current	Research Assistant Professor
2013-2014	*Assistant Research Scientist*, Georgia Regents University, Augusta GA, 30912
2011-2013	*Postdoctoral Fellow*, Georgia Regents University, Augusta GA, 30912
2009-2011	*Postdoctoral Fellow*, School of Pharmacy, University of Georgia, Athens GA, 30602
2008-2009	*Research Assistant*, Central Zoo Authority, Ministry of Environment and Forests Indian Veterinary Research Institute, Izatnagar, Uttar Pradesh, India

Honors:

- AAPS Exceptional Abstract & Podium Presentation Award, AAPS Workshop on Drug Transporters, Washington DC-2011.

- Qualified Indian Council of Agricultural Research (ICAR)-National Eligibility Test (ICAR-NET) as an eligibility for teaching Life Sciences- (2008).
- Awarded Senior Research Fellowship (SRF) at the Indian Veterinary Research Institute (IVRI)- (2004- 2008).
- Awarded Junior Research Fellowship (JRF) by the Indian Council of Agricultural Research (ICAR)- (2001- 2004).
- Awarded Indian Council of Agricultural Research (ICAR) State Education Fellowship- (1996-2001).

Publications Last 3 Years:

1. Bhutia, Y.D., Babu, E., and Ganapathy, V. (2014). Interferon-γ induces a tryptophan-selective amino acid transporter in human colonic epithelial cells and mouse dendritic cells. *Biochim Biophys Acta.* 1848(2): 453- 462.
2. Bhutia, Y.D., Babu, E., Prasad, P.D., and Ganapathy, V. (2014). The amino acid transporter SLC6A14 in cancer and its potential use in chemotherapy. *Asian Journal of Pharmaceutical Sciences.* Review Article.
3. Ananth, S., Gnana-Prakasam, J. P., Bhutia, Y. D., Martin, P. M., Smith, S. B., and Ganapathy, V. (2013) Regulation of the cholesterol efflux transporters ABCA1 and ABCGl in retina in hemochromatosis and by the endogenous siderophore 2,5-dihydroxybenzoic acid. *Biochim Biophys Acta.* 1842(4): 603-12.
4. Hung, S.W., Mody, H., Marrache, S., Bhutia, Y.D., Davis, F., Cho, J.H., Zastre, J., Dhar, S., Chu, C.K., and Govindarajan, R. (2013) Pharmacological reversal of histone methylation presensitizes pancreatic cancer cells to nucleoside drugs: In vitro optimization and novel nanoparticle delivery studies. *PLoS One* 8(8): e71196.
5. Bhutia, Y.D., Hung, S.W., Krentz, M., Patel, D., Lovin, D., Manoharan, R., Thomson, M., and Govindarajan, R. (2013) Differential processing of *let-7a* precursors influences RRM2 expression and chemosensitivity in pancreatic cancer: Role of LIN-28 and SET oncoprotein. *PLoS One* 8:e53436.

Abstracts

1. Coothankandaswamy, V., Cao, S., Xu, Y., Ganapathy, V. and Bhutia, Y. 2014. "The amino acid transporter SLC6A14 is an effective drug target for treatment of pancreatic cancer". *AACR Annual Meeting*, San Diego, CA, April 5- 9.
2. Ellappan, B., Bhutia, Y.D., Thangaraju, M., Prasad, P.D. and Ganapathy, V. 2014. "Genetic deletion or pharmacologic blockade of the amino acid transporter Slc6a14 in mice suppresses breast cancer induced by Polyoma middle T oncogene". *AACR Annual Meeting*, San Diego, CA, April 5- 9.
3. Hung, S.W., Mody, H., Marrache, S., Bhutia, Y.D., Davis, F., Cho, J.H., Dhar, S., Chu, K.K. and Govindarajan, R. 2013. "Optimized DZNep exposure presensitizes pancreatic cancer cells to anticancer nucleoside analogues: potential clinical implications". *AACR Annual Meeting*, San Diego, CA, April 5- 9.

In: Medicine Research Summaries. Volume 17
Editors: Zhongwen Liáng and Bibao Zhang

ISBN: 978-1-53612-751-5

Chapter 2

Raquel Munhoz da Silveira Campos

Affiliation:

Post-graduate Program of Nutrition, Universidade Federal de São Paulo, São Paulo-SP, Brazil

Address:

Rua Cardeal Arcoverde, 1183 apto. 43, Pinheiros, CEP: 05407-001 São Paulo/SP Brazil

Date of Birth:

5/26/1983

Education:

Master degree (Msc)

Publications Last 3 Years:

1. Campos, Raquel M.S.; Masquio, Deborah Cristina Landi; Corgosinho, Flavia Campos; Carvalho-Ferreira, J. P.; Netto, B. D. M.; Ackel-Delia, C.; Tock, L.; Tufik, Sergio; Mello, Marco Túlio De; Damaso, A. Low Vitamin D Intake is Associated with Increase in Cardiovascular Risk Factors in Obese Adolescents. *Endocrine Regulations* (Print), v. 49, p. 11-19, 2015.
2. Carvalho-Ferreira, J. P.; Masquio DCL; Campos, RMS; Netto, B. D. M.; Corgosinho, Flavia; Sanches, P. L.; Tock, Lian; Tufik, S; Mello, MT; Finlayson G; Dâmaso, Ana R. Is there a role for leptin in the reduction of depression symptoms during weight loss therapy in obese adolescent girls and boys? *Peptides* (New York, N.Y. 1980), v. 25, p. 20-28, 2015.
3. Masquio DCL; de Piano, A; Campos, RMS; Sanches, P. L.; Corgosinho, F. C.; Carantti DA; Tock, L.; Mello, M. T.; Tufik, Sergio; Damaso, A. R. . Cut-off values of waist circumference to predict metabolic syndrome in obese adolescents. *Nutrición Hospitalaria*[JCR], v. 31, p. 1540-1550, 2015.
4. Campos, RMS; Mello, MT; Tock, Lian; Silva, Patricia L.; Masquio, Deborah C.L.; de Piano, A; Carnier, J.; Sanches, Priscila L.; Corgosinho, Flavia; Foschini, D.; Tufik, S; Dâmaso, Ana R. Aerobic Plus Resistance Training Improves Bone

Metabolism and Inflammation in Adolescents who Are Obese. *Journal of Strength and Conditioning Research*, v. 28, p. 758-766, 2014.

5. Netto, B. D. M.; Masquio, Deborah C.L.; CAMPOS, RMS; Sanches, Priscila L.; Corgosinho FC; Tock, L.; Oyama LM; de Mello, Marco Túlio; Tufik S; Dâmaso, Ana R. The High Glycemic Index Diet Was An Independent Predictor To Explain Changes In Agouti -Related Protein In Obese Adolescents. *Nutrición Hospitalaria*^{JCR}, v. 29, p. 305-314, 2014.
6. Damaso, A.; Campos, RMS; Carantti DA; de Piano, A; Fisberg, M.; Foschini, D.; Sanches PL; Tock, L.; Lederman, H. M.; Tufik, S; Mello, MT. Aerobic plus Resistance Training was more effective in improving the visceral adiposity, metabolic profile and inflammatory markers than Aerobic Training in Obese Adolescents. *Journal of Sports Sciences* (Print)^{JCR}, v. 32, p. 1435, 2014.
7. Ackel-D'elia, Carolina; Campos, RMS; Masquio DCL; Netto, B. D. M.; Sanches PL; Corgosinho FC; Clemente, A. P.; Carvalho, J.; Tock, L.; Tufik S; Mello M T; Damaso, A. . Aerobic plus resistance training on pro-anti-inflammatory adipokinesin obese adolescents. European Journal of Sports and Exercise Science, v. 1, p. 1, 2014.
8. Inoue, Daniela Sayuri; De Mello, Marco Túlio; Foschini, Denis; Lira, Fabio Santos; De Piano Ganen, Aline; Da Silveira Campos, Raquel Munhoz; De Lima Sanches, Priscila; Silva, Patrícia Leão; Corgosinho, Flávia Campos; Rossi, Fabrício Eduardo; Tufik, Sergio; Dâmaso, Ana R. . Linear and Undulating Periodized Strength Plus Aerobic Training Promote Similar Benefits and Lead to Improvement of Insulin Resistance on Obese Adolescents. *Journal of Diabetes and its Complications*, v. 1, p. 01-07, 2014.
9. Masquio DCL; de Piano, A; Sanches PL; Corgosinho FC; Campos, RMS; CARNIER, J.; Silva PL; Carantti DA; Tock, L.; Oyama LM; Oller do Nascimento CM; Mello M T; Tufik S; Dâmaso A R . The effect of weight loss magnitude on pro-/anti-inflammatory adipokines and carotid intima-media thickness in obese adolescents engaged in interdisciplinary weight loss therapy. *Clinical Endocrinology* (Oxford. Print), v. 19, p. n/a-n/a, 2013.
10. Campos, RMS; Mello M T; Silva PL; Corgosinho, Flavia Campos; Carnier, June; de Piano, A; Sanches PL; Masquio DCL; Tufik S; Dâmaso, Ana R. . Interaction of Bone Mineral Metabolism, adipokine and hormones in obese adolescents girls submitted in an interdisciplinary therapy. *Journal of Pediatric Endocrinology & Metabolism*, v. 1, p. 1-6, 2013.
11. Silva, A; Queiroz, SS; Andersen, ML; Mônico-Neto, M; Campos, RM; Roizenblatt, S; Tufik, S; Mello, MT. Passive body heating improves sleep patterns in female patients with fibromyalgia. *Clinics* (USP. Impresso), v. 68, p. 135-139, 2013.
12. Corgosinho, F. C.; Damaso, A. R.; Ganen, A. P.; Campos, RMS; Silva, P. L.; Sanches, P. L.; Ackel-Delia, C.; Carnier, J.; Tock, L.; Andersen, M. L.; TUFIK, S.; Mello, M. T. Short sleep time increases lipid intake in obese adolescents. *Sleep Science* (Impresso), v. 6, p. 26-31, 2013.
13. Ackel-Delia, C.; Bueno, C. R.; Campos, RMS; Sanches PL; Clemente, A. P.; Tufik, Sergio; Mello, M. T.; Damaso, A. . Effects of Different Physical Exercises on Leptin Concentration in Obese Adolescents. *International Journal of Sports Medicine*, v. 1, p. 1, 2013.

14. Carnier, June; Mello, Marco Túlio De; Ackel-D'elia, Carolina; Corgosinho, Flavia; Da Silveira Campos, Raquel Munhoz; De Lima Sanches, Priscila; MASQUIO, Deborah Cristina Landi; Bueno Júnior, Carlos Roberto; Ganen, Aline De Piano; Martins, Aniela C.; Caranti, Danielle Arisa; Tock, Lian; Clemente, Ana Paula Grotti; Tufik, Sergio; Dâmaso, Ana R. Aerobic training (AT) is more effective than aerobic plus resistance training (AT+RT) to improve anorexigenic/orexigenic factors in obese adolescents. *Appetite* (London. Print), v. 1, p. 1, 2013.
15. Sanches PL; Mello, MT; Elias, N.; Fonseca, F.; Campos, RMS; Carnier, J.; de Piano, A; Masquio DCL; Silva PL; Oyama LM; Corgosinho FC; Oller do Nascimento CM; Tock, L.; Ackel-Delia, C.; Tufik S; DAMASO, A. Hyperleptinemia: Implications on the Inflammatory State and Vascular Protection in Obese Adolescents Submitted to an Interdisciplinary Therapy. *Inflammation*, p. 1, 2013.
16. Damaso, A.; de Piano, A; Campos, RMS; Corgosinho, Flávia C.; Siegfried, W.; Caranti, Danielle Arisa; Masquio DCL; Carnier, June; Sanches PL; Silva PL; Nascimento, Claudia Maria Oller do; Oyama, Lila Missae; Dantas, A. D. A.; Mello, M. T.; Tufik, Sergio; Tock, Lian . Multidisciplinary Approach to the Treatment of Obese Adolescents: Effects on Cardiovascular Risk Factors, Inflammatory Profile, and Neuroendocrine Regulation of Energy Balance. *International Journal of Endocrinology*, v. 2013, p. 1-10, 2013.

In: Medicine Research Summaries. Volume 17
Editors: Zhongwen Liáng and Bibao Zhang
ISBN: 978-1-53612-751-5

Chapter 3

HENRY VICTOR DOCTOR

Affiliation:
United Nations Office on Drugs and Crime

Address:
United Nations Office on Drugs and Crime, Plot 617-618
Diplomatic Zone, Central Area, Abuja, Nigeria

Date of Birth:
May 18, 1973

Education:
University of Pennsylvania, (PhD in Demography, 2003)

Research and Professional Experience:

Dr. Henry Doctor, a Research Officer at the United Nations Office on Drugs and Crime (UNODC), graduated in 2003 with a doctoral degree in demography from the University of Pennsylvania. His thesis was entitled "Mortality in twentieth-century Malawi." He took up a postdoctoral research fellowship (sponsored by the Mellon Foundation) based at the Navrongo Health Research Centre in the Upper East Region, Ghana. He has 15 years of experience as a population scientist and also worked at the Universities of Malawi, Western Cape (South Africa), Columbia University, and Statistics South Africa. From mid-2009 to mid-2013, he worked as a resident operations research advisor for a program to revitalize routine immunization, maternal, newborn, and child health in northern Nigeria. Currently, he is coordinating UNODC's research activities in the Country Office for Nigeria (Abuja). His research interests include Mortality; Fertility Transitions; Religion and Demographic Behavior; Survey Research Design and Implementation; Demographic Surveillance and Longitudinal Health Research; and Health Systems Operations Research. He is also the Secretary General of the Union for African Population Studies.

Professional Appointments:

1. West Media Consultants, Malawi - Market Research Assistant
2. Standard Bank of Malawi - Graduate Trainee

3. Navrongo Health Research Centre, Ghana and Population Council, New York - Mellon Foundation Demography Research Fellow
4. University of the Western Cape – Senior Lecturer
5. Statistics South Africa – Demographer
6. Columbia University, Mailman School of Public Health – Associate Research Scientist
7. University of Basel, Swiss Tropical Institute of Public Health – Scientific Project Leader
8. United Nations Office on Drugs and Crime – Research Officer

Publications Last 3 Years:

1. Doctor, H.V. 2013. "Variations in under-five mortality estimates in Nigeria: explanations and implications for program monitoring and evaluation." *Maternal and Child Health Journal* 17(8): 1355-1358; doi: 10.1007/s10995-012-1161-1
2. Doctor, H.V., S.E. Findley, G. Cometto, and G.Y. Afenyadu. 2013. "Awareness of critical danger signs of pregnancy and delivery, preparations for delivery and utilization of skilled birth attendants in Nigeria." *Journal of Health Care for the Poor and Underserved* 24(1): 152-170; doi: 10.1353/hpu.2013.0032
3. Doctor, H.V., E. Sakeah, and J.F. Phillips. 2013. "Religious affiliation among the Kassena-Nankana of northern Ghana: do switching trends differ by gender." Chapter 5. In. *Religion and Ethics*, edited by Gloria Simpson and Spencer Payne. New York: Nova Science Publishers, Inc. ISBN: 978-1-62257-813-9
4. Doctor, H.V. 2013. "Layers of socio-economic vulnerability in Malawi in the context of the Millennium Development Goals." *ISRN Economics*, Volume 2013, Article ID 346750, 7 pages; http://dx.doi.org/10.1155/2013/346750
5. Ashir, G.M., H.V. Doctor, and G. Afenyadu. 2013. "Performance based financing and uptake of maternal and child health services in Yobe State, Nigeria." *Global Journal of Health Science* 5(3): 34-41; http://dx.doi.org/10.5539/gjhs.v5n3p34
6. Wablembo, S.M. and H.V. Doctor. 2013. "The influence of age cohort differentials on antenatal care attendance and supervised deliveries in Uganda." *Journal of Nursing Education and Practice* 3(11): 101-110; http://dx.doi.org/10.5430 /jnep.v3n11p101
7. Sibanda, A. and H.V. Doctor. 2013. "Measuring health gaps between the rich and the poor: a review of the literature and its implications for health research in Africa." *Journal of Public Health in Africa* 4(e3): 12-18; doi:10.4081/jphia.2013.e3
8. Peters, G., H. Doctor, G. Afenyadu, S. Findley, and A. Ager. 2013. "Mobile clinic services to serve rural populations in Katsina State, Nigeria: Perceptions of services and patterns of utilization. *Health Policy and Planning* doi:10.1093/heapol/czt052
9. Wablembo, S.M. and H.V. Doctor. 2013. "Intergenerational differences in current contraceptive use among married women in Uganda." *International Journal of Population Research,* Volume 2013, Article ID 329390, 7 pages; http://dx.doi.org/10.1155/2013/329390
10. Findley, S.E., O.T. Uwemedimo, H.V. Doctor, C. Green, F. Adamu, and G. Afeyadu. 2013. "Comparison of high and low intensity community health worker intervention to promote maternal and child health in Northern Nigeria." *International Journal of*

Women's Health 5: 717-728; http://dx.doi.org/10.2147/IJWH.S49785; PMID: 24194649.

11. Findley, S.E., O.T. Uwemedimo, H.V. Doctor, C. Green, F. Adamu, and G. Afeyadu. 2013. "Early results of an integrated maternal, newborn, and child health program, Northern Nigeria, 2009 to 2011." *BMC Public Health* 2013, 13:1034; doi: 10.1186/1471-2458-13-1034
12. Doctor, H.V., S.E. Findley, G.Y. Afenyadu, C. Uzondu, and G.M. Ashir. 2013. "Awareness, use, and unmet need for family planning in rural Northern Nigeria." *African Journal of Reproductive Health* 17(4): 107-117.
13. Doctor, H.V., O.A. Idowu, A. Olatunji, and A. Jumare. 2013. "Orphanhood and living arrangements in northern Nigeria: An analysis of Nahuche Health and Demographic Surveillance System baseline census data." *Dounia: Journal of Strategic Intelligence and International Relations* 7: 51-66.
14. Sakeah, E., H.V. Doctor, L. McCloskey, J. Bernstein, K. Yeboah-Antwi, and S. Mills. "Using the community-based health planning and services program to promote skilled delivery in rural Ghana: Socio-demographic factors that influence women utilization of skilled attendants at birth in Northern Ghana." *BMC Public Health* 2014, 14:344; doi: 10.1186/1471-2458-14-344

In: Medicine Research Summaries. Volume 17
Editors: Zhongwen Liáng and Bibao Zhang
ISBN: 978-1-53612-751-5

Chapter 4

Gilles Duvoisin

Affiliation:

Department of Gastroenterology, Sydney Children's Hospital Randwick, Sydney, Australia

Department of Paediatrics (Département Médico-Chirurgical de Pédiatrie), Lausanne University Hospital (CHUV), Lausanne, Switzerland

Address:

Sydney Children's Hospital, High Street, Randwick NSW 2031 Australia

Education:

MBBS (equivalent), Dip Paed (equivalent), MD, Master of advance studies in Health Organisation.

Research and Professional Experience:

Dr Duvoisin is the Fellow of Gastroenterology at the Sydney Children's Hospital, Sydney, Australia. Dr Duvoisin areas of interest are general gastroenterology and paediatric pancreatitis. Dr Duvoisin is conducting several international multicentric studies in the field of Paediatric Gastroenterology. Dr Duvoisin obtained his MD in studying the field of risks of early-onset neonatal sepsis and the use of IV antibiotics.

Publications Last 3 Years:

1. Duvoisin, G, C Fischer, D Maucort-Boulch, and E Giannoni. "Reduction in the Use of Diagnostic Tests in Infants with Risk Factors for Early-Onset Neonatal Sepsis Does Not Delay Antibiotic Treatment." *Swiss Medical Weekly,* June 25, 2014. doi:10.4414/smw.2014.13981.

In: Medicine Research Summaries. Volume 17
Editors: Zhongwen Liáng and Bibao Zhang

ISBN: 978-1-53612-751-5

Chapter 5

OLDØICH FARSA

Affiliation:

Department of Chemical Drugs, Faculty of Pharmacy, University of Veterinary and Pharmaceutical Sciences Brno, Brno, Czech Republic.

Address:

Department of Chemical Drugs, Faculty of Pharmacy, University of Veterinary and Pharmaceutical Sciences Brno, Palackého 1-3, 612 42 Brno, Czech Republic

Date of Birth:

December 3rd, 1971

Education:

Master of Pharmacy 1995 (Charles University in Prague, Faculty of Pharmacy in Hradec Králové, Czech Republic)

Doctor of Pharmacy (PharmDr.) and Ph.D. in Bioorganic Chemistry 2000 (Charles University in Prague, Faculty of Pharmacy in Hradec Králové, Czech Republic)

Research and Professional Experience:

- design and synthesis of potential cognitive enhancers
- design and synthesis of transdermal penetration enhancers
- QSAR regression methods
- teaching of Medicinal Chemistry and related disciplines

Professional Appointments:

Associate Professor in Medicinal Chemistry since 2010 (University of Veterinary and Pharmaceutical Sciences Brno, Brno, Czech Republic)

Publications Last 3 Years:

1. Kubínová R., Poøízková R., Navrátilová A., Farsa O., Hanáková Z., Baèinská A., Čížek A, Valentová, M.: Antimicrobial and enzyme inhibitory activities of the constituents of Plectranthus madagascariensis (Pers.) Benth. *Journal of Enzyme Inhibition and Medicinal Chemistry* **29**, 749-752 (2014), (ISSN 1475-6366).

2. Farsa O., Sedláková S., Podlipná J. Maxa, J.: Aminopeptidase N inhibition could be involved in the anti-angiogenic effect of dobesilates. *Journal of the Serbian Chemical Society* **79**, 1-12 (2014), (ISSN 0352-5139).
3. Farsa O.: Therapeutic monoclonal antibodies in treatment and development. *Chem. Listy* **107**, 464-470 (2013), (ISSN 0009-2770).
4. Farsa O.: Chromatographic behaviour predicts the ability of potential nootropics to permeate the blood-brain barier. *Scientia Pharmaceutica* **81**, 81-91 (2013), (ISSN 0036-8709).
5. Kubínová R., Švajdlenka E, Schneiderová K., Hanáková Z., Dall'Acqua S., Farsa O.: Polyphenols and diterpenoids from Plectranthus forsteri 'Marginatus'. *Biochemical Systematics and Ecology* **49**, 39-42 (2013), (ISSN 0305-1978).

In: Medicine Research Summaries. Volume 17
Editors: Zhongwen Liáng and Bibao Zhang
ISBN: 978-1-53612-751-5

Chapter 6

THIALLY BRAGA GONÇALVES

Affiliation:
Universidade Federal do Ceará

Address:
Avenue Carapinima 2298, Brazil

Date of Birth:
April 27, 1989

Education:
Doctor in biotechnology, assistant professor clinical microbiology

Publications Last 3 Years:

1. Oliveira, F. F. M.; Torres, A. F.; Gonçalves, T. B.; Santiago, G. M. P.; Carvalho, C B M; Braga, M.A; Camara, L. M. C.; Rabenhorst, S. H.; Martins, A. M. C.; Valenca Junior, O. T.; Nagao-Dias, A. T. . Efficacy of Plectranthus amboinicus (Lour.) Spreng in a Murine Model of Methicillin-Resistant Staphylococcus aureus Skin Abscesses. *Evidence-Based Complementary and Alternative Medicine* (Online), v. 2013, p. 1-9, 2013.
2. Cabral, Paula Brito E; Júnior, José Evandro Cunha; Macedo, Alexandre Casimiro De; Alves, Alexandre Rodrigues; Gonçalves, Thially Braga; Cabral, Tereza Cristina Brito E; Gondim, Ana Paula Soares; Pinto, Maria Isabel Moraes; Oseki, Karen Tubono; Camara, Lilia Maria Carneiro; Rabenhorst, Silvia Helena Barem; Nagao-Dias, Aparecida Tiemi. Anti-PGL1 salivary IgA/IgM, serum IgG/IgM, and nasal Mycobacterium leprae DNA in individuals with household contact with leprosy. *International Journal of Infectious Diseases*, v. 17, p. e1005-e1010, 2013.
3. Santos, N. O.; Gonçalves, T. B. Microbiological Evaluation of the Hands of Food Handlers In Kindergartens In The City Of Juazeiro Do Norte, CE. *Revista Saúde em Dílogo*, v. IV, p. 6-86, 2013.

In: Medicine Research Summaries. Volume 17
Editors: Zhongwen Liáng and Bibao Zhang

ISBN: 978-1-53612-751-5

Chapter 7

CHIN-CHANG HUANG

Affiliation:
Department of Neurology,
Chang Gung Memorial Hospital and Chang Gung University

Address:
No.91, Xueshi Rd., North Dist.,
Taichung City 404, Taiwan (R.O.C.)

Date of Birth:
Feb-16-1953

Education:
China Medical University

Research and Professional Experience:
Neurotoxicology

Professional Appointments:
Professor of Chang Gung Memorial Hospital and University

Publications Last 3 Years:

1. Hsuan-Min Wang, Chien-Ming Yang, Wan-Chin Kuo, Chin-Chang Huang, Hung-Chou Kuo*. Use of a Modified Spatial-Context Memory Test to Detect Amnestic Mild Cognitive Impairment. *PLoS ONE* 2013;8:e57030. (SCI)
2. Kuo-Hsuan Chang, Mu-Yun Tseng, Long-Sun Ro, Rong-Kuo Lyu, Yu-Han Tai, Hong-Shiu Chang, Yih-Ru Wu, Chin-Chang Huang, Wen-Chuin Hsu, Hung-Chou Kuo, Chun-Che Chu, Chiung-Mei Chen. Analyses of haptoglobin level in the cerebrospinal fluid and serum of patients with neuromyelitis optica and multiple sclerosis. *Clinica Chimica Acta* 2013;417:26-30. (SCI)
3. Ser-Chen Fu, Hung-Chou Kuo, Chun-Che Chu, Yih-Ru Wu, Long-Sun Ro, Chin-San Liu, Chin-Chang Huang*. Long-term Follow-up of Spinal and Bulbar Muscular Atrophy in Taiwan. *J Formos Med Assoc* 2013;112: 326-331. (SCI)

4. Kuo-Hsuan Chang, Chiung-Mei Chen, Yi-Chun Chen, Ya-Chin Hsiao, Chin-Chang Huang, Hung-Chou Kuo, Hsuan-Chu Hsu, Guey-Jen Lee-Chen, Yih-Ru Wu. Association between *GRN* rs5848 polymorphism and Parkinson¡¦s disease in Taiwanese population. *PLoS ONE* 2013;8:e54448. (SCI)
5. Chi-Hung Liu, Kun-Ju Lin, Hsuan-Min Wang, Hung-Chou Kuo, Wen-Li Chuang, Yi-Hsin Weng, Tung-Sheng Shih, Chin-Chang Huang*. Brain Fluorodeoxyglucose-positron emission tomography (^{18}FDG-PET) study in patients with acute thallium intoxication. *Clinical Toxicology* 2013;51:167-173. (SCI)
6. Kuo-Lun Huang, Kun-Ju Lin, Ing-Tsung Hsiao, Hung-Chou Kuo, Wen-Chun Hsu, Wen-Li Chuang, Mei-Ping Kung, Chia-Ju Hsieh, Daniel M. Skovronsky, Yau-Yau Wai, Tzu-Chen Yen, Chin-Chang Huang*. Regional Amyloid Deposition in Amnestic Mild Cognitive Impairment and Alzheimer¡¦s Disease Evaluated by [18F]AV-45 Positron Emission Tomography in Chinese Population. *PLoS ONE* 2013;8:e58974. (SCI)
7. Ing-Tsung Hsiao*, Chin-Chang Huang*, Chia-Ju Hsieh, Shiaw-Pyng Wey, Mei-Ping Kung, Tzu-Chen Yen, Kun-Ju Lin. Perfusion-like template and standardized normalization-based brain image analysis using 18F-florbetapir (AV-45/Amyvid) PET. *Eur J Nucl Med Mol Imaging* 2013; 40:908-920. (SCI)
8. Kuo-Hsuan Chang, Rong-Kuo Lyu, Chiung-Mei Chen, Yih-Ru Wu, Hong-Shiu Chang, Chin-Chang Huang, Hung-Chou Kuo, Chun-Che Chu, Wen-Chuin Hsu and Long-Sun Ro. Distinct features between longitudinally extensive transverse myelitis presenting with and without anti-Aquaporin 4 antibodies. *Multiple Sclerosis Journal (MSJ)* 2013; 19: 299-307. (SCI)
9. Chih-Hsien Hung, Kuo-Hsuan Chang, Yi-Ming Wu, Yao-Liang Chen, Rong-Kuo Lyu, Hong-Shiu Chang, Yih-Ru Wu, Chiung-Mei Chen, Chin-Chang Huang, Chun-Che Chu, Ming-Feng Liao, Yau-Yau Wai, Shih-Pin Hsu, Long-Sun Ro. A comparison of benign and inflammatory manifestations of Tolosa-Hunt syndrome. *Cephalalgia* 2013; 33: 842-852. (SCI)
10. Yi-Chia Wei, Chi-Hung Liu, Jainn-Jim Lin, Kun-Ju Lin, Ko-Lun Huang, Tsong-Hai Lee, Yeu-Jhy Chang, Tsung-I Peng, Kuang-Lin Lin, Ting-Yu Chang, Chien-Hung Chang, Hung-Chou Kuo,Kuo-Hsuan Chang, Mei-Yun Cheng, Chin-Chang Huang. Rapid progression and brain atrophy in anti-AMPA receptor encephalitis. *J Neuroimmunol* 2013;261:129-133. (SCI)
11. Hung-Chou Kuo*, Hsiu-Chuan Yen, Chin-Chang Huang, Wen-Chuin Hsu1, Hsing-Ju Wei, Chih-Lung Lin. Cerebrospinal fluid biomarkers for neuropsychological symptoms in early stage of late-onset Alzheimer¡¦s disease. *Int J Neurosci* 2014; Early Online: 1¡V8. (SCI)
12. Wei-Chia Tsao, Rong-Kuo Lyu, Long-Sun Ro, Ming-Fen Lao, Chiung-Mei Chen, Yih-Ru Wu, Chin-Chang Huang, Hong-Shiu Chang, Hung-Chao Kuo, Chun-Che Chu, Kuo-Hsuan Chang. Clinical Correlations of Motor and Somatosensory Evoked Potentials in Neuromyelitis Optica. *PLoS One* 2014; 9(11): e113631. (SCI) doi:10.1186/s12883-014-0218-8.
13. Ming-Feng Liao, Kuo-Hsuan Chang, Rong-Kuo Lyu, Chin-Chang Huang, Hong-Shiu Chang, Yih-Ru Wu, Chiung-Mei Chen, Chun-Che Chu, Hung-Chou Kuo, Long-Sun Ro. Comparison between the cranial magnetic resonance imaging features

of neuromyelitis optica spectrum disorder versus multiple sclerosis in Taiwanese patients. *BMC Neurol* 2014;14:218. (SCI)

14. Chi-Lin Wu, Long-Sun Ro, Shih-Ming Jung, Zung-Chang Tsai, Chun-Che Chu, Rong-Kuo Lyu, Chin-Chang Huang, Hung-Chou Kuo*. Clinical presentation and electrophysiological findings of porphyric neuropathies: a follow-up study. *Muscle Nerve* 2015; 51:363-369. (SCI)
15. Chih-Hsien Hung, Kuo-Hsuan Chang, Yao-Liang Chen, Yi-Ming Wu, Chiou-Lian Lai, Hong-Shiu Chang, Rong-Kuo Lyu, Yih-Ru Wu, Chiung-Mei Chen, Chin-Chang Huang, Chun-Che Chu, Chun-Hung Chen, Long-Sun Ro. Clinical and Radiological Findings Suggesting Disorders OtherThan Tolosa¡VHunt Syndrome Among Ophthalmoplegic Patients: A Retrospective Analysis. *Headache* 2015;55:252-264. (SCI)
16. Huang HL, Shyu YIL*, Chen MC, Huang CC, Kuo HC, Chen ST, Hsu WC. Family caregivers¡¦ role implementation at different stages of dementia. *Clin Interv Aging* 2015;10:135-46.
17. Chu-Yun Huang, Chi-Hung Liu, Eusden Tsao, Chia-Ju Hsieh, Yi-Hsin Weng, Ing-Tsung Hsiao, Tzu-Chen Yen, Kun-Ju Lin, Chin-Chang Huang*. Chronic manganism: a long-term follow-up study with a new dopamine terminal biomarker of 18F-FP(+)-DTBZ(18F-AV-133) brain PET scan. *J Neurol Sci* 2015;353:102-106. (SCI)
18. Kuo-Hsuan Chang*, Ya-Jen Chiu, Shu-Ling Chen, Chen-Hsiang Huang, Chih-Hsin Lin, Te-Hsien Lin, Chi-Mei Lee, Chintakunta Ramesh, Chung-Hsin Wu, Chin-Chang Huang, Hon-Chung Fung, Yi-Chun Chen, Jung-Yaw Lin, Ching-Fa Yao, Hei-Jen Huang, Guey-Jen Lee-Chen, Ming-Chung Lee, Hsiu Mei Hsieh-Li. The potential of synthetic indolylquinoline derivatives for Ab aggregation reduction by chemical chaperone activity. *Neuropharmacology* 2016; 101: 309-319. (SCI)

In: Medicine Research Summaries. Volume 17
Editors: Zhongwen Liáng and Bibao Zhang
ISBN: 978-1-53612-751-5

Chapter 8

Hyasinta Jaka

Affiliation:
Catholic University of Health and Allied Sciences, Bugando, Mwanza, Tanzania

Address:
PO Box 1464, Bugando, Mwanza, Tanzania

Date of Birth:
4/27/1974

Education:
MD, MMED, MHPE

Research and Professional Experience:
Currently I am doing a project on Helicobacter mutations and resistance pattern in Tanzania

Professional Appointments:
Internist in the gastroenterology and hepatology unit, Bugando Hospital and Senior Lecturer at Catholic University of Health and Allied Sciences

Publications Last 3 Years:

Book Chapters:

1. Hyasinta Jaka; Gastrointerstinal bleeding: Diagnosis and outcomes chapter 1. In Ahmed Kamel and Souheil Saddekni: *Gastrointerstinal bleeding: symptoms, treatment and prognosis* (2nd ed). New York. NOVA Publisher 2014.
2. Hyasinta Jaka; Epidemiology, pathogenesis and clinical features. In Adriana Erica Miele: *Schistosomiasis Epidemiology, Diagnosis and Treatment*. New York. NOVA Publisher. 2014.
3. Hyasinta Jaka; The diagnosis, treatment options and prevention. In Adriana Erica Miele: *Schistosomiasis Epidemiology, Diagnosis and Treatment*. New York. NOVA Publisher. 2014.

Research articles:

1. Hyasinta Jaka, Stephan E, Mshana, Peter Rambau, Nestory Masalu, Phillipo Chalya, samuel kalluvya; Hepatocellular carcinoma: clinical profile and challenges of management in Resource limited setting. *World Journal of surgical Oncology* 2014.12:246.
2. Hyasinta M. Jaka, Mariam Mirambo, Lambauand Phillipo Leo Diffuse benign gastric inflammatory hyperplastic polyps in adolescent man Case report. *TJMR* 2013.
3. Hyasinta Jaka Mabula D Mchembe Peter F Rambau Phillipo L Chalya Gastric outlet obstruction at Bugando Medical Centre in Northwestern Tanzania: a prospective review of 184 cases; *BMC Surgery* 2013, 13:41.

In: Medicine Research Summaries. Volume 17
Editors: Zhongwen Liáng and Bibao Zhang
ISBN: 978-1-53612-751-5

Chapter 9

NOBUTADA KIMURA

Affiliation:

Bioproduction research Institute, National Institute of Advanced Industrial Science and Technology (AIST)

Address:

Central 6, 1-1-1 Higashi, Tsukuba-City, Ibaraki, 305-8566 Japan

Date of Birth:

02/12/1968

Education:

Entered Faculty of Agriculture, Kyushu University, April 1988, and graduated, March, 1992, with the degree of Bachelor of Agriculture. Obtained an M.S. ("Nogaku Shushi", literal translation is Master of Agriculture) March, 1994. Received a Ph.D. ("Nogaku Hakase", literal translation is Doctor of Agriculture) in March, 1997 from Kyushu University for a thesis entitled: "Studies on the Functional and structural analysis of Biphenyl/Polichlorinated biphenyl (PCB) metabolic genes".

Research and Professional Experience:

Nobutada Kimura interests include the Microbiology, the molecular biology of environmental microbes, and the environmental biotechnology.

Professional Appointments:

In 1997 Nobutada Kimura joined at National Institute of Advanced Industrial Science and Technology as a Research Scientist. From 2004 to 2006, Nobutada Kimura was a Visiting Fellow in the Department of Plant Pathology at the University of Wisconsin-Madison, USA. Since 2006, Nobutada Kimura has been a Senior Research Scientist of the Bioproduction research Institute at National Institute of Advanced Industrial Science and Technology.

Honors:

Best Paper Award, *Journal of Bioscience and Bioengineering*. 2002

Publications Last 3 Years:

1. Hirose J, Yamazoe A, Hosoyama A, Kimura N, Suenaga H, Watanabe T, Fujihara H, Futagami T, Goto M, Furukawa K.: Draft genome sequence of the polychlorinated biphenyl-degrading bacterium *comamonas testosterone.* KF712 (NBRC 110673). *Genome Announcements.* Vol. 3, No.5, pp. e01214-15, 2015.
2. Fujihara H, Yamazoe A, Hosoyama A, Suenaga H, Kimura N, Hirose J, Watanabe T, FutagamiT, Goto M, Furukawa K: Draft genome sequence of *Pseudomonas aeruginosa* KF702 (NBRC110665), a polychlorinated biphenyl-degrading bacterium isolated from biphenyl-contaminated soil. *Genome Announcements*, Vol.3, No.3, pp.e00517-15, 2015.
3. Kanno M, Tamaki H, Mitani Y, Kimura N, Hanada S, Kamagata Y: pH-Induced change in cell susceptibility to butanol in a high butanol-tolerant bacterium, *Enterococcus faecalis* strain CM4A, *Biotechnology for Biofuels*, Vol.8, No.1, pp.69, 2015.
4. Fujihara H, Yamazoe A, Hosoyama A, Suenaga H, Kimura N, Hirose J, Watanabe T, FutagamiT, Goto M, Furukawa K: Draft genome sequence of *Pseudomonas abietaniphila* KF701 (NBRC110664), a polychlorinated biphenyl-degrading bacterium isolated from biphenyl-contaminated soil. *Genome Announcements*, Vol.3, No.3, pp.e00473-15, 2015.
5. Suenaga H, Yamazoe A, Hosoyama A, Kimura N, Hirose J, Watanabe T, Fujihara H, Futagami T, Goto M, and Furukawa K: Draft genome sequence of the polychlorinated biphenyl-degrading bacterium *Pseudomonas putida* KF703 (NBRC 110666) isolated from biphenyl-contaminated soil. *Genome Announcements*, Vol.3, No.2, pp.e00142-15, 2015.
6. Suenaga H, Yamazoe A, Hosoyama A, Kimura N, Hirose J, Watanabe T, Fujihara H, Futagami T, Goto M, and Furukawa K: Draft genome sequence of the polychlorinated biphenyl-degrading bacterium *Cupriavidus bacilensis* KF708 (NBRC 110671). *Genome Announcements*, Vol.3, No.2, pp.e00143-15, 2015.
7. Kimura N, Yamazoe A, Hosoyama A, Hirose J, Watanabe T, Suenaga H, Fujihara H, Futagami T, Goto M, and Furukawa K: Draft genome sequence of *Pseudomonas abietaniphila* KF717 (NBRC 110669) isolated from biphenyl-contaminated soil in Japan. *Genome Announcements*, Vol.3, No.2, pp.e00059-15, 2015.
8. Watanabe T, Yamazoe A, Hosoyama A, Fujihara H, Suenaga H, Hirose J, Futagami T, Goto M, Kimura N, and Furukawa K: Draft Genome Sequence of *Pseudomonas toyotomiensis* KF710, a Polychlorinated Biphenyl-Degrading Bacterium Isolated from Biphenyl-Contaminated Soil, *Genome Announcements*, Vol.3, No.2, pp.e00223-15, 2015.
9. Watanabe T, Yamazoe A, Hosoyama A, Fujihara H, Suenaga H, Hirose J, Futagami T, Goto M, Kimura N, and Furukawa K: Draft Genome Sequence of *Cupriavidus pauculus* Strain KF709, a Biphenyl-Utilizing Bacterium Isolated from Biphenyl-Contaminated Soil, *Genome Announcements*, Vol.3, No.2, pp.e00222-15, 2015.
10. Narihiro T, Suzuki A (equally contributed 1st author), Yoshimune K, Hori T, Hoshino T, Yumoto I, Yokota A, Kimura N, Kamagata Y: The combining functional metagenomics and oil-fed enrichment strategy revealed the phylogenetic diversity of lipolytic bacteria overlooked by cultivation-based method. *Microbes Environ.* Vol.29, No.2, pp.154-161, 2014.

11. Y Yasutake, H Kusada, T Ebuchi, S Hanada, Y Kamagata, N Kimura, Structural studies of β-lactam antibiotic degrading enzyme, MacQ, *Photon Factory Activity* Report, #31, 2014.
12. Kusada H, Hanada S, Kamagata Y, Kimura N.: The effects of N-acylhomoserine lactones, β-lactam antibiotics and adenosine on biofilm formation in the multi-β-lactam antibiotic-resistant bacterium Acidovorax sp. strain MR-S7. *J Biosci Bioeng*, Vol.118, No.1, pp.14-19, 2014.
13. Miura T, Kusada H, Kamagata Y, Hanada S, Kimura N: Genome Sequence of the Multiple-Β-Lactam-Antibiotic-Resistant Bacterium *Acidovorax* sp. Strain MR-S7. *Genome Anouncements*, Vol.1, pp.e00412-13, 2013.
14. Kanno M, Katayama T, Tamaki H, Mitani Y, Meng X-Y, Hori T, Narihiro T, Morita N, Hoshino T, Yumoto I, Kimura N, Hanada S, Kamagata Y: Isolation of butanol- and isobutanol-tolerant bacteria and physiological characterization of their butanol tolerance. *Appl Environ Microbiol*, Vol.79, pp.6998-7005, 2013.
15. Takasaki K, Miura T, Kanno M, Tamaki H, Hanada S, Kamagata Y, Kimura N: Discovery of glycoside hydrolase enzymes from an avicel-adapted forest soil eukaryotic community revealed by a metatranscriptomic approach, *PLoS One*, Vol.8, pp.e55485, 2013.

In: Medicine Research Summaries. Volume 17
Editors: Zhongwen Liáng and Bibao Zhang
ISBN: 978-1-53612-751-5

Chapter 10

PETER KUBISZ, MD, DSC

Affiliation:

National Centre of Haemostasis and Thrombosis, Department of Haematology and Transfusiology, Comenius University in Bratislava, Jessenius Faculty of Medicine in Martin, Martin University Hospital, Martin, Slovak Republic

Address:

National Centre of Haemostasis and Thrombosis, Department of Haematology and Transfusiology, Comenius University in Bratislava, Jessenius Faculty of Medicine in Martin, Martin University Hospital, Kollarova 2, 036 59 Martin, Slovak Republic

e-mail: kubisz@jfmed.uniba.sk, telephone: +421434203233, fax: +421434132061

Education:

Scientific titles and degrees:

1966 Doctor of Medicine Degree, Faculty of Medicine, Palacky University, Olomouc, Czech Republic

1975 Philosophy Doctor Degree, Faculty of Medicine, Comenius University, Bratislava, Slovakia

1976 Habilitation Thesis, Faculty of Medicine, Charles University, Prague, Czech Republic

1990 D.Sc. Degree, Faculty of Medicine, Comenius University, Bratislava, Slovak Republic

1992 Professor of Medicine, Jessenius Faculty of Medicine, Comenius University, Martin, Slovakia

Research and Professional Experience:

Current research interest:

- haemophilia and inhibitors
- immune tolerance induction (ITI)
- activated factor VIIa (FVIIa) related to management of bleeding in haemophilic and non-haemophilic patients
- monitoring of the effectiveness of new oral anticoagulants
- genetic polymorphisms asssociated with thrombophilia

- expression of platelet glycoprotein receptors in thrombophilic thrombocytopathies
- monitoring of dual antiplatelet treatment (patients with acute coronary syndrome)
- haemostasis and cellular therapy
- endothelial and platelet dysfunction in vascular disorders (preeclampsia, hypertension, diabetes mellitus, haemodialysed patients)

Main professional field:
- haemophilia and inhibitors
- immune tolerance induction (ITI)
- activated factor VIIa (FVIIa) related to management of bleeding in haemophilic and non-haemophilic patients
- monitoring of the effectiveness of new oral anticoagulants
- monitoring of dual antiplatelet treatment
- inherited and acquired thrombophilia
- haemostasis in vascular disorders (preeclampsia, hypertension, diabetes mellitus, haemodialysed patients)
- haemostasis and cellular therapy
- haemostasis and tumours

Professional Appointments:

1966-1969	Fellow, Dept. of Internal Medicine, General Hospital, Cadca, Slovakia
1969-1970	Assistant, Research Institute of Blood Diseases, Paris, France
1970-1975	Senior Assistant, Dept. of Clinical Biochemistry and Hematology, General Hospital, Cadca, Slovakia
1975-1992	Assistant Professor, Head of Dept., Dept. of Haematology, University Hospital, Oran, Algeria
1992-2014	Professor, Head of Dept., Dept. of Haematology and Blood Transfusion, Faculty Hospital, Martin, Slovakia
2015-ongoing	Professor, Deputy Head of Dept. for educational purposes, Dept. of Haematology and Blood Transfusion, Faculty Hospital, Martin, Slovakia

Honors:

The Award of the Board of the Slovak Medical Society – Jessenius Award – 1972

The Award of the Presidium of the Czech-Slovak Medical Society of Jan Evangelista Purkyně – Hynek Award – 1977

Dérer Award of the Slovak Medical Society – 1987

Award for the Best Publication of the Publishing House – 1987

Award of the International Biographical Centre Cambridge for Haematology – 2001

Award of the American Biographical Institute – Biomedical Research – 2002, 2007

Award of the XVI. Czech-Slovak Conference on Haemostasis and Thrombosis in Hradec Kralove –Rokytansky Lecture - 2009

Award of the Institute for Haematology and Blood Transfusion in Prague - Neuwirth Lecture - 2010

Gold Medal for the Individual Achievement of the Slovak Medical Society – 2011

Purkyně Medal of the Czech Medical Society of Jan Evangelista Purkyně – May 2012

Medal of the Establishment of the Society Medical-Slavic in Budapest – November 2012

Publications Last 3 Years:

1. Kubisz P, Hollý P, Staško J, Plameňová I. The use of intravenous immunoglobulin in immune tolerance induction in inherited haemophilia A: a single-centre experience and a review of literature. *Blood Coagul Fibrinolysis*. 2015;26(6):604-12. DOI: 10.1097/MBC.0000000000000304.
2. Simurda T, Stanciakova L, Stasko J, Dobrotova M, Kubisz P. Yes or no for secondary prophylaxis in afibrinogenemia? *Blood Coagul Fibrinolysis*. 2015;26(8):978-80. DOI: 10.1097/MBC.0000000000000392.
3. Stanciakova L, Simurda T, Stasko J, Snahnicanova Z, Loderer D, Lasabova Z, Kubisz P. Novel fibrinogen bbeta chain mutation as an underlying mechanism of afibrinogenemia? *Semin Thromb Hemost*. 2015; 41(8):901-2. DOI: 10.1055/s-0035-1564802.
4. Simurda T, Snahnicanova Z, Loderer D, Sokol J, Stasko J, Lasabova Z, Kubisz P. Fibrinogen Martin: A Novel Mutation in FGB (Gln180Stop) Causing Congenital Afibrinogenemia. *Semin Thromb Hemost*. 2016; 42(4):455-8.
5. Kubisz P, Holly P, Stasko J, Plamenova I. The use of intravenous immunoglobulin in immune tolerance induction in inherited haemophilia A: a single-centre experience and a review of literature. *Blood Coagul Fibrinolysis* 2015; 26(6):604-612
6. Kubisz P, Stanciakova L, Stasko J, Dobrotova M, Skerenova M, Ivankova J, Holly P. Sticky platelet syndrome: an important cause of life-threatening thrombotic complications. *Expert Rev Hematol*. 2016;9(1):21-35. DOI: 10.1586/17474086.2016.1121095.
7. Simurda T, Stanciakova L, Stasko J, Dobrotova M, Kubisz P. “Afibrinogenaemia in Slovakia“. *18th International Meeting Danubian League against Thrombosis and Haemorrhagic Disorders* [electronic source] Sarajevo: 2015. S. 24
8. Holly P, Lisa L, Plamenova I, Dobrotova M, Kubisz P. Recombinant activated factor VII as an additional agent in the management of bleeding in patients with chemotherapy-induced thrombocytopenia. *Blood Transfusion* 2013; 11(3): 466-468.
9. Samoš M, Fedor M, Kovář F, Duraj L, Stančiaková L, Galajda P, Staško J, Kubisz P, Mokáň M. Ticagrelor: A safe and effective approach for overcoming clopidogrel resistance in patients with stent thrombosis? *Blood Coagul Fibrinolysis*. 2016;27(2):117-20. DOI: 10.1097/MBC.0000000000000406.
10. Hamzik J, Chudej J, Dzian A, Sokol J, Kubisz P. Endovascular stenting in malignant obstruction of superior vena cava. *Int J Surgery Case Reports* 2015; 13:84-87.
11. Dobrotova M, Plamenova I, Necas L, Stasko J, Kubisz P. The perioperative management of haemophilic patients. 22. Czech Slovak conference on haemostasis and thrombosis. *Hradec Kralove* 2015; S. 54.
12. Stasko J, Holly P, Plamenova I, Ivankova J, Sokol J, Stanciakova L, Kubisz P. Inhibitors and hemophilia. *18th International Meeting Danubian League against Thrombosis and Haemorrhagic Disorders* [electronic source] Sarajevo. 2015; S. 50.
13. Stanciakova L, Stasko J, Dobrotova M, Holly P, Sokol J, Kubisz P. Haemophilia and arterial thrombosis. *18th International Meeting Danubian League against Thrombosis and Haemorrhagic Disorders* [electronic source] Sarajevo : 2015. S. 124.
14. Stanciakova L, Holly P, Dobrotova M, Plamenova I, Stasko J, Kubisz P. Hot topic - new perspectives on care management and treatment of patients with bleeding

disorders. *18th International Meeting Danubian League against Thrombosis and Haemorrhagic Disorders* [electronic source] Sarajevo : 2015. S. 113.

15. Fedor M, Chudy P, Pavlenkova O, Kubiz P. Rare bleeding disorders in the region of northern Slovakia. *18th International Meeting Danubian League against Thrombosis and Haemorrhagic Disorders* [electronic source] Sarajevo : 2015. S. 98.
16. Simurda T, Stanciakova L, Stasko J, Dobrotova M, Kubisz P. Afibrinogenaemia - just a rare disease or therapeutic challenge? 22. Czech-Slovak conference on thrombosis and haemostasis. *Hradec Kralove* 2015. S. 39.
17. Skornova I, Stasko J, Holly P, Dobrotova M, Kubisz P. Use of von Willebrand factor multimers analysis in diagnostics and treatment of von Willebrand disease. *18th International Meeting Danubian League against Thrombosis and Haemorrhagic Disorders* [electronic source] Sarajevo : 2015. S. 20.
18. Stasko J, Holly P, Plamenova I, Sokol J, Stanciakova L, Kubisz P. Immune tolerance induction in haemophilia a with inhibitors. *Bilten za Transfuziologiju* 2014; 60(1-2): 156.
19. Samoš M, Stančiaková L, Ivanková J, Staško J, Kovář F, Dobrotová M, Galajda P, Kubisz P, Mokáň M. Monitoring of dabigatran therapy using Hemoclot® Thrombin Inhibitor assay in patients with atrial fibrillation. *J Thromb Thrombolysis*. 2015; 39(1):95-100. doi: 10.1007/s11239-014-1125-y.
20. Chudy P, Chuda D, Hudecek J, Fedorova J, Sinak I, Talapkova R, Laca L, Kubisz P. Therapeutic angiogenesis for the critical limb ischemia decreases platelet activation. *Platelets* 2014; 25(2):132-134.

In: Medicine Research Summaries. Volume 17
Editors: Zhongwen Liáng and Bibao Zhang

ISBN: 978-1-53612-751-5

Chapter 11

Liang Qin Liu

Affiliation:
Middlesex University, London, United Kingdom

Address:
Adult, Child & Midwifery, School of Health and Education, Middlesex University, Hendon Campus, Williams Building Room WG36, Tel: 02084112893, Email: L.Q.Liu@mdx.ac.uk.

Date of Birth:
08/09/1966

Education:

PhD. in Clinical Physiology, University College London, London. UK, 2007

Bachelor degree in Clinical Medicine, Southeast University Medical School, Nanjing, P. R. China. Medicine degree was awarded in July 1990 with 1st class honour.

Research and Professional Experience:

Research Fellow (Grade 7), Department of Adult, Child and Midwifery, School of Health and Education, Middlesex University, June 2013-present

During this period, I have consolidated my research supported by the following evidence:

- Successfully securing external and internal research grant as a principle or co-investigator with a total of £385,810 to conduct primary (experimental & observational studies) and secondary (systematic review, meta-analysis and service evaluations) research projects in a variety of patient population.
- As a principle investigator, I successfully secured an external grant of £2,000 from the Hospital Saturday Funds in February 2015: The project is entitled 'Using motion sensor to monitor pressure relief exercise at home in people living with spinal cord injury. The vision of this project is to improve lifetime fitness/ reduce cardiac risk in people living with spinal cord injury. We introduce the non-invasive motion sensor to quantify the magnitude of disabled patient's motions after they are discharged

from hospital. The project is in collaboration with Spinal injury unit, Royal National Orthopaedic Hospital.

- As a principle investigator, I successfully secured an internal grant of £11,050 in November 2014: The project is entitled as 'An exploration of the extent and role of adherence to 'pressure relief' regimen for pressure ulcer prevention in people living with spinal cord injury'. The project involves a survey of members from 2 Spinal cord injury associations (SIA & ASPIRE) and a systematic review of 'pressure relief' exercise in spinal cord injuries The vision of this project is to gather initial data for future designing new interventions to reduce long-term complications following spinal cord injuries.
- As a co-investigator, an international collaboration grant application to 'Global Innovation Initiative Grant, USA has been submitted in October 2014. This joint international proposal is collaborated with Queen Mary University, London, UK & Ohio State University, USA. Currently it is under the review process. The final results will be announced in July 2015. The project is entitled 'micro-wearable epidermal textile sensors for low cost deep tissue monitoring for people at-risk'. The objective of the project is to develop a portable and non-invasive carefree sensor to image the human cross-section and monitor chest fluids or dielectric changes in human tissues. It aims to prevent unneeded hospitalizations, and provide early diagnosis of congestion heart failure, cancer or deep tissue injuries for people-at-risk while living at home.
- As a principle investigator and a mentor for teaching staff, I supervised a number of staff (Julie Moody) to engage the research and completed a systematic review and meta-analysis of electrical stimulation in pressure ulcer prevention in spinal cord injuries. The results were published as a full paper in a peer reviewed leading journal in spinal cord injury (JSCIM), and .were presented in high profile conferences in spinal cord injury society and tissue viability. My presentations were well received and through attending conferences, several new research collaborations have been established, thus increased Middlesex University visibility in a broad research area, which has a strong synergy with the research strategy set out by the university.
- Successfully securing an external grant of a total £330k funded by Local Education and Training Boards (LETBs) as a co-investigator with Professors Michael Traynor and Sue Dyson in Oct 2013 (the project covered 4 parts, Middlesex University secured 'Sage and Thyme' part). The 1-year project completed in October 2014.

As a principle investigator securing an internal funding £5,951 in November 2013, I completed the research project in collaboration with Royal National Orthopaedic Hospital in August 2014. The project was entitled as 'Effect of sacral nerve root stimulation implant versus conventional surface FES on tissue blood volume in spinal cord injury.

Completed 1-year project as a co-investigator with a secured internal funding £6,625 in October 2013. The project was entitled as 'Building social capital through volunteerism: an exploration of the extent and role of student volunteering in the undergraduate student population: a pilot project'.

Published 4 journal papers (first author) with overall impact factor over 2.8; two additional papers are under authors' revision.

Attended and presented papers in several high profile international conferences (ISCOS 2014, EPUAP 2014 & EWMA 2015) on behalf of nursing Department, MDX.

Entered REF 2014 in Biomed area (UoA--Professor Richard Bayford), Middlesex University.

Professional Appointments:

- Research Associate/ academic consultant, Centre for Evidence in Transplantation (directed by Sir Peter Morris), Royal College of Surgeons, London, Jan 2010–March 2013
- Research Associate, Surgery Unit, UCL Institute of Child Health, London. Sept 2007- December 2010
- Research Fellow/PhD student, Spinal Research Centre, Royal National Orthopaedic Hospital, Stanmore, University College London, May 2003- August 2007
- Research Assistant, Department of Physiological Medicine, Division of Cardiac & Vascular Medicine, St. George's, University of London, Sept 2000 – April 2003
- Research Assistant, Department of Cardiovascular Science, Queen Elizabeth Hospital, University of Birmingham. Jun 1999 – Sept. 2000.
- Visiting Scholar, Bristol Royal Infirmary, Bristol. UK. Oct 1996- Jan 1998.
- Registrar in histopathology, the Second Affiliated Hospital, Nanjing Medical University, and Nanjing, China. July 1990 – June 1996.

Honors:

Membership of Professional bodies

- Member of British Hypertension Society (Sept 2000-Sep 2006);
- Member of the European Society for Microcirculation (Sept 2001-Sep 2012);
- Member of International Spinal Cord Society (June 2003 –Jan 2008);
- Member of British Transplantation Society (Feb 2012 - Feb 2013);
- Member of European Wound Management Association (February 2015-present).

Learned societies

- Editorial member of Journal of Physical Medicine, Rehabilitation & Disabilities
- Editorial member of Jacobs Journal of Physical Rehabilitation Medicine
- Editorial member of & SM Journal of Orthopaedics
- Reviewer of Journal of Rehabilitation and Research Development
- Reviewer of Journal of Spine,
- Reviewer of Journal of Gerontology & Geriatric Research
- Reviewer of journal of International Neuro-rehabilitation
- Reviewer of Journal of Clinical & Experimental Cardiology

External and Internal Academic Leadership or Evidence of Academic Standing

- Awarded for best research posters prize in cardiovascular research symposium (March 2002).
- Awarded for a PhD research fellowship at Royal National Orthopaedic Hospital (May 2003);

- Awarded for the best clinical paper prize at 29th Annual EPOS Meeting, Zagreb (Croatia) (April 2010);
- Awarded with research prize of £400 for the best abstract submitted to British Transplantation Society (Jan 2012).

Publications Last 3 Years:

1. Liu LQ, Moody J, Gall A. A meta-analysis and systematic review of electrical stimulation on pressure ulcer healing in spinal cord injuries. *Ostomy wound management.* Under review.
2. Liu LQ, Ferguson-Pell M. Pressure Changes under the Ischial Tuberosities during Gluteal Neuromuscular Stimulation in Spinal Cord Injury: a Comparison of Sacral Nerve Root Stimulation with Surface Functional Electrical Stimulation. *Archives of Physical Medicine and Rehabilitation.* 2015 Apr; 96(4):620-6.
3. Liu LQ, Moody J, Dyson S, Traynor M, Gall A.. A systematic review of Electrical Stimulation for Pressure Ulcer Prevention and Treatment in people with Spinal Cord Injury. Submitted to *Journal of Spinal Cord Medicine* 2014 Nov; 37(6):703-18.
4. Liu LQ, Pengel LH, Morris PJ. CONSORT compliance and methodological quality of Randomized Controlled Trials in solid organ transplantation, a 3-year overview. *Transpl Int.* 2013 Mar; 26(3):300-6.
5. Andreas Roposch, Liang Q. Liu, Evangelia Protopapa. Variations in the Use of Diagnostic Criteria for Developmental Dysplasia of the Hip. *Clin Orthop Relat Res* (2013) 471:1946–1954.

In: Medicine Research Summaries. Volume 17
Editors: Zhongwen Liáng and Bibao Zhang
ISBN: 978-1-53612-751-5

Chapter 12

KAREN J. MILLER, PHD

Affiliation:
UCLA Longevity Center
David Geffen School of Medicine at UCLA
Semel Institute for Neuroscience & Human Behavior

Address:
Peter V. Ueberroth Building
10945 Le Conte Avenue
Los Angeles, CA 90095-6980, US

Date of Birth:
12/9/1969

Education:
PhD in Clinical Psychology
Fuller Seminary, School of Psychology

Research and Professional Experience:
Early detection of cognitive decline, aging and memory, brain fitness

Professional Appointments:
Health Sciences Associate Clinical Professor of Psychiatry and Biobehavioral Sciences, Clinical Compensated Series, Step II, UCLA Semel Institute, Department of Psychiatry and Biobehavioral Sciences, Division of Geriatric Psychiatry

Honors:

- Exceptional Educator, Women In Leadership, National Academy of Neuropsychology
- American Psychological Association, Division 40, Blue Ribbon Award for Research
- Outstanding Housestaff Teaching Award, UCLA Medical School, Dept of Psychiatry
- Semel Scholar Award, UCLA – Semel Institute
- Judith Braun Excellence in Research Award, National Gero Nurses Association

· Outstanding Graduate Teaching Award, UCLA Medical School, Department of Psychiatry

Publications Last 3 Years:

1. Kaiser NC, Miller KJ, Siddarth P, Ercoli LM, Small GW. The impact of age and Alzheimer's disease risk factors on memory performance over time. *Aging Health.* 2013; 9(1):1-10.
2. Miller KJ, Dye RV, Kim J, Jennings JL, O'Toole E, Wong J, Siddarth P. The Effect of a Computerized Brain Exercise Program on Cognitive Performance in Older Adults. *American Journal of Geriatric Psychiatry.* 2013. Jul;21(7):655-63. doi: 10.1016/j.jagp.2013.01.077. Epub 2013 Apr 18.
3. Merrill DA, Siddarth P, Kepe V, Raja PV, Saito N, Ercoli LM, Miller KJ, Lavretsky H, Bookheimer SY, Barrio JR, Small GW. Vascular Risk and FDDNP-PET influence cognitive performance. *Journal of Alzheimer's Disease.* 2013:35;147-157.
4. Smid LM, Kepe V, Vinters HV, Bresjanac M, Toyokuni T, Satyamurthy N, Wong KP, Huang SC, Silverman DH, Miller K, Small GW, Barrio JR. Postmortem 3-D brain hemisphere cortical tau and amyloid-β pathology mapping and quantification as a validation method of neuropathology imaging. *Journal of Alzheimer's Disease.* 2013:336(2):261-74.
5. Chen ST, Siddarth P, Saito N, Rueda F, Haight T, Ercoli LM, Miller KJ, Lavretsky H, Barrio JR, Bookheimer SY, Small GW, Merrill D. Psychological well-being and regional brain amyloid and tau in mild cognitive impairment. *Am J Geriatr Psychiatry.* 2014; 22(4):362-9.
6. Baerresen KM, Miller KJ, Hanson ER, Miller JS, Dye RV, Hartman RE, Vermeersch D, Small GW. Neuropsychological tests for predicting cognitive decline in older adults. *Journal of Neurodegenerative Disease Management (in press).*

In: Medicine Research Summaries. Volume 17
Editors: Zhongwen Liáng and Bibao Zhang
ISBN: 978-1-53612-751-5

Chapter 13

Professor Conor C Murphy

Affiliation:

Professor of Ophthalmology, Royal College of Surgeons in Ireland

Consultant Ophthalmic Surgeon and Medical Director, Royal Victoria Eye and Ear Hospital, Dublin

Address:

123 St Stephen's Green, Dublin 2, Ireland

Research and Professional Experience:

Profiling Toll-like receptor responses in patients with primary Sjögren's syndrome (Supervising MD student 2013-15)

Evasion of the innate immune response by HSV-1 in the cornea: molecular mechanisms mediating interferon downregulation and virus survival (Supervised MD student 2011-14, thesis in preparation)

Effect of corneal Herpes Simplex Virus-1 infection on Toll-Like Receptor expression in human peripheral blood mononuclear cells (Supervised MSc - awarded 2012)

Acute anterior uveitis in an Irish Cohort: clinical characteristics and molecular mechanisms (in collaboration with SVUH, supervising PhD student 2012-15)

Giant cell arteritis – PI on a multi-centred study aimed at Improving outcomes in giant cell arteritis through clinical collaboration including studies in imaging and pathogenic mechanisms using an ex-vivo temporal artery culture model (in collaboration with SVUH, 2011 -)

Corneal tissue engineering (with NICB DCU & Tissue Engineering Research Group, RCSI, 2010 -)

Proteomics of uveal melanoma (in collaboration with NICB DCU, supervised MD student 2011-13, thesis submitted)

Genetic analysis of patients with congenital hereditary endothelial corneal dystrophy (in collaboration with UCC, 2012 -).

Professional Appointments:

- Medical Director of the Royal Victoria Eye and Ear Hospital

- Consultant Ophthalmic surgeon with a special interest in cornea, external eye disease and uveitis
- Undergraduate and postgraduate Professor of Ophthalmology at RCSI
- Principle Investigator, Department of Molecular and Cellular Therapeutics, RCSI
- Chief examiner of the MRCSI (Ophth) and FRCSI(Ophth) examinations
- Academic member of Irish College of Ophthalmologists Manpower and Training Committee
- Founding committee member of the Irish Regional Ophthalmic Anaesthesia Society

Honors:

2014 Health Research Board/ Medical Research Charities Group "Restoring immune balance in patients with primary Sjögren's syndrome by modulating microRNA expression" (€40,000)

2014 RCSI Seed funding call "Modulating microRNA expression as a means to restore immune function in patients with primary Sjogrens Syndrome" (€30,000)

2013 Irish College of Ophthalmologists/Pfizer Research Fellowship "Acute anterior uveitis in an Irish Cohort: clinical characteristics and molecular mechanisms" (€35,000)

2013 EU FP7 grant Award. Partner in VISICORT: Adverse Immune Signatures and their Prevention in Corneal Transplantation (Personal award €400,000 (total consortium: €6 million))

2012 Health Research Board/ Medical Research Charities Group: "Profiling Toll-like receptor responses in patients with primary Sjögren's syndrome" (€50,000)

2011 Royal Victoria Eye and Ear Hospital Research Foundation: "Acute anterior uveitis in an Irish Cohort: clinical characteristics and molecular mechanisms" (€30,000)

2011 Irish College of Ophthalmologists/Pfizer Research Fellowship: "Targeting toll-like receptor pathways in the treatment of HSV-1 keratitis" (€35,000)

2010 Royal Victoria Eye and Ear Hospital Research Foundation: "Evasion of the innate immune response by HSV-1 in the cornea: molecular mechanisms mediating interferon downregulation and virus survival" (€20,000)

2007 Foundation for the Prevention of Blindness, UK "Determining the minimum inhibitory concentration of topical ophthalmic antimicrobials and their concentration and biological activity in the cornea in vitro" (£33,000)

Publications Last 3 Years:

1. Pilson Q., Jefferies C.A., Gabhann J.N., Murphy C.C. (2015) Isolation of microRNA from conjunctival impression cytology. *Exp Eye Res*. 2015 Jan 10 [Epub ahead of print] PubMed PMID: 25584869.
2. Gallagher C, Clarke C, Aherne ST, Katikireddy KR, Doolan P, Lynch V, Shaw S, Bobart-Hone A, Murphy C, Clynes M, Power W, O'Sullivan F. Comparative transcriptomic analysis of cultivated limbal epithelium and donor corneal tissue reveals altered wound healing gene expression. *Invest Ophthalmol Vis Sci*. 2014 Aug 14;55(9):5795-805. PubMed PMID: 25125605.

3. Haroon M, O'Rourke M, Ramasamy P, Murphy CC, FitzGerald O. A novel evidence-based detection of undiagnosed spondyloarthritis in patients presenting with acute anterior uveitis: the DUET (Dublin Uveitis Evaluation Tool). *Ann Rheum Dis.* 2014 Jun 13. [Epub ahead of print] PubMed PMID: 24928841.
4. Rahman N, Murphy CC. Impact of intracameral cefuroxime on the incidence of postoperative endophthalmitis following cataract surgery in Ireland. *Ir J Med Sci.* 2014 May 21. [Epub ahead of print] PubMed PMID: 24846749.
5. Ramasamy P, Murphy CC, Clynes M, Horgan N, Moriarty P, Tiernan D, Beatty S, Kennedy S, Meleady P. Proteomics in uveal melanoma. *Exp Eye Res.* 2014 Jan;118:1-12. PubMed PMID: 24056206.
6. O'Rourke M, Haroon M, Murphy C.C., FitzGerald O. Anterior Uveitis in Spondyloarthropathy: The ophthalmologist's role in earlier recognition Book chapter in *Ankylosing spondylitis; symptoms, treatment and complications.* Nova Publishers. 2013, ISBN: 978-1-62618-362-9
7. Treacy MP, Treacy MG, Dimitrov BD, Seager FE, Stamp MA, Murphy CC. A method for prescription of inexpensive spectacles by non-specialist healthcare workers: S-Glasses. *Eye* 2013 Apr;27(4):474-9
8. Stylianides A, Jones MN, Stewart RM, Murphy CC, Goodson NJ, Kaye SB. Rheumatoid Arthritis-Associated Corneal Ulceration: Mortality and Graft Survival. *Ophthalmology.* 2013 Apr;120(4):682-6

In: Medicine Research Summaries. Volume 17
Editors: Zhongwen Liáng and Bibao Zhang
ISBN: 978-1-53612-751-5

Chapter 14

Carla Duarte Nunes

Affiliation:

CQB, Departamento de Química e Bioquímica, Faculdade de Ciências da Universidade de Lisboa (FCUL), Portugal

Address:

C8 bld., DQB-FCUL, Campo Grande, 1749-016 Lisboa, Portugal

Date of Birth:

08/01/1970

Education:

BSc in Chemistry (1998) – Faculdade de Ciências da Universidade de Lisboa, Portugal; PhD in Chemistry (2003) – Universidade de Aveiro, Portugal

Research and Professional Experience:

Research on materials chemistry for application in heterogeneous catalysis. Development of drug delivery systems based on inorganic materials. Development of magnetic nanostructures for highly recoverable catalysts.

Professional Appointments:

2000 – Research assistant (Universidade de Aveiro, Portugal);
2004 – Post-doctoral research associate (FCUL, Portugal);
2008 – Assistant researcher (FCUL, Portugal);
2013 – Associate researcher (FCUL, Portugal).

Honors:

FCT PhD grant (2001);
FCT post-doctoral fellowship (2004);
Ciencia2007 tenure-track fellowship (2008);
iFCT Senior researcher (2012)

Publications Last 3 Years:

1. Cristina I. Fernandes, Maria Deus Carvalho, Liliana P. Ferreira, Carla D. Nunes, Pedro D. Vaz, Organometallic Mo complex anchored to magnetic iron oxide nanoparticles as highly recyclable epoxidation catalyst, *J. Organomet. Chem.*, 760 (2014), 2-10.
2. Pedro Florindo, Ines J. Marques, Carla D. Nunes, Ana C. Fernandes, Synthesis, characterization and cytotoxicity of cyclopentadienyl ruthenium(II) complexes containing carbohydrate-derived ligands, *J. Organomet. Chem.*, 760 (2014), 240-247.
3. Marta S. Saraiva, Cristina I. Fernandes, Teresa G. Nunes, Carla D. Nunes, Maria Jose Calhorda, New Mo(II) complexes in MCM-41 and silica: Synthesis and catalysis, *J. Organomet. Chem.*, 760 (2014), 443-452.
4. Inês J. Marques, Pedro D. Vaz, Ana C. Fernandes, Carla D. Nunes, Advantageous delivery of Nifedipine from inorganic materials showing increased solubility and biocompatibility, *Microporous Mesoporous Mater.*,183 (2014), 192-200.
5. Cristina I. Fernandes, Marta S. Saraiva, Teresa G. Nunes, Pedro D. Vaz, Carla D. Nunes, Highly enantioselective olefin epoxidation controlled by helical confined environments, *J. Catal.,* 309 (2014), 21-32.
6. Isabel Ribeiro da Costa, P. C. R. Rodrigues, F. J. A. S. Barriga, P. A. Rona, Carla D. Nunes, Pedro D. Vaz, Colorless aegirine in metamorphic rocks from Bayan Obo (Inner Mongolia): lack of charge transfer transitions as possible explanation, *Eur. J. Mineral.*, 25 (2013), 987-993.
7. Gomes, A. Videira, O. C. Monteiro, C. D. Nunes, M. L. Carvalho, A. B. Lopes, Pulsed current electrodeposition of Zn-Ag2S/TiO2 nanocomposite films as potential photoelectrodes, *J. Solid St. Electrochem.*, 17 (2013), 2349-2359.
8. Marta S. Saraiva, Cristina I.Fernandes, Teresa G. Nunes, Carla D. Nunes, Maria Jose Calhorda, Mo(II) complexes of 8-aminoquinoline and their immobilization in MCM-41, *Applied Catal A – Gen.*, 455 (2013), 172-182.
9. Cristina I. Fernandes, Carla D. Nunes, Pedro D. Vaz, Clays in organic synthesis – preparation and catalytic applications, *Curr. Org. Synth.*, 9 (2012), 670-694.
10. Newton L. Dias Filho, Fátima C. M. Portugal, J. M. F. Nogueira, Paula Brandão, Vitor Félix, Pedro D. Vaz, Carla D. Nunes, Luis F. Veiros, Maria J. Villa de Brito, Maria José Calhorda, An oligosilsesquioxane cage functionalized with molybdenum(II) organometallic fragments, *Organometallics*, 31 (2012), 4495–4503.
11. Marco Araújo, Joana R. Xavier, Carla D. Nunes, Pedro D. Vaz, Madalena Humanes, Marine sponge melanin: a new source of an old biopolymer, *Struct. Chem.*, 23 (2012), 115-122.
12. Nuno U. Silva, Teresa G. Nunes, Marta S. Saraiva, Mohammad S. Shalamzari, Pedro D. Vaz, Olinda C. Monteiro, Carla D. Nunes, Photocatalytic degradation of rhodamine B using Mo heterogeneous catalysts under aerobic conditions, *Applied Catal. B: Environm.* 113-114 (2012), 180-191.
13. Pedro D. Vaz, Carla D. Nunes, The versatility of immobilized Mo complexes in organic transformations – epoxidation and metathesis reactions, *Curr. Org. Chem.* (Sp. Iss. *Mo chemistry*), 16 (2012), 89-114.
14. Nuno U. Silva, Cristina I. Fernandes, Teresa G. Nunes, Marta S. Saraiva, Carla D. Nunes, Pedro D. Vaz, Performance evaluation of mesoporous host materials in olefin

epoxidation using Mo(II) and Mo(VI) active species – inorganic vs. hybrid matrix, *Applied Catal. A: Gen.,* 408 (2011), 105-116.

15. Ana Carina Ventura, Cristina I. Fernandes, Marta S. Saraiva, Teresa G. Nunes, Pedro D. Vaz, Carla D. Nunes, Tuning the surface of mesoporous materials towards hydrophobicity – effects in olefin epoxidation, *Curr. Inorg. Chem.* (Sp. Iss. *Recent advances on oxidation chemistry*), 1 (2011), 156-165.
16. Maria Vasconcellos-Dias, Sara Raquel M. M. de Aguiar, Carla D. Nunes, Pedro D. Vaz, Teresa G. Nunes, Maria José Calhorda, Pyridine carboxylate complexes of Mo(II) as active catalysts in homogeneous and heterogeneous olefin epoxidation, *Curr. Inorg. Chem.* (Sp. Iss. *Recent advances on oxidation chemistry*), 1 (2011), 146-155.

In: Medicine Research Summaries. Volume 17
Editors: Zhongwen Liáng and Bibao Zhang

ISBN: 978-1-53612-751-5

Chapter 15

DAVID PADILLA-VALVERDE, MD, PHD

Affiliation:

Head of Section of Digestive and General Surgery .Department of Surgery. University General Hospital, Ciudad Real, Spain

Chief of Traslacional Research Unit, University General Hospital, Ciudad Real, Spain

Professor of Surgery .Faculty of Medicine, Castilla La Mancha University, Spain

Address:

University General Hospital, Ciudad Real, Spain
Avd Obispo Torija s/n
13005 Ciudad Real, Spain

Date of Birth:

8/11/1969

Education:

Grade of Medicine and Surgery, Medicine Faculty, Autonoma University, Madrid 1987-1993

Medicine and Surgery, Medicine Faculty, Autonoma University, Madrid 1995-1997.

Medicine and Surgery, University of Cordoba, Spain 1998- 2001

Research and Professional Experience:

- "Test of safety and effectiveness in hemodynamic monitoring, fluid and drug distribution during the development of a model of laparoscopic access for cytoreductive surgery and hyperthermic intra-abdominal chemotherapy through a closed recirculating CO2 in a porcine experimental model system" Foundation Eugenio Rodriguez Pascual, 2014. PI: David Padilla
- Usefulness of hyperthermic chemotherapy using intraabdominal gemcitabine for inhibiting tumor progression in an experimental model of pancreatic peritoneal carcinomatosis, and their behavior respect to CD133 + CXCR4 + cancer stem cells. Fundacion Eugenio Rodriguez Pascual. Madrid 12/26/2012. PI: Dr David Padilla

- FIS Project of Health Research, Institute of Health, Carlos III, Madrid, Spain. 2011. "Value of 18-FDG-PET-CT with intravenous contrast in the post-neoadjuvant restaging of patients with liver metastases" PI: Dr Ana Garcia Vicente.
- Development of independent clinical research, Department of Pharmacy and Health Products of the Ministry of Health, Social and Equality Policy . SAS / 2377/2010 and SAS / 2039/2009. Intraperitoneal chemohyperthermia closed with paclitaxel in the treatment of ovarian carcinomatosis" PI: Dr Pedro Villarejo.
- Project of Health Research. Foundation for Health Research in Castilla La Mancha (DOCM No 124 of 16 June 2008): "Analysis of the prognosis- therapeutic utility of serum determination by polymerase chain reaction, PCR, and histologically by in situ, FISH, miR-21, microRNA21 in patients with colorectal cancer "(number PI-2008/16) hybridization PI: Dr David Padilla.
- Project: GEDI (Global Volume diastolic) versus PVC (Central Pressure Vein) In Control Blood Loss during Liver Resection of Colorectal Metastasis who have received preoperative chemotherapy. IP: Dr Javier Redondo Calvo. Funding by Mutua Madrileña, Madrid, Spain .PI: DR Javier Redondo.2013
- "Selected advanced therapy for ovarian cancer using isolation, diagnosis and treatment of CD133 + CD44 + ovarian cancer stem cells after intra-abdominal citorreductive surgery and closed recirculation with CO2 chemotherapy". Funding by AMUMA, Ciudad Real, 2014. PI: David Padilla-Valverde
- "Individualized therapy in ovarian and pancreatic cancer by isolation, diagnosis and treatment of cancer stem cells after cytoreductive surgery and intraabdominal chemohyperthermia closed recirculating with CO2 chemotherapy ". Funding by Roche Fundacion. 2014-2015. PIs: David Padilla-Valverde / Pedro Villarejo-Campos
- Research project: "Technical and functional validation in animal model PRS equipment for treatment of peritoneal chemo-hyperthermia" .2009-2011.Departament of Animal Medicine and Surgery Autonomous University, Barcelona. Funding by: BIOSURGICAL, SL. 2011.PI: Alberto Martinez
- Research project: "Technical and functional validation in an animal model of the PRS equipment for chemo-hyperthermia bladder treatment" .2009-2011.Departament of Animal Medicine and Surgery .Autonomous University. Funding by: BIOSURGICAL, SL.2011. PI: Alberto Martinez
- Principal co-investigator of the International Liver Met Survey Project "Multidisciplinary treatment of colorectal liver metastases," 2007-2012. Funding by: Safonis Aventis. PI: Dr René Adams.2007-2013

Honors:

- Top 20 awards, General Surgery and Digestive Diseases. Hospital Complex, Ciudad Real. Health and Consumer Affairs Ministry, 2004.
- Award for Best Scientific Communication in Medicine, "Angiogenesis and lymphangiogenesis in gastric cancer", presented at the XXI National Meeting of the Spanish Chapter of the ISDE (Madrid, April 2009).
- 2005 "Research projects Fiscam Award" , "Serum growth factor of vascular endothelium in patients with colorectal cancer and its prognostic significance." 2005.
- Golden badge for David Padilla Valverde, as a member of hyperthermia Group, University General Hospital, Ciudad real.

- Best Oral Communication Award, XVII National Meeting of the Spanish Association of Coloproctology, Mallorca, 2013, "Prognostic Utility of serum determination of microRNA-21 in patients with colorectal scanner functions"
- Prize for the best publication in 2013 in HGUCR: Villarejo-Campos P, D Padilla-Valverde, Martin RM, Menedez-Sanchez P, Cubo-Cintas T, Bondia-Navarro JA, Martín J. Serum VEGF and VEGF-C values before and after surgery postoperative treatment in gastric cancer. Clin Transl Oncol 2012.
- "Dionisio Daza Chacon Award", 2013, for the study: Menendez p, Villarejo P, D Padilla Menendez JM, JA Rodriguez-Montes. "Diagnostic and prognostic utility of microRNA-21 in colorectal cancer.2013
- Best research work in health, University General Hospital, Ciudad Real, 2014, Development of an Experimental intraabdominal Chemohyperthermia Model with Closed Technique and CO2 Recirculation System by Means of Combat @ PRS-I.0
- Accesit best oral communication "Utility of hyperthermic intra-abdominal chemotherapy by gemcitabine for inhibiting tumor progression in an experimental model of pancreatic peritoneal carcinomatosis, concerning their behavior with CD133 + CXCR4 + cancer stem cells ". Biomedicina 2014, Ciudad Real, HGUCR, Spain
- Accesit to best oral communication, "Utility of hyperthermic intra-abdominal chemotherapy by gemcitabine for inhibiting tumor progression in an experimental model of pancreatic peritoneal carcinomatosis, concerning their behavior with CD133 + CXCR4 + cancer stem cells .XX National Meeting of the Spanish Association of Surgeons, Granada 2015
- Best communication, "Utility of hyperthermic intra-abdominal chemotherapy by gemcitabine for inhibiting tumor progression in an experimental model of pancreatic peritoneal carcinomatosis, concerning their behavior with CD133 + CXCR4 + cancer stem cells ". IV National Congress of Surgical Oncology .SEOQ. Madrid, 2015

Publications Last 3 Years:

1. Garcia-Santos EP, Padilla-Valverde D, Villarejo-Campos P, Murillo-Lazar C, Fernandez-Grande E, Palomino-Muñoz T, Rodriguez-Martinez M, Amo-Salas M, Nuñez-Guerrero P, Sanchez-García S, Puerto-Puerto A, Martin-Fernandez J.The utility of hyperthermic intra-abdominal chemotherapy with gemcitabine for the inhibition of tumor progression in an experimental model of pancreatic peritoneal carcinomatosis in relation to their behavior with pancreatic cancer stem cells CD133+CXCR4+*Pancreatologya*, 2016.In Press
2. Intraperitoneal Hyperthermia Chemotherapy (HIPEC) for Peritoneal carcinomatosis of Ovarian Cancer Origin Fluids and CO2 by a Recirculation Closed-Abdomen Technique (Combat PRS-1.0) Sanchez Garcia S, P Villarejo Campos, Padilla Valverde D, Martin J. *International Journal of Hyperthermia*, 2016 ; 7: 1-8.Articulo
3. Sanchez Garcia S, D Padilla Valverde, Villarejo Campos P, Martin Fernandez J, M Rojo Garcia, Rodriguez Martinez M, Experimental development of an intra-abdominal chemohyperthermia model with closed abdominal technique and CO2 recirculation system by Means of PRS-I.0 Combat. *Surgery*, 2014; 155 (4): 719-25. Article.
4. Pascual-Ramirez J, Sánchez García S, Gonzalez Ruiz de la Herran F, Villarejo Campos P, the Manzanara Cano Lopez C, Beech Palazuelo J, Valverde D Padilla,

Martin Fernandez J. Security and efficiency of a closed-system, turbulent-intraperitoneal hyperthermic flow circuit for ovarian cytoreductive chemotherapy after surgery: perioperative outputs. *Arch Gynecol Obstet*, 2014, Feb 1.DOI 10.1007 / s00404-014-3153-4. Article.

5. P Menendez, D Padilla, Villarejo P, Palomino T, P Nieto Menendez JM, JA Rodriguez-Montes. Prognostic Implications of serum microRNA-21 in colorectal cancer. *J Surg Oncol.* 2013 Nov; 108 (6): 369-73. Article.
6. Menendez P, Villarejo P, D Padilla Menendez JM, JA Rodriguez Montes. Implications of the histological determination of microRNAs in the screening, diagnosis and prognosis of colorectal cancer. *J Surg Oncol*, 2013; 108: 70-3. Article.
7. Menendez P, P Villarejo, Padilla D, Menedez J, Morales J. Diagnostic and prognostic significance of serum microRNAs in colorectal cancer. *J Surg Oncol* 2013; 107: 217-2. Article
8. Garcia-Santos EP, MC Manzanares-Campillo, Padilla-Valverde D, et al. Nesidioblastosis. A case of hyperplasia of the islets of Langerhans in the adult. *Pancreatology* 2013; 13: 544-8. Article.
9. Villarejo-Campos P, D Padilla-Valverde, Martin RM, Menedez-Sanchez P, Cube. Tapes T, Bondia-Navarro JA, JM Fernandez. Serum VEGF and VEGF-C values before surgery and postoperative treatment after Transl Oncol in gastric cancer.*Clin* 2013; 15: 265-70. Article.
10. New Roles of lymphangiogenesis in Cancer Spread. Villarejo-Campos P, D Padilla-Valverde, J. Sanchez Redondo-In *The lymphatic System: Components, functions and diseases*. Ramirez C, Editor.Nova Science Publishers, 2016. Chapter Book
11. Villarejo Campos P, D Padilla Valverde, Eds. fatores gastric cancer and vascular endothelial growth. Prognostic value of serum levels of VEGF and VEGF-C. Saarbrucken, Alemania.*Editorial Academic Spanish*, 2013. Complete Book.
12. Padilla D, JM Cano Garcia Red M, Palomar A. gastrointestinal stromal tumors (GIST). In: *Protocols Multidisciplinary Oncology. Espinosa Arranz J. Aran Ediciones*, Madrid 2013.pp 510-15. CL

In: Medicine Research Summaries. Volume 17
Editors: Zhongwen Liáng and Bibao Zhang
ISBN: 978-1-53612-751-5

Chapter 16

GIORGIA PASTORIN

Affiliation:
National University of Singapore

Address:
3 Science Drive 2, Block S15#5-PI-03,Singapore 117543

Date of Birth:
13 May 1976

Education:
PhD in Medicinal Chemistry (2000-2004)

Research and Professional Experience:
Medicinal Chemistry:

- Potent antagonists towards different adenosine receptors' subtypes.
- Novelmulti -targeting chemical entities for the treatment of Parkinson's disease. Molecular modeling studies to investigate ligand-receptor interactions.

Nano-bio-technologies:

- Targeted drug delivery, through strategic functionalizations of nanodevices. Transdermal vaccine delivery through aligned nano-needles systems. Toxicological evaluation of drug delivery systems for biomedical applications.
- Lab-on-a-chip devices for selective detection of rare circulating tumor cells (started recently).

Professional Appointments:

2014-present	Assistant Head at the Department of Pharmacy, NUS
2011-present	Associate Professor at the Department of Pharmacy, NUS
2006-2011	Assistant Professor at the Department of Pharmacy, NUS
2004-2006	Research Fellow at the Laboratoire d'Immunologie et Chimie Therapeutiques, CNRS in Strasbourg (France)

Honors:

Excellence Young Teacher Award AY 2010/2011

Publications Last 3 Years:

1. Priyankar Paira, Chow Mun Juinn, Gopalakrishnan Venkatesan, Vamsi Krishna Kosaraju, Siew Lee Cheong, Karl-Norbert Klotz, Wee Han Ang*, Giorgia Pastorin*. Organoruthenium Antagonists of Human A3 Adenosine Receptors. *Chemistry: A European Journal,* 2013, *19(25},* 8321-8330.
2. Jun Hu, Yuancai Dong, Giorgia Pastorin*, Wai Kiong Ng*, Reginald B. H. Tan. Spherical agglomerates of pure drug nanoparticles for improved pulmonary delivery in dry powder inhalers. *Journal of Nanoparticle Research,* 2013, *15,* 1560.
3. Xiao Chen, Ce-Belle Chen, Chammika N.B. Udalagama, Minqin Ren, Kah Ee Fong, Lin Vue Lanry Yung, Pastorin Giorgia, Andrew Anthony Bettiol, Frank Watt. High-Resolution 3D Imaging and Quantification of Gold Nanoparticles in a Whole Cell Using Scanning Transmission ton Microscopy. *Biophysical Journal,* 2013, *104,* 1419-1425.
4. Zhuolin Xiang, Wang Hao, Aakanksha Pant, Giorgia Pastorin*, Chengkuo Lee* Vertical SU-8 Microtubes Integrated with Dissolvable Tips for Transdermal Drug Delivery. *Biomicrofluidics,* 2013, *7.* 026502.
5. Zhuolin Xiang, Wang Hao, Aakanksha Pant, Giorgia Pastorin*, Chengkuo Lee*. Development of vertical SU-8 microneedles for transdermal drug delivery by double drawing lithography technology. *Biomicrofluidics,* 2013, 7 *{6),* 6501.
6. Jan Gruber, Sheng Fong, Ce-Belle Chen, Sialee Yoong, Giorgia Pastorin, Sebastian Schaffer, Irwin Cheah, Barry Halliwell*. Mitochondria-targeted Antioxidants and Metabolic Modulators as Pharmacological Interventions to slow Ageing. *Biotechnology Advances* 2013, 31(5): 563-92.
7. Panczyk, Tomasz; Jagusiak, Anna; Pastorin, Giorgia; Ang, Wee Han; Narkiewicz-Michalek, Jolanta. Molecular Dynamics Study of Cisplatin Release from Carbon Nanotubes Capped By Magnetic Nanoparticles. *The Journal of Physical Chemistry.* Part C: Energy Conversion and Storage, Optical and Electronic Devices, Interfaces, Nanomaterials, and Hard Matter. Section: C: Physical Processes in *Nanomaterials and Nanostructures.* 2013, 117 (33), 17327-17336.
8. Bin Sheng Wong , Sia lee Yoong, Anna Jagusiak, Tomasz Panczyk, Han Kiat Ho, Wee Han Ang, Giorgia Pastorin . Carbon Nanotubes for Delivery of Small Molecule Drugs. *Advanced Drug Delivery Reviews,* 2013, *65,* 1964-2015.
9. Hao Wang, Zhuolin Xiang, Chih-Fan Hu, Aakanksha Pant, Weileun Fang, Sylvie Alonso, Giorgia Pastorin* and Chengkuo lee*. Development of Stretchable Membrane Based Nanofilters Using Patterned Array of Vertically Grown Carbon Nanotubes. *Nanoscale,* 2013, *5,* 8488-8493
10. Chunyan Zhao, Aaron Tan, Giorgia Pastorin*, Han Kiat Ho*. Nanomaterial scaffolds for stem cell proliferation and differentiation in tissue engineering. *Biotechnology Advances,* 2013, *31{5),* 654-668.
11. Sia lee Yoong, Bin Sheng Wong, Qi lin Zhou, Chee Fei Chin, Jian li, Thirumalai Venky Venkatesan, Han Kiat Ho, Victor Chun Kong Yu, Wee Han Ang*, Giorgia Pastorin*. Enhanced Cytotoxicity to Cancer Cells by Mitochondria-targeting

MWCNTs Containing Platinum(IV) Prodrug of Cisplatin. *Biomaterials,* 2014, *35{2),* 748-759.

12. Jian li, Aakansha Pant, Chee Fei Chin, Wee Han Ang*, Cecilia Menard-Moyon, Tapas R. Nayak, Dan Gibson, Sundara Ramaprabhu. Tomasz Panczyk, Alberto Bianco*, and Giorgia Pastorin*. *In vivo* biodistribution of platinum-based drugs encapsulated into multi-walled carbon nanotubes. *Nanomedicine,* 2014, *10{7),* 1465-1475.
13. Tomasz Panczyk·, Tatiana Da os, Giorgia Pastorin, Anna Jagusiak, Jolanta Narkiewicz-Michalek. Role of Intermolecular Interactions in Assemblies of Nanocontainers Composed of Carbon Nanotubes and Magnetic Nanoparticles. A Molecular Dynamics Study. *The Journal of Physical chemistry,* Part C, 2014, *118* (2), 1353-1363.
14. Chee Fei Chin, Siew Qi Yap, Jian li, Giorgia Pastorin* and Wee Han Ang*. Ratiometric Delivery of Cisplatin and Doxorubicin using Tumour-Targeting Carbon-Nanotubes Entrapping Platinum (IV) Prodrugs. *Chemical Science,* 2014, *5,* 2265-2270.
15. Stephanie Federico, Antonella Ciancetta, Nicola Porta, Sara Redenti, Giorgia Pastorin, Barbara Cacciari, Karl Norbert Klotz, Stefano Moro, * and Giampiero Spalluto*. Scaffold Profiling on Adenosine Receptors: A Preliminary SAR Study. *Journal of Medicinal Chemistry,* 2014, *57(14},* 6210-6225.
16. Hao Wang, Zhuolin Xiang, Chih-Fan Hu, Giorgia Pastorin, Weileun Fang, and Chengkuo lee. Microneedle Array Integrated with CNT Nanofilters for Controlled and Selective Drug Delivery. *IEEE Journal of Microelectromechanical Systems.*2014, 23{5), 1036-1044. {October)
17. Zhuolin Xiang, Hao Wang, Suresh Kanna Murugappan, Shih-Cheng Yen, Giorgia Pastorin* and Chengkuo lee*. Dense vertical SU-8 microneedles drawn from a heated mold with precisely controlled volume. *J. Micromech.Microeng.*2015, 25, 025013 {10 pp).
18. G. Venkatesan, P. Paira, S.L. Cheong, S. Federico*, K.N. Klotz, G. Spalluto*, G. Pastorin*. A facile and novel synthesis of N 2 C6-substituted pyrazolo[3, 4-d]pyrimidine-4 carboxylate derivatives as adenosine receptor antagonists. *European Journal of Medicinal Chemistry*, 2015, *92,* 784-798.
19. Chow, Mun Juinn; Licona, Cynthia; Wong, Daniel Yuan Qiang; Pastorin G, Gaiddon C., Ang Wee Han. Discovery and Investigation of Anticancer Ruthenium-Arene Schiff-Base Complexes via Water-Promoted Combinatorial Three-Component Assembly. *Journal of Medicinal Chemistry,* 2014, *57 (14),* 6043 6059.
20. Laura Muzi, Cecilia Menard-Moyon, Julie Russier, Jian li, Chee Fei Chin, Wee Han Ang, Giorgia Pastorin·, Gianfranco Risuleo, Alberto Bianco·. Diameter-dependent release of a cisplatin pro- drug from small and large functionalized carbon nanotubes. *Nanoscale,* 2015, accepted.

In: Medicine Research Summaries. Volume 17
Editors: Zhongwen Liáng and Bibao Zhang
ISBN: 978-1-53612-751-5

Chapter 17

MEGAN A. RECH

Affiliation:
Loyola University Medical Center

Address:
3422 N Seminary Ave. Chicago IL, 60657, US

Date of Birth:
11/30/1984

Education:

2014 – Present	Clinical Research Methods Master Program Loyola University Chicago, Maywood, Illinois
2006 – 2009	Doctor of Pharmacy Lake Erie College of Osteopathic Medicine (LECOM) School of Pharmacy, Erie, Pennsylvania
2003 – 2006	Pre-Pharmacy and Spanish Studies The University of Toledo Toledo, Ohio

Research and Professional Experience:

March 2013 – Present	Emergency Medicine Clinical Pharmacist Loyola University Medical Center, Maywood, Illinois
Aug 2011 – Feb 2013	Critical Care/Transplant Clinical Pharmacist Henry Ford Hospital, Detroit, Michigan

Professional Appointments:

March 2013 – Present	Emergency Medicine Clinical Pharmacist

Honors:

2014	Magis Award, Loyola University Medical Center

2013 – 2014	Preceptor of the Year PGY-1 Pharmacy Residency Class Loyola University Medical Center
2013	Magis Award, Loyola University Medical Center

Publications Last 3 Years:

1. Rech MA, To L, Tovbin A, et al. Heavy Metal in the ICU: A Review of Current Literature on Trace Element Supplementation in Critically Ill Patients. *Nutr Clin Pract.* 2014; 29 (1): 78-89.
2. Bauman ZM, Killu K, Rech MA, et al. Racial Differences in Vasopressor Requirements for Septic Shock. *Shock.* 2014; 41 (3): 188-192.
3. Rech MA, Fleming JN, Moore CL. 25-Hydroxyvitamin D Deficiency Predicts Incidence of Opportunistic Viral Infections after Kidney Transplantation. *Exp Clin Transplant.* 2014; 2:95-100.
4. Rech MA, Hunsaker T, Rodriguez J. 25-Hydroxyvitamin D Deficiency Predicts 30-Day Mortality in Patients with Severe Sepsis and Septic Shock. *Am J Crit Care.* 2014; 23 (5): e72-9.
5. Rech MA, Donahey E, Cappiello-Dziedzic J, et al. *New Illicit Drugs of Abuse. Pharmacotherapy.* 2015; 35 (2):189-97.
6. Rech MA, Day SA, Kast, JA, et al. Major publications in the critical care pharmacotherapy literature: January 2013 through December 2013. *Am J Health Syst Pharm.* 2015; 72 (3): 224-36.

In: Medicine Research Summaries. Volume 17
Editors: Zhongwen Liáng and Bibao Zhang
ISBN: 978-1-53612-751-5

Chapter 18

Lucia de Fatima Sobral Sampaio

Affiliation:

Federal University of Pará. Belém, PA. Brazil

Address:

Av. Augusto Corrêa No. 1. UFPA, ICB. Belém, PA. Brazil. CEP: 66075-110

Date of Birth:

4/29/1964

Education:

PhD at University of the São Paulo (USP), São Paulo, SP. Brazil.

Research and Professional Experience:

Biochemistry Professor since 2002 and heard of the research group Biochemical of the Neurodevelopment since 2004.

Professional Appointments:

Biochemistry Lectures and Project management

Honors:

2013 Best Poster Award, FASEB Science Research Conference. Melatonin Biology Actions and Therapeutics

Publications Last 3 Years:

1. Sampaio, Lde F; MESQUITA, F. P.; de Sousa, PRM; SILVA, J. L.; Alves, CN. NRH: Quinone Reductase activity results in the accumulation of endogenous dopamine in the retina. *Neurotransmitter*, v. 2, p. 2015 2: e505, 2015.
2. Sampaio, Lucia de Fatima Sobral; Mesquita, Felipe Pantoja ; Sousa, Paulo Robson Monteiro De; Silva, Jerônimo Lameira ; Alves, Claudio Nahum . The melatonin analog 5-MCA-NAT increases endogenous dopamine levels by binding NRH: Quinone reductase enzyme in the developing chick retina. *International Journal of Developmental Neuroscience*, v. 38, p. 119-126, 2014.

3. SILVA, R. N.; Sampaio, L de F. Immunoreactivity of Mel1a-like melatonin receptor and NRH: Quinone reductase enzyme (QR2) in testudine whole embryo and in developing whole retinas. *Trends in Developmental Biology*, v. 8, p. 39-46, 2014.
4. Sampaio, L. F. S.; Nogueira, R. C.; Ferreira, M. A. P., Forskolin Embryotoxicity in Initial Stages of the Embryonic Development in Chick. In: Marty H. Walker. (Org.). Forskolin: Sources, *Mechanisms of Action and Health Effects*. 1 ed. New York: Nova Science Publishers, Inc., 2015, v. 1, p. 51-66.
5. Sampaio, L. F. S. By Receptors, Binding Sites or Free Radical Scavenger Action: Is There a Pivotal Action Mechanism for Melatonin in Retinal Pathologies? In: Dario Acuña-Castroviejo; Iryna Rusanova; Germaine Escames. (Org.). *New Developments in Melatonin Research*. 1ed. New York: NOVA Publishers, 2013, v., p. 193-204.
6. Sampaio, L. F. S. Catecholquinones as Substrates of the NRH: Quinone Oxidoreductase 2 in the Brain and Retina. In: Ervin R. Price, Smith C. Johnson. (Org.). *Quinones: Occurrence, Medicinal Uses and Physiological Importance*. 1ed.New York: NOVA Publishers, 2013, v., p. 141-156.

In: Medicine Research Summaries. Volume 17
Editors: Zhongwen Liáng and Bibao Zhang
ISBN: 978-1-53612-751-5

Chapter 19

HAIPENG SHAO

Affiliation:
Moffitt Cancer Center

Address:
12902 Magnolia Dr, MCC-LAB, Tampa, Fl, US

Date of Birth:
09/07/1970

Research and Professional Experience:

2010-Present	Assistant Member Department of Hematopathology and Laboratory Medicine Moffitt Cancer Center (MCC}, Tampa, FL Assistant Professor Department of Oncologic Sciences Department of Pathology & Cell Biopsy College of Medicine, University of South Florida, Tampa, FL
2003-2004	Postdoctoral Fellow Department of Physiology and Neuroscience
2000-2003	Medical University of South Carolina, Charleston, SC Postdoctoral Associate Department of Genetics Yale University, New Haven, CT

Professional Appointments:
Assistant Member

Publications Last 3 Years:

1. Wu H, Bui MM, Leston DG, Shao H, Sokol L, Sotomayor EM, Zhang L. Clinical characteristics and prognostic factors of bone lymphomas: focus on the clinical significance of multifocal bone involvement by primary bone large B-celllymphomas. *BMC Cancer*. 2014 Dec 2;14:900. PMID: 25465716

2. Dalia S, Shao H, Sagatys E, Cualing H, Sokol L. Dendritic cell and histiocytic neoplasms: Biology, Diagnosis, and Treatment. *Cancer Control.* 2014 Oct;21(4):290-300. PMID:25310210.
3. Harrington L1, Sokol L, Holdener S, Shao H, Zhang L. Cutaneous Gamma-delta (yo) T-cell Lymphoma with Central Nervous System {CNS) Involvement: Report of a Rarity with Review of Literature. *J Cutan Pathol.* 2014 Oct 8. PMID: 25292289.
4. You Y, Shao H, Bui K, Bui M, Klapman J, Cui Q, Coppola D. Epstein-barr virus positive inflammatory pseudotumor of the liver: report of a challenging case and review of the literature. *Ann Clin Lab Sci.* 2014 Fall;44(4):489-98. PMID: 25361938.
5. Wu H, Zhang L, Shao H, Sokol L, Sotomayor E, Letson D, Bui MM. Prognostic significance of soft tissue extension, International Prognostic Index, and multifocality in primary bone lymphoma: a single institutional experience. *Br J Haematol.* 2014 Jul;166{1):60-8. PMID: 24673481.
6. Zhang L, Shao H. Primary cutaneous CD4 positive small/medium T-celllymphoma with high proliferation index and CD30-positive large lymphoid cells. *J Cutan Pathol.* 2013 Aug;40{8):720-4. PMID: 23672694.
7. Zhang X, Sun M, Zhang L, Shao H. Primary hepatosplenic COS-positive diffuse large B-cell lymphoma: a case report with literature review. *Int J Clin Exp Pathol.* 2013 Apr 15;6{5):985-9. PMID: 23638236
8. Shao H, Calvo KR, Gronborg M, Tembhare PR, Kreitman RJ, Stetler-Stevenson M, Yuan CM. Distinguishing hairy cell leukemia variant from hairy cell leukemia: Development and validation of diagnostic criteria. *Leuk Res.* 2013 Apr;37{4):401-9. PMID: 23347903
9. Zhang L, Sotomayor EM, Papenhausen PR, Shao H, Moscinski LC, Sandin RL, Caceres G, Valenica H, Malafa M, List AF, Sokol L. Unusual concurrence of T-celllarge granular lymphocytic leukemia with Franklin disease (gamma heavy chain disease) manifested with massive splenomegaly. *Leuk Lymphoma.* 2013 Jan;54(1):205-208. PMID: 22694793.
10. Setoodeh R, Schwartz S, Papenhausen P, Zhang L, Sagatys EM, Moscinski LC, Shao H. Double-hit mantle cell lymphoma with MYC gene rearrangement or amplification: a report of four cases and review of the literature. *Int J Clin Exp Pathol.* 2013;6(2):155-67. PMID:23330001

In: Medicine Research Summaries. Volume 17
Editors: Zhongwen Liáng and Bibao Zhang
ISBN: 978-1-53612-751-5

Chapter 20

IANA SIMOVA, MD, PHD

Affiliation:

Department of Noninvasive Cardiovascular Imaging and Functional Diagnostics, National Cardiology Hospital, Sofia, Bulgaria

Address:

65 Koniovitsa Str, Sofia 1309, Bulgaria

Education:

1995	Mathematical High School, Sofia
1996-2002	MD - Medical University, Sofia
2006 – 2009	PhD - Medical University, Sofia
03.2003	Internal Disease residency started
11.2008 – 11.2012	Cardiology residency, Basal and expert degree Echocardiography
October 2005	Basic Cardiology - Niguarda Hospital, Milan, Italy -
September 2013	Noninvasive coronary flow reserve - Department of Medical Translational Sciences, University of Naples Federico II, Naples, Italy

Research and Professional Experience:

04.2015 –	Associate professor at Department of Noninvasive Cardiovascular Imaging and Functional Diagnostics, National Cardiology Hospital
01.2015 -	Head of Scientific Department at MHAT “Doverie”; consulting physician at MC “Doverie”
03.2011 –	Senior research associate at Department of Noninvasive Cardiovascular Imaging and Functional Diagnostics, National Cardiology Hospital
01.2009 - 03.2011	Appointed physician and research associate at Department of Noninvasive Cardiovascular Imaging and Functional Diagnostics, National Cardiology Hospital
03.2006 – 12.2008	PhD procedure at the Clinic of Cardiology, University Hospital “Alexandrovska”;

03.2003 – 10.2004 Appointed physician at the University Hospital Losenetz, clinic of Cardiology

Professional Appointments:

- EACVI Educational Committee member 2015-2016
- Member of Scientific Council at National Cardiology Hospital from 03.2015
- Ambassador for Bulgaria for EACVI Club 35 2012-2014
- EACVI Club 35 Committee member 2013-2014
- Working group on e-Cardiology of the European Society of Cardiology
- Working group on Acute Cardiac Care of the European Society of Cardiology
- Working group on Myocardial Function of the European Society of Cardiology

Honors:

- Awarded "Best poster" at XIV National Congress of Cardiology with international participation, Varna, Zlatni piasutsi, 02-05.10.2014;
- Awarded "Best poster" at XIII National Congress of Cardiology with international participation, Sofia, 04-07.10.2012;
- Certificate for best achievement in "Competition for high scientific achievements for 2010", organized by Bulgarian Union of Scientists
- Awarded "Best poster in cardiac imaging" at XII National Congress of Cardiology with international participation, Albena, 07-10.10.2010;
- Certificate for best achievement in the "Competition for scientific achievements for PhD students, graduated 2008", organized by Bulgarian Union of Scientists
- Certificate of achievement for the best research work in the "Young researcher 2006" and " Young researcher 2007" competitions in the scientific field of Medicine, medico-clinical branch
- Second best in the Physionet/Computers in Cardiology Challenge "QT interval measurement" 2006 in:
    - Division 1: Manual and semi-automated methods
    - Division 3: Fully automated methods with source code submitted
- "Golden Hypocrate" award for highest GPA (6.00) on Medical University graduation, 2002
- Gold medal for GPA (Grade Point Average) on Mathematical High School graduation, 1995

Publications Last 3 Years:

International journals

Clinical research

1. Simova1 I., Christov I., Bortolan G., Abächerli R., Kambova L., Jekova I. Hemodialysis-induced ST-segment Deviation. *Computing in Cardiology* 2015; 42:1133-1136 IF-Scopus(2011)=0.39.
2. Christov I., Simov D., Dotsinsky I., Simova I. Increase of electrical impedance following hemodialysis is not the reason for QRS augmentation. *Annals of Noninvasive Electrocardiology*. Accepted IF (2014) = 1.131.

3. Simova I, Bortolan G, Kambova L, Christov I, Katova T. Episodes of T-wave and QRS Complex Alternans in Haemodialysis Patients. *EC Cardiology* 2015; 2 (1):60-67.
4. The EchoNoRMAL (Echocardiographic Normal Ranges Meta-Analysis of the Left Heart) Collaboration. Ethnic-Specific Normative Reference Values for Echocardiographic LA and LV Size, LV Mass, and Systolic Function. The EchoNoRMAL Study. *JACC: Cardiovascular Imaging* 2015; 8 (6): 656-665. IF (2013) = 6.986.
5. Simova I, Katova T, Santoro C, Galderisi M. Comparison between regional and local pulse wave velocity data. Echocardiography – *A Journal of Cardiovascular Ultrasound and Alied technoques*. Accepted IF (2013) = 1.254.
6. Bortolan G, Christov I, Simova I, Dotsinsky I. Noise processing in exercise ECG stress test for the analysis and the clinical characterization of QRS and T wave alternans. *Biomedical Signal Processing and Control*. 2015; 18:378-385 IF(2013)=1.68.
7. Simova I, Christov I, Kambova L, Bortolan G, Katova T. QRS and T Loops Area Changes During Haemodialysis. *Computing in Cardiology* 2014; 41:409-412 IF-Scopus(2011)=0.39.
8. Christov I, Batchvarov VN, Simova I, Dimitrov N, Behr ER. Comparative Study of Signal Decomposition Methods for Enhancement of the Accuracy of T-wave End Localisation. *Computing in Cardiology* 2014; 41:1073-1076 IF-Scopus(2011)=0.39.
9. Christov I., Simova I., Abächerli R. Extraction of the fetal ECG in noninvasive recordings by signal decompositions. *Physiological Measurement* 2014; 35:1713-1721 Impact Factor 1.7 citations: 6.
10. Dimitrov N, Simova I, Boichev B, Mateev H. Early or selective invasive strategy in patients with non-ST-segment elevation acute coronary syndrome according to the risk factors at presentation? An outcome study. *Cardiology and Angiology: an International Journal* 2014; 2 (4):205-222.
11. Simova I, Katova T, Nesheva A, Hristova K, Kostova V, Boyadzhiev L, Dimitrov N. Echocardiographic predictors of early postoperative atrial fibrillation in coronary artery bypass surgery patients. *World Heart J* 2014; 6 (3): 163-170.
12. Simova I, Katova T, Kostova V. Effects of combined antihypertensive treatment with ramipril and amlodipine on blood pressure and arterial stiffness parameters. *Experimental and Clinical Cardiology* 2014; 20 (1):3495-3502 http://www.cardiologyacademicpress.com/?p=20475.
13. Christov I., Simova I., Abächerli R. Cancellation of the maternal and extraction of the fetal ECG in noninvasive recordings. *Computing in Cardiology*, 2013, 40, 153-156, ISSN: 2325-8861. *IF-Scopus(2011)=0.39 citations: 4.*
14. Christov I., G. Bortolan, I. Simova. Load dependent changes of cardiac depolarization and repolarization during exercise ECG test. *Computing in Cardiology*, 2013, 40, 547-550, ISSN: 2325-8861. IF-Scopus(2011)=0.39.
15. A meta-analysis of echocardiographic measurements of the left heart for the development of normative reference ranges in a large international cohort: the EchoNoRMAL study. The Echocardiographic Normal Ranges Meta-Analysis of the Left heart (EchoNoRMAL) Collaboration. *Eur Heart J Cardiovasc Imaging* 2013; doi: 10.1093/ehjci/jet240 First published online: November 17, 2013

http://ehjcimaging.oxfordjournals.org/content/early/2013/11/17/ehjci.jet240.full.html ?papetoc *Impact Factor - 2.394 citations: 4.*

16. Simova I, Mateev H, Katova T, Haralanov L, Dimitrov N. Telemonitoring boosts atrial fibrillation detection in cryptogenic stroke patients – preliminary findings. *Cardiology and Angiology: An International Journal* 2013; 1 (2): 47-57, Article no.CA.2013.002 *citations: 1.*

Letter to the Editor

1. Christov I., Simov D., Dotsinsky I., Simova I. Increase of electrical impedance following hemodialysis is not the reason for QRS augmentation. *Ann Noninvasive Electrocardiol 2015*;00(0):1.

Reviews

1. Simova I. Role of tilt-table testing in syncope diagnosis and management. An article from the e-journal of the *ESC Council for Cardiology Practice*, Vol 13 No 35, 10 Nov 2015.
2. Simova I. Coronary flow velocity reserve assessment with transthoracic Doppler echocardiography. *European Cardiology Review*, 2015;10(1):12-8.
3. Simova I. Intima-media thickness: Appropriate evaluation and proper measurement, described. An article from the e-journal of the *ESC Council for Cardiology Practice*, Vol 13, No 21, 05 May 2015.
4. Simova I., Christov I., Bortolan G. A review on electrocardiographic changes in diabetic patients. Current Diabetes Review 2015; 11 (4): 102-106.

Local journals

Clinical research

1. Simova I., Dimitrov N., Gesheva N., Ognianov S. Efficacy and safety of Romazic for addressing dyslipidemy in aortic atheromatosis patients. *Cardio D* 2015; 4 (30):36-38.
2. Simova I., Katova T., Tsonev S., Vasilev D., Ognianov S. Molsidomine improves coronary flow reserve and endothelial function in patients with microvascular angina. *Cardio D* 2015; 3 (29):17-20.
3. Simova I., Katova T., Kostova V. Combined antihypertensive therapy olmesartan / amlodipine decreases blood pressure and improves ventricular-arterial coupling. *Cardio D* 2015; 3 (29):14-16.
4. Katova T., Simova I., Kostova V. Antihypertensive efficacy of Egiramlon - effects in time. *Cardio D* 2015; 3 (29):10-12.
5. Dimitrov N, Simova I, Mateev H, Iliev R. Influence of renal function on management of patients with non-ST segment elevation acute coronary syndrome. *Bulgarian Cardiology* 2014; 4 (XX):37-47.
6. Simova I, Katova T, Zerdeva E, Dasheva A, Levunlieva E, Kuneva A. Role of tilt-table testing in the diagnostic work-up of syncope in children. *Bulgarian Cardiology* 2014; 3 (XX):35-40.

7. Katova T, Simova I, Kostova V. Egiramlon - antihypertensive efficacy and effects on arterial stiffness. *Cardio D* 2014; 3 (25):25-28.
8. Boychev B., Simova I., Dimitrov N. Telecardiology in Bulgaria - follow-up data of more than 3 000 patients. *Cardiovascular Diseases* 2014; 2014; 3:10-16
9. Dimitrov N, Simova I, Mateev M, Kalpachka M, Pavlov P, Tasheva I. Timing of invasive strategy in diabetic and non-biabetic patients with non-ST-segment elevation acute coronary syndrome. *Folia Medica* 2013; 55(2):16-25. *citations: 2*
10. Simova I, Katova T, Kostova V. Egiramlon in the treatment of arterial hypertension. *Cardio D* 2013; 3 (21):22-24.
11. Kostova V, Simova I, Katova T, Bojadjiev L, Hristova K. Patient-prosthesis mismatch and left ventricular function in aortic valve replacement patients. *Diagnostic and Therapeutic Ultrasound* 2013; 1 (21):51-56.

Case reports

12. Simova I. Contemporary antihypertensive strategy - Combine initially and wisely for better results. *Cardio D* 2015; 4 (30):53-56.
13. Simova I. Exforge HCT – the power of easy solutions. *Cardio D* 2015; 4 (30):29-32.
14. Simova I. Exforge HCT - when we need a little more added power. *Cardio D* 2015; 3 (29):26-29.
15. Simova I. Natrixam - when we need the right solution. *Cardio D* 2015; 2 (28):16-18.
16. Simova I., Katova T. Effects of Molsidomin on endothelial function and coronary flow reserve in a patient with microvascular angina. *Cardio D* 2014; 4 (26):47-50.
17. Simova I. Exforge HCT - when we need a prompt and secure effect. *Cardio D* 2014; 3 (25):56-59.
18. Simova I. Clinical case: Exforge HCT in high-risk patients. *Cardio D* 2014; 2(24):36-38.
19. Simova I. Antihypertensive efficacy of Exforge HCT - a clinical case. *Cardio D* 2014; 1(23):43-46.

Reviews

20. Simova I. Antihypertensive and additional cardiovascular protective effects of combined therapy zofenopril + HCT. Cardio D Д 2015; 4 (30):33-35.
21. Simova I. Benefits of adding ezetimibe to statin therapy. *Cardio D* 2015; 4 (30):39-40.
22. Simova I. Update from European Cardiology Congress, London 2015. *Cardio D* 2015; 4 (30):22-29.
23. Simova I. Echocardiographic evaluation of prosthetic valves. *Cardio D* 2015; 4 (30):5-13.
24. Simova I. Residual cardiovascular risk after myocardial infarction. *Cardio D* 2015; 3 (29):56-59.
25. Simova I. Importance of blood pressure variability and possibilities to influence it. *Cardio D* 2015; 3 (29):32-36.
26. Simova I. Echocardiographic evaluation of the aorta. *Cardio D* 2015; 3 (29):65-72.
27. Simova I. ACE inhibitors and HCT - one of the favoured antihypertensive combinations. *Cardio D* 2015; 3 (29):29-30.

28. Simova I. Heart failure with reduced left ventricular ejection fraction. *MD* 2015; 3 (XII):23-30.
29. Simova I. Update from ACC/AHA Scientific sessions 2015. *Cardio D* 2015; 2(28): 38-45.
30. Simova I. Aortic regurgitation - echocardiographic evaluation. *Cardio D* 2015; 2 (28): 30-36.
31. Simova I. Evidence supporting Exforge HCT application in contemporary clinical practice. *Cardio D* 2015; 2 (28):23-26.
32. Simova I. Olmesartan/amlodipine - stable and smooth antihypertensive effect, with added value in hypertensive patients with high cardiovascular risk. *Cardio D* 2015; 2 (28):20-22.
33. Simova I. Combined antihypertensive treatment - advantages of fixed combination ramipril/amlodipine. *MD* 2015; 2 (XII): 37-38.
34. Simova I. Olmesartan/amlodipine - appropriate and powerful combination for patients with arterial hypertension and obesity. *Cardio D* 2015; 1 (27):42-45.
35. Simova I. Valsartan effects on left ventricular hypertrophy in patients with arterial hypertension and diabetes mellitus. *Cardio D* 2015; 1 (27):33-36.
36. Simova I. Cardiology update - Davos 2015. *Cardio D* 2015; 1 (27):20-32.
37. Simova I. Aortic stenosis - echocardiographic assessment. *Cardio D* 2015; 1 (27): 10-16.
38. Simova I. Advances in cardiology and angiology during 2014. MD; *Medicine Today in Bulgaria* 2015; 1 (85):110-114.
39. Simova I. Importance of antihypertensive therapy tolerability - advantages of the different calcium channel blocker lercanidipine. *Cardio D* 2014; 4 (26):8-10.
40. Simova I. Lercanidipine effects blood pressure and total cardiovascular risk. *CardioD* 2014; 3 (25):29-31.
41. Simova I. Bisoprolol in the treatment of chronic heart failure. *CardioD* 2014; 3 (25):49-52.
42. Simova I. Lercanidipine in arterial hypertension treatment. MD 2014; 5 (XI):44-47
43. Simova I. Protecting the brain with lercanidipine in hypertensive patients. *Cardio D* 2014; 2(24):40-42.
44. Simova I. Comparison between American and European guidelines for management of dyslipidemy. *MD* 2014; 2 (80):23-26.
45. Simova I. Low-dose rosuvastatin application in primary prevention. Cardio D 2014; 1(23):5-8.
46. Simova I. Nephroprotection with calcium channel blockers? Why not, when using lercanidipine. *Cardio D* 2014; 1(23):47-48.
47. Simova I. Relief or confusion for hypertensive patients and their doctors - two new guidelines for management of arterial hypertension in USA. *MD Bulgaria* 2014 1(79):88-91.
48. Simova I. Choice and titration of antilipemic therapy for cardiovascular risk management. *Cardio D* 2013; 4(22):5-6.
49. Simova I. Zofenopril – effective in a wide specter of hypertensive conditions. *Cardio D* 2013; 3 (21):26-28.
50. Simova I. Application of Lipanthyl for the management of residual cardiovascular risk. *Cardio D* 2013; 3 (21):28-30.

51. Simova I. Combination bisoprolol + ASA (Betapres) in cardiology. *Cardio D* 2013; 3 (21):33-34.
52. Simova I, Dimitrov N, Iliev R. Application of dabigatran in atrial fibrillation patients. *Cardio D* 2013; 3 (21):42-47.
53. Simova I. Benefits of statin treatment outweigh the risk for diabetes mellitus. *DoctorD* 2013; 2(62): 5-8.
54. Kostova V, Simova I, Katova T. Left ventricular twist mechanics: general principles and application. *Bulgarian cardiology* 2013; 1 (XIX):5-11.
55. Simova I, Dimitrov N. Antiaggregant therapy in the prevention and treatment of atherothrombosis. *Cardio D* 2013; 2 (20): 10-14.

In: Medicine Research Summaries. Volume 17
Editors: Zhongwen Liáng and Bibao Zhang
ISBN: 978-1-53612-751-5

Chapter 21

Petr Štourač, MD, PhD

Affiliation:

Department of Anaesthesiology and Intensive Care Medicine of Faculty Hospital in Brno and Medical Faculty of Masaryk University

Address:

Brno Jihlavska 20, 62500 Brno, Czech Republic

Date of Birth:

7/22/1977

Education:

2012: PhD Degree, Anaesthesia and analgesia options in the peripartum period

2008: Second Degree Specialty in Anaesthesiology and Resuscitation

2005: First Degree Specialty in Anaesthesiology and Resuscitation

2002: Medicinae Universae Doctor, Faculty of Medicine in Hradec Králové of Charles University in Prague

Research and Professional Experience:

Member of Czech Ministry of Health Committee for Anaesthesiology Nurses Competencies

Chair of Simulation in Medicine Committee of Medical Faculty

Ordinary for Obstetric Anaesthesia

Coordinator of Acute Pain Service for University Hospital

Internal Auditor of Quality Management

Assistant Professor

Professional Appointments:

2006 - today	Faculty of Medicine Masaryk University, Department of Anaesthesiology and Intensive Care Medicine
2003 - today	University Hospital in Brno, Department of Anaesthesiology and Intensive Care Medicine
2002 - 2003	Hospital in Trebic, Department of Anaesthesiology

Publications Last 3 Years:

1. Štourač P., Suchomelová H, et al. Comparison of Parturient-Controlled Remifentanil with Epidural Bupivacain and Sufentanil for Labour Analgesia: Randomised Controlled Trial. *Biomed Pap Med Fac Univ Palacky Olomouc Czech Repub.* 2014, 158(2):227-232. IF=1,661
2. Schwarz D, Štourač P, Komenda M, Harazim H, Kosinová M, Gregor J, Hůlek R, Smékalová O, Křikava I, Štoudek R, Dušek L: Interactive Algorithms for Teaching and Learning Acute Medicine in the Network of Medical Faculties MEFANET. *J Med Internet Res* 2013;15(7):e135 DOI:10.2196/jmir.2590 IF=4.669
3. Stourac P, Krikava I, Seidlova J, Strazevska E, Huser M, Hruban L, Janku P, Gal R. Sugammadex in a parturient with myotonic dystrophy. *Br J Anaesth.* 2013 Apr;110(4):657-8. doi: 10.1093/bja/aet037. IF=4.354
4. Stružková K., Štourač P., Kaňovský J., Křikava I., Ťoukálková M., Ševčík P.: An Unusual Reason of Severe Bradycardia Leading to Cardiac Arrest During General Anaesthesia - Case Report. *Biomed P* 2013; 1 DOI: 10.5507/bp. In print IF=1.661

In: Medicine Research Summaries. Volume 17
Editors: Zhongwen Liáng and Bibao Zhang ISBN: 978-1-53612-751-5

Chapter 22

MILAN TERZIC

Affiliation:
Clinic of Obstetrics and Gynecology, Clinical Center of Serbia & Medical Faculty University of Belgrade

Address:
Dr. Koste Todorovica 26, 11000 Belgrade, Serbia

Date of Birth:
January 29th, 1962

Education:

1986 September	MD, Medical Faculty University of Belgrade
1990 May	MSc, Medical Faculty University of Belgrade
1992 December	PhD, Medical Faculty University of Belgrade
1993 December	Consultant Ob/Gyn, Clinic of Ob/Gyn, Clinical Center of Serbia & Medical Faculty, University of Belgrade, Serbia

Research and Professional Experience:

- Education course of laparoscopic and hysteroscopic surgery organized by Clinic for Ob/Gyn Clinical Center of Serbia and Olimpus Winter and IBE, November 1997.
- Basic course in laparoscopic surgery, March 1998.
- Basic cource in laparoscopic gynecology, May 1998.
- Advanced workshop in gynecological oncological laparoscopy, may 2006.
- Advanced workshop in laparoscopic surgery in gynecology organized by Faculty of Medicine, University of Belgrade, April 2009.
- Participated in the Urogynecological Surgery Course in Paris May 2013, organised by Dr Richard Villet, Groupe Hospitalier Diaconesses Croix Saint Simon.
- Clinical Attachment: Consultant Ob/Gyn on expertise in operative laparoscopy, Department of Ob/Gyn, University Clinic Offenbach, Germany, 1996/1997.

- Clinical Attachment: Consultant Ob/Gyn on expertise in laparoscopy in gynecological oncology, Department of Gynecology, West Kent Gynecological Oncology Centre, Maidstone, United Kingdom, 2004/2005.

CO-LEADER IN RESEARCH PROJECTS:

- "Thymus endocrine function in human reproduction" in period of 1991-1996.
- "Diagnosis of the severe forms of fetal hemolytic disease and their treatment by intrauterine transfusions under ultrasound control" in period of 1996 - 2000.
- "Applications of MRI imaging and ultrasonography in the assessment of fetal malformations" joint research project Greece and Serbia in period of 2003 - 2005.
- "Diagnosis of preeclampsia by means of new laboratory diagnostic markers (Elecsys sFlt-1 and PlGF)", Roche Diagnostics GmbH, Clinical Trials Centralized Diagnostics, in period of 2008 – 2010.
- "Prima trial: Primary mesh closure of abdominal midline wounds – double blind randomized controlled trial" in period of 2010 – present.
- "Cellular and molecular pathogenetic mechanisms of reproduction disorders and genital organ diseases in prevention, diagnosis and therapy" in period of 2011 – 2014.
- "Regenerative and modulatory potential of adult stem cells" in period of 2011 – present.

Professional Appointments:

- Research Post - Elective Year of Specialist Training: 1 year (Oct 1986–Oct 1987).
- Senior House Officer Post - Basic Specialist Training: 2 yrs (Oct 1987–Oct 1989).
- Specialist Registrar Post - Higher Specialist Training, Core Specialist Training: 2 yrs (Oct 1989-Oct 1991).
- Specialist Registrar Post - Higher Specialist Training, Advanced Specialist Training 2 yrs (Oct 1991–Dec 1993).
- Consultant Ob/Gyn: Dec 1993 – June 2001.
- Consultant Ob/Gyn, Chief – General Gynecology Department, June 2001 – June 2009.
- Consultant Ob/Gyn, Head – Gynecological Surgery Department, July 2009 – June 2013.
- Consultant Ob/Gyn, Head – Reproductive Surgery & Infertility Department, July 2013 – present.
- Board Member - License Exam Board for Specialist Training in Ob/Gyn, Serbian Ministry of Health and School of Medicine, University of Belgrade, Jan 2003 – present.
- Board Member - License Exam Board for Specialist Training in Family Medicine, United Nations University for Peace, UNDP, Belgrade, Serbia and Montenegro, June 2004 – present.
- Board Member - License Exam Board for Specialist Training in General Medicine, Serbian Ministry of Health and School of Medicine, University of Belgrade, Oct 2008 – present.

Honors:

- Consultant Ob/Gyn, Head: Reproductive Surgery & Infertility Department, Clinic of Obstetrics and Gynecology, Clinical Center of Serbia, Medical Faculty, University of Belgrade, Serbia
- Senior Professor of Obstetrics and Gynecology: Clinic of Obstetrics and Gynecology, Clinical Center of Serbia & Medical Faculty, University of Belgrade, Serbia
- Expert and Lecturer: United Nations University for Peace, UNDP, Belgrade, Serbia

Publications Last 3 Years:

1. Terzic MM, Dotlic J, Likic I, Ladjevic N, Brndusic N, Arsenovic N, Maricic S, Mihailovic T, Andrijasevic S. Current diagnostic approach to patients with adnexal masses: which tools are relevant in routine praxis? *Chin J Cancer Res* 2013; 25: 55-62.
2. Likic Ladjevic I, Terzic M, Ladjevic N, Dotlic J, Pilic I, Bila J, Knezevic N, Milenkovic S, Maricic S, Arsenovic N, Brndusic N, Nikolic B. Introduction of new Tumor Marker Age Score in clinical practice: Validity evaluation for differentiation benignant from malignant adnexal masses. *ACI* 2013; 59: DOI: 10.2298/ ACI1203049L.
3. Terzic M, Dotlic J, Likic I, Ladjevic N, Brndusic N, Mihailovic T, Andrijasevic S, Pilic I, Bila J. Predictive factors of malignancy in patients with adnexal masses. *Eur J Gynaec Oncol* 2013; 34: 65-69.
4. Vujovic S, Pala A, Isakovic A, Terzic M. Use of the first-trimester biochemical markers to predict intrauterine growth retardation. *HealthMED* 2013; 7: 190-197.
5. Dotlic J, Terzic M, Babic D, Vasiljevic N, Janosevic S, Janosevic Lj, Pekmezovic T. The Influence of Body Mass Index on the Perceived Quality of Life during Pregnancy. *Applied Research Quality Life* 2013 DOI 10.1007/s11482-013-9224-z.
6. Terzic M, Bila J, Pilic I, Kocijancic D. Bilateral ampulary pregnancy after clomifen citrate and intrauterine insemination – a unique case report. *Gynecol Endocrinol* 2013; 29: 619-621.
7. Trivanovic D, Kocic J, Mojsilovic S, Krstic A, Ilic V, Okic Djordjevic I, Santibanez JF, Jovcic G, Terzic M, Bugarski D. Mesenchymal Stem Cells Isolated from Peripheral Blood and Umbilical Cord Wharton's Jelly. *Srp Arh Celok Lek* 2013; 141: 178-186.
8. Okic-Djordjevic I, Trivanovic D, Krstic J, Jaukovic A, Mojsilovic S, Santibanez JF, Terzic M, Vesovic D, Bugarski D. GE132+Natural: Novel promising dietetic supplement with antiproliferative influence on prostate, colon, and breast cancer cells. *JBUON* 2013; 18: 504-510.
9. Terzic M, Dotlic J, Likic I, Brndusic N, Pilic I, Ladjevic N, Maricic S, Arsenovic N, Maricic Z. Risk of malignancy index validity assessment in premenopausal and postmenopausal women with adnexal tumors. *Taiwan J Obstet Gynecol* 2013; 52: 253e257.
10. Terzic M, Maricic S, Dotlic J. Vaginal Removal of Very Large Nascent Uterine Myoma – Case Report and Literature Review. *Geburtsh Frauenheilk* 2013; 73: 724–726.

11. Terzic M, Dotlic J, Brndusic N, Arsenovic N, Likic I, Ladjevic N, Maricic S, Andrijasevic S. Histopathological adiagnoses of adnexal masses: which parameters are relevant in preoperative assessment? *Ginekol Pol* 2013: 84: 700-708.
12. Ladjevic N, Durutovic O, Likic-Ladjevic I, Lalic N, Mimic A, Dencic N, Sreckovic S, Dzamic Z, Terzic M, Vuksanovic A, Milenkovic-Petronic D. Epidural anesthesia can block the negative effects of prostaglandin mediators during prostate surgery. *Can J Urol* 2013; 20: 7021-7027.
13. Terzic M, Dotlic J, Likic I, Nikolic B, Brndusic N, Pilic I, Bila J, Maricic S, Arsenovic N. Diagnostic value of serum tumor markers evaluation for adnexal masses. *Cent Eur J Med* 2014; 9: 210-216.
14. Andrijasevic S, Dotlic J, Aksam S, Micic J, Terzic M. Impact of Conception Method on Twin Pregnancy Course and Outcome. *Geburtsh Frauenheilk* 2014; 74: 933–939.

In: Medicine Research Summaries. Volume 17
Editors: Zhongwen Liáng and Bibao Zhang
ISBN: 978-1-53612-751-5

Chapter 23

KINGSLEY NNANNA UKWAJA

Affiliation:
Department of Internal Medicine, Federal Teaching Hospital Abakaliki, Ebonyi State, Nigeria

Address:
FMC Rd, Abakaliki, Nigeria

Date of Birth:
01/01/1983

Education:

- Usmanu Danfodiyo University Sokoto Nigeria (MD); Faculty of Internal Medicine, National Postgraduate Medical College of Nigeria (AFMCP)
- MPH© London School of Hygiene and Tropical Medicine, U.K (2014 to present)

Research and Professional Experience:

- Extensive experience in clinical and epidemiological research related to infectious diseases (Lassa fever, Tuberculosis, HIV, TB/HIV etc.) and it control

Professional Appointments:

- Resident Physician, Department of Internal Medicine, Federal Teaching Hospital Abakaliki, Ebonyi State, Nigeria

Honors:

- 10 Research / Training Grants and Scholarships,
- International Grant Reviewer (MRC-UK),
- Editor of Frontiers in BioScience
- Peer Reviewer of 30 International Journals including (Bulletin of the WHO, Tropical Medicine and International Health, BMC Infectious Diseases, Infectious Diseases of Poverty, BMJ, BMJ Case Reports, Journal of Infection in Developing Countries, PlosOne, Plos Medicine etc.)

Publications Last 3 Years:

1. The GBD 2013 Incidence and Prevalence Collaborators. Global, regional, and national incidence, prevalence, and YLDs for 301 acute and chronic conditions and injuries for 188 countries, 1990-2013: a systematic analysis for the Global Burden of Disease Study 2013. *Lancet* (in press)
2. Abimbola SA, Ukwaja KN, Onyedum CC, Negin J, Jan S, Martiniuk AL. Transaction costs of access to health care: Implications of the care-seeking pathways of tuberculosis patients for health system governance in Nigeria. *Global Public Health* (in press)
3. Oshi DC, Oshi SN, Alobu I, Ukwaja KN. Gender-related factors influencing women's health seeking for tuberculosis care in Ebonyi State, Nigeria. *Journal of Biosocial Science* (in press)
4. Ukwaja KN. Interactions between leprosy and human immunodeficiency virus: more questions than answers. *Journal of Neurosciences in Rural Practice* 2015; 6(2) :135-6.
5. Oshi SN, Alobu I, Ukwaja KN, Oshi DC. Investigating gender disparities in the profile and treatment outcomes of tuberculosis in Ebonyi State, Nigeria. *Epidemiology & Infection* 2015; 143 (5): 932 – 942
6. Ogbudebe C, Chukwu JN, Nwafor CC, Meka AO, Ekeke N, Madicihie N, Anyim MC, Onyeonoro UU, Osakwe C, Ukwaja KN, Oshi DC. Reaching the underserved: active tuberculosis case finding in urban slums in South-Eastern Nigeria. *International Journal of Mycobacteriology* 2015; 4: 18 – 24
7. Ukwaja KN, Oshi SN, Alobu I, Oshi DC. Six- versus eight-month antituberculosis regimen for pulmonary tuberculosis under programme conditions. *International Journal of Tuberculosis & Lung Disease* 2015; 19 (3): 295 – 301
8. The Global Burden of Disease 2013 Mortality and Causes of Death Collaborators. Global, regional and national levels of age-specific mortality and 240 causes of death, 1990-2013: A systematic analysis for the Global Burden of Disease Study 2013. *Lancet* 2015; 385: 117–71
9. Ajayi NA, Ukwaja KN, Ifebunandu NA, Nnabu R, Onwe F, Asogun D. Lassa fever – full recovery without ribavarin treatment: a case report. *African Health Sciences* 2014; 14: 1074 – 1077
10. Alobu I, Oshi SN, Oshi DC, Ukwaja KN. Risk factors of treatment default and death among tuberculosis patients in a resource-limited setting. *Asian Pacific Journal of Tropical Medicine* 2014;7:977-984
11. Oshi DC, Oshi SN, Alobu I, Ukwaja KN. Profile, outcomes and determinants of unsuccessful tuberculosis treatment outcomes among HIV-infected tuberculosis patients in a Nigerian state. *Tuberculosis Research and Treatment* 2014; 2014: 202983
12. Oshi DC, Oshi SN, Alobu I, Ukwaja KN. Profile and treatment outcomes of tuberculosis in the elderly in Southeastern Nigeria, 2011-2012. *PloS One* 2014; 9: e111910.
13. The Global Burden of Disease 2013 Malaria, TB and HIV Collaborators. Global, regional and national incidence and mortality for HIV, tuberculosis and malaria 1990-2013: a systematic analysis for the Global Burden of Disease Study 2013. *Lancet* 2014; 384(9947): 1005-70.

14. The Global Burden of Disease 2013 Maternal Mortality Collaborators. Global, regional, and national levels and causes of maternal mortality during 1990-2013: a systematic analysis for the Global Burden of Disease Study 2013. *Lancet* 2014;384(9947):980-1004
15. Ukwaja KN, Oshi DC, Oshi SN, Alobu I. Profile and treatment outcome of smear-positive TB patients who failed to smear convert after 2 months of treatment in Nigeria. *Transactions of the Royal Society of Tropical Medicine and Hygiene* 2014; 108 (7): 431–438.
16. Alobu I, Oshi DC, Oshi SN, Ukwaja KN. Profile and determinants of treatment failure among smear-positive pulmonary tuberculosis patients in Ebonyi, Southeastern Nigeria. *International Journal of Mycobacteriology* 2014; 3(2):127–131.
17. Ukwaja KN, Onyedum CC. The performance of a tuberculosis control programme in a high burden country – the Nigeria situation. *Annals of Tropical Medicine and Public Health* 2013; 6(5):500–502.
18. Ukwaja KN, Abimbola SA. A trial of mass isoniazid preventive therapy for tuberculosis control. *New England Journal of Medicine* 2014;370:1661
19. Onyedum CC, Desalu OO, Ukwaja KN, Chukwuka C, Nwosu NI, Ezeudo C. Out-of-Pocket Costs of Asthma Follow-Up Care in Adults in a Sub-Saharan African Country. *Journal of Respiratory Medicine* 2014; 2014: 768378.
20. Onyedum CC, Desalu OO, Nwosu NI, Chukwuka CJ, Ukwaja KN, Ezeudo C. Evaluation of inhaler techniques among asthma patients seen in Nigeria: an observational cross-sectional study *Annals of Medicine and Health Sciences Research* 2014; 4: 67–73.
21. Ukwaja KN, Onyedum CC. Design of pragmatic trials of tuberculosis interventions. *Lancet* 2014; 383: 214
22. Ukwaja KN. Tuberculosis treatment default among TB-HIV co-infected patients in Nigeria. *Annals of Tropical Medicine and Public Health* 2013; 6: 382 – 383
23. Ajayi NA, Nwigwe CG, Azuogu BN, Onyire BN, Nwonwu EU, Ogbonnaya LU, Onwe FI, Tobin E, Gunther S, Ukwaja KN. Containing a Lassa fever epidemic in a resource-limited setting: outbreak description and lessons learned from Abakaliki, Nigeria (January—March 2012). *International Journal of Infectious Diseases* 2013; 17: e1011 - e1016
24. Ukwaja KN, Alobu I, Onu EM. Nigerian frontline healthcare workers' knowledge of tuberculosis disease, treatment and infection control. *African Journal of Respiratory Medicine* 2013; 9: 7 – 10
25. Ukwaja KN. Comment on "Community-Wide Isoniazid Preventive Therapy Drives Drug-Resistant Tuberculosis: A Model-Based Analysis". *Science Translational Medicine* 2013; 5, 204le3.
26. Ukwaja KN, Alobu I, Abimbola S, Hopewell PC. Household catastrophic payments for tuberculosis care in Nigeria: incidence, determinants and policy implications for universal health coverage. *Infectious Diseases of Poverty* 2013; 2:21
27. Ukwaja KN, Alobu I, Ifebunandu NA, Osakwe C, Igwenyi C. Trend in case detection rate for all tuberculosis cases notified in Ebonyi, Southeastern Nigeria during 1999 – 2009. *Pan African Medical Journal* 2013;16:11

28. Onyedum CC, Ukwaja KN, Desalu OO, Ezeudo C. Challenges in the management of bronchial asthma among adults in Nigeria: a systematic review. *Annals of Medicine and Health Sciences Research* 2013; 3: 324-329
29. Ukwaja KN, Alobu I, Igwenyi C, Hopewell PC. The high cost of free tuberculosis services: patient and household costs associated with tuberculosis care in Ebonyi State, Nigeria. *PloS One* 2013; 8: e73134.
30. Ajayi NA, Ukwaja KN Possible artemisinin-based combination therapy resistant malaria in Nigeria: a report of three cases. *Journal of the Brazilian Society of Tropical Medicine* 2013; 46 :525– 527
31. Ukwaja KN, Onyedum CC. High dose rifampicin and moxifloxacin for tuberculous meningitis. *Lancet Infectious Diseases* 2013; 13 : 569 – 570
32. Ukwaja KN, Ifebunandu NA, Osakwe PC, Alobu I. Tuberculosis treatment outcome and its determinants in a tertiary care setting in southeastern Nigeria. *Nigerian Postgraduate Medical Journal* 2013; 20: 125 – 129
33. Ukwaja KN, Onyedum CC. Reaction to Ilesanmi OS et al. The managed hypertensive: the costs of blood pressure control in a Nigerian town. Pan Afr Med J. 2012;12:96. *Pan African Medical Journal* 2013; 14:85
34. Ukwaja KN, Alobu I, Ogbodo NC. Onyenwe CE. Healthcare-seeking behavior, treatment delays and its determinants among pulmonary tuberculosis patients in rural Nigeria: a cross-sectional study. *BMC Health Services Research* 2013; 13: 25
35. Ukwaja KN. Socioeconomic impact of tuberculosis on patients: further study needed. *Lung India* 2013; 30(1): 77 – 78
36. Ukwaja KN. Acute rhinosinusitis, and systemic corticosteroids. *CMAJ* 2013; 185: 62

In: Medicine Research Summaries. Volume 17
Editors: Zhongwen Liáng and Bibao Zhang

ISBN: 978-1-53612-751-5

Chapter 24

GENTIAN VYSHKA

Affiliation:
Faculty of Medicine, University of Medicine in Tirana, Albania

Address:
Lagja 1 Rr Kostaq Cipo, Pall. 2/19, Tirana, Albania

Date of Birth:
10/22/1970

Education:
Medicine, Neurology and Psychiatry

Research and Professional Experience:

- Specialist in neurology, electromyography and evoked potentials; lecturer of human physiology and pharmacology; expertise in forensic psychiatry.

Professional Appointments:

- Associated Professor of Human Physiology, Faculty of Medicine, University of Tirana; Expert at the Institute of Forensic Medicine, Tirana, Albania; Neurologist at the UHC Mother Theresa and Hygeia Hospital, Tirana; Albania.

Honors:

- DAAD Alumni; Fulbright Alumni Member; Editorial Board Member at Insight Knowledge (UK), Omics Anthropology; OA Medicine London; International Journal of Clinical Toxicology.

Publications Last 3 Years:

1. Sulaj Z, Drishti A, Çeko I, Gashi A, Vyshka G. Fatal aluminum phosphide poisonings in Tirana (Albania), 2009 - 2013. *Daru.* 2015 Jan 25;23(1):8. doi:10.1186/s40199-015-0090-0. PubMed PMID: 25618461; PubMed Central PMCID: PMC4308883.

2. Myftari K, Vyshka G. Mission impossible: upholding successfully a charge of infanticide in the Albanian legal practice. *J Med Ethics Hist Med.* 2014 Feb 18;7:4. eCollection 2014. PubMed PMID: 25512825; PubMed Central PMCID: PMC4263390.
3. Vyshka G, Seferi A, Myftari K, Halili V. Last call for informed consent: confused proxies in extra-emergency conditions. *Indian J Med Ethics.* 2014 Oct-Dec;11(4):252-4. PubMed PMID: 25377040.
4. Devor M, Vaso A, Adahan HM, Vyshka G. PNS origin of phantom limb sensation and pain: reply to letter to the editor regarding Foell et al., peripheral origin of phantom limb pain: is it all resolved? *Pain.* 2014 Oct;155(10):2207-8. doi: 10.1016/j.pain.2014.08.018. Epub 2014 Aug 26. PubMed PMID: 25168666.
5. Vyshka G, Vacchiano G. Severe flaccid paraparesis following spinal anaesthesia: a sine materia occurrence. *BMJ Case Rep.* 2014 May 15;2014. pii: bcr2013202071. doi: 10.1136/bcr-2013-202071. PubMed PMID: 24832705.
6. Vaso A, Adahan HM, Gjika A, Zahaj S, Zhurda T, Vyshka G, Devor M. Peripheral nervous system origin of phantom limb pain. *Pain.* 2014 Jul;155(7):1384-91. doi: 10.1016/j.pain.2014.04.018. Epub 2014 Apr 21. PubMed PMID: 24769187.
7. ilaca A, Vyshka G, Pepa A, Shytaj K, Shtjefni V, Boçari A, Beqiri A, Kraja D. A Neglected Zoonosis in Albania: why Echinococcosis is Becoming a Surgeon's Exclusivity? *Mediterr J Hematol Infect Dis.* 2014 Feb 16;6(1):e2014013. doi: 10.4084/MJHID.2014.013. eCollection 2014. PubMed PMID: 24678390; PubMed Central PMCID: PMC3965721.
8. Seferi A, Alimehmeti R, Vyshka G, Bushati T, Petrela M. Case study of a spinal epidural capillary hemangioma: a 4-year postoperative follow-up. *Global Spine J.* 2014 Feb;4(1):55-8. doi: 10.1055/s-0033-1354251. Epub 2013 Aug 22. PubMed PMID: 24494182; PubMed Central PMCID: PMC3908985.
9. Vyshka G, Kruja J. Clinical variability of the cerebral autosomal-dominant arteriopathy with subcortical infarcts and leukoencephalopathy phenotype in two siblings of a large family showing the same mutation. *Int Med Case Rep J.* 2013 Oct 1;6:59-63. doi: 10.2147/IMCRJ.S51875. eCollection 2013. PubMed PMID: 24124395; PubMed Central PMCID: PMC3794843.
10. Shkurti K, Vyshka G, Velo E, Boçari A, Kokici M, Kraja D. Imported malaria in Albania and the risk factors that could allow its reappearance. *Malar J.* 2013 Jun 12;12:197. doi: 10.1186/1475-2875-12-197. PubMed PMID: 23758911; PubMed Central PMCID: PMC3691593.
11. Vyshka G, Troshani B, Bozaxhiu D, Mitrushi A. Rotational head trauma with callosal contusion and C6 fracture: a high-speed motorcycle accident. *Ulus Travma Acil Cerrahi Derg.* 2013 Jan;19(1):77-9. doi: 10.5505/tjtes.2013.40374. PubMed PMID: 23588986.
12. Vacchiano G, Vyshka G. Balkans syndrome: a potential link between multiple sclerosis and hypervaccination. *J R Army Med Corps.* 2012 Dec;158(4):338-40. PubMed PMID: 23402075.
13. Nikolla J, Nanushi M, Vyshka G, Hafizi H. A six-month study of pulmonary cancer in Albanian women. ISRN *Prev Med.* 2013 Mar 4;2013:824670. doi: 10.5402/2013/824670. eCollection 2013. PubMed PMID: 24977098; PubMed Central PMCID: PMC4062866.

In: Medicine Research Summaries. Volume 17
Editors: Zhongwen Liáng and Bibao Zhang
ISBN: 978-1-53612-751-5

Chapter 25

NATALIE LYNN YANCHAR, MD, MSC, FRCSC

Affiliation:
Associate Professor in Surgery (Pediatric), Emergency Medicine and Community Health and Epidemiology, Dalhousie University; Medical Director IWK Trauma Care Program, IWK Health Centre, Halifax, Nova Scotia, Canada

Address:
Division of Pediatric Surgery, IWK Health Centre, 5850 University Avenue, Halifax, NS, Canada, B3K 6R8

Date of Birth:
9/13/1963

Education:
- Master of Science (MSc) in Community Health and Epidemiology, Dalhousie University, Halifax, NS., April 2007
- Residency in Pediatric General Surgery, Children's Hospital of Eastern Ontario, University of Ottawa, Ottawa, Ontario, . January 1997 - December 1998.
- Master of Science in Experimental Surgery, University of Alberta, Edmonton, AB. Supervisor, Dr. D.L. Sigalet. November 1994
- Residency in General Surgery, University of Alberta, Edmonton, Alberta. July 1991 - June 1996.
- Rotating Internship, Charles Camsell Provincial General Hospital, University of Alberta Edmonton, Alberta. July 1990 -June 1991.
- Doctorate of Medicine, Queen's University, Kingston, Ontario. Sept. 1986 - June 1990.
- B.Sc., Honors in Biochemistry, University of Alberta, Edmonton, Alberta. September 1981 - May 1986.

Research and Professional Experience:
Natalie Yanchar is an Associate Professor in Pediatric General Surgery at Dalhousie University and the Medical Director of the Trauma Program at the IWK Health Centre, the

Level I Pediatric Trauma Centre for the Maritimes. She has MSc degrees in both Experimental Surgery (University of Alberta) and in Community Health and Epidemiology (Dalhousie University) and holds cross-appointments with the Dalhousie Departments of Emergency Medicine and Community Health and Epidemiology. In addition to her clinical role, Natalie has a strong research interest in clinical management of trauma, pediatric trauma systems and primary injury prevention. This interest allows her to co-lead work on Pediatric Trauma Systems and access to Pediatric Trauma Care within the Scope of the CIHR funded STAIR Team in Child and Youth Injury Prevention. Collaborative links as Chair of the TAC Working Group for the new Canadian Trauma Registry (CaNTR) and Executive member of the Trauma Association of Canada provide opportunities to engage other experts and stakeholders in her field of research. Finally, she is also a strong advocate for evidence-informed policy development in the areas of childhood injury prevention, chairing the Injury Prevention Committee of the Canadian Pediatric Society and being the founding President of Injury Free Nova Scotia.

Professional Appointments:

Associate Professor in Pediatric General Surgery at Dalhousie University and the Medical Director of the Trauma Program at the IWK Health Centre. President-elect, Trauma Association of Canada

Honors:

- The Tom Pashby Sports Safety Award, November 2012
- Canadian Paediatric Society Victor Marchessault Award for Advocacy, June 2010
- Doctors Nova Scotia Award For Health Promotion, June 2010

Publications Last 3 Years:

1. Yanchar NL, Young JB, Langille DB. Knowledge and practice of childhood motor vehicle restraint use in Nova Scotia: phase II. *Accid Anal Prev.* 2015 Jan;74:150-6.
2. Hynick N, Brennan M, Schmit P, Noseworthy S, Bettoli M, Yanchar NL. Identification of blunt abdominal injuries in children. *J Trauma Acute Care Surg.* 2014 Jan;76(1):95-100.
3. Ornstein A, Bowes M, Shouldice M, Yanchar NL. *The Importance of Child and Youth Death Review Paediatr Child Health.* 2013 Oct;18(8):425-32.
4. Yanchar NL, Woo K, Brennan M, Palmer C, Ee, Crameri J, Sweeney B. Chest X-ray as a Screening Tool for Blunt Thoracic Trauma in Children. *J Trauma Acute Care Surg.* 2013 Oct;75(4):613-9.

PART II

RESEARCH SUMMARIES

In: Medicine Research Summaries. Volume 17
Editors: Zhongwen Liáng and Bibao Zhang
ISBN: 978-1-53612-751-5

Chapter 26

Concepts of Periodontal Regeneration and Regenerative Medicine: Mechanisms that Modulate Cells and Matrices[#]

Mena Soory [*]
Periodontology, King's College London Dental Institute,
Denmark Hill, London, UK

Research Summary

Regenerative medicine and dentistry combine applications of molecular biology, material science, bioengineering and nanoscience in order to repair, regenerate and replace missing tissue. Diverse technologies have emerged in recent times to streamline applications of more predictable materials and methods; in order to attain the elusive goal of periodontal regeneration. In addition to grafting materials and barrier membranes to exclude epithelial down growth and promote mesenchymal elements, the environment of the cell is pivotal to events that follow. These include cell-based-, gene-based, protein and peptide therapy, application of scaffolds, lasers, harnessing bone anabolic activity and the resolution of inflammation. Recommendations embrace suitable targets for patient outcome, based on clinical applications of scientific principles for more predictable and consistent results, in regenerating hard and soft tissues of a functional periodontium.

Various approaches have evolved, including autologous tissue, growth factors, platelet concentrates and scaffolds. Appropriate manipulation of stem cells using sophisticated technology, makes them versatile for a range of applications. Decellularised extracellular matrices containing a complex assembly of relevant growth factors, matrix macromolecules and fibrillar proteins that mimic the natural ECM; have significant biomedical applications for coating scaffolds, as adhesive cell culture substrates and tissue engineered products.

[#] This chapter was previously published as a book: *Concepts of Periodontal Regeneration and Regenerative Medicine: Mechanisms that Modulate Cells and Matrices,* by Mena Soory, New York: Nova Publishers Inc., 2015.

[*] Corresponding Author Email: mena.soory@kcl.ac.uk.

Interactions of extracellular vesicles (EV) with ECM/relevant cells, affect cell signalling, differentiation and proliferation. This has potential for the development of a focal cell phenotype with applications in regenerative medicine; including stem-cell based therapeutic interventions. Incorporation of EV in regenerative therapy, includes combination with hydrogels and applications for scaffold coatings, by linking with cell- and ECM-interactive fibrin gels.

The endogenous, highly conserved small, non-coding microRNA molecules, have applications in regulating post-transcriptional gene expression by binding to their target mRNAs. Periosteal cell sheets are effective in enhancing bone formation. Autologous cell sheets are readily translated for clinical applications. Endothelial and mesenchymal 3D printing have evolved as the cutting edge of tissue engineering research. 3D printing enables the synthesis of multi-material and cell-laden biomimetic and nanostructured scaffolds more effectively, with less effort. These concepts are reviewed in the context of a coordinated strategy for effective combinations to deliver more consistent applications and outcome.

In: Medicine Research Summaries. Volume 17
Editors: Zhongwen Liáng and Bibao Zhang

ISBN: 978-1-53612-751-5

Chapter 27

TRENDS IN THE BIRTH PREVALENCE OF BOYS WITH ISOLATED HYPOSPADIAS AND UNDESCENDED TESTIS IN HUNGARY DURING THE LAST 50 YEARS: A POPULATION-BASED STUDY[#]

Stelios Mavrogenis[1] and Andrew E. Czeizel[2,*]
[1]National Institute of Oncology,
Department of Uro-Oncology, Budapest, Hungary
[2]Foundation for the Community
Control of Hereditary Diseases, Budapest, Hungary

RESEARCH SUMMARY

Previously an increasing birth prevalence of hypospadias and undescended testis was recorded in some countries, including in the Hungarian Congenital Abnormality Registry, 1962-2011, i.e., during the last 50 years. However, the critical evaluation of cases with recorded isolated hypospadias (IHS) and isolated undescended testis (IUT), particularly to compare with the so-called reference birth prevalence of IHS (2.25 $\pm$ 0.30 per 1000 live-births) and IUT (6.86 $\pm$ 0.62 per 1000 live-births) determined in a Hungarian clinical-epidemiological study based on the physical examination of newborns with well-defined diagnostic criteria did not indicate a real increase in the birth prevalence of IHS and IUT. Thus, the increase of recorded cases with IHS and IUT can be explained by the more complete reporting of cases and a larger proportion of mild subgroup of IHS and the lack of differentiation between birth IUT (with many postnatal descents of testes) and true IUT (diagnosed at 3,5 months after birth). In conclusion, birth defect-registries are not appropriate for the estimation of real birth prevalence of IHS and IUT. In addition the socio-demographic

---

[#] This chapter was previously published in *Advances in Medicine and Biology. Volume 87,* edited by Leon V. Berhardt, New York: Nova Publishers Inc., 2015.

[*] Corresponding Author: Foundation for the Community Control of Hereditary Diseases, Budapest, 1026, Budapest, Törökvész lejtő 32, Hungary. Tel/Fax 36 1 3944 712. E-mail: czeizel@interware.hu.

variables of mothers were also analyzed without significant association of changes in birth prevalence of recorded IHS and IUT. Finally maternal risk factors were evaluated in the large population-based Hungarian Case-Control Surveillance of Congenital Abnormalities, 1980-1996, some of them showed association with the risk of IHS and IUT but without connection of the trend in the birth prevalence of cases with IHS and IUT.

In: Medicine Research Summaries. Volume 17
Editors: Zhongwen Liáng and Bibao Zhang
ISBN: 978-1-53612-751-5

Chapter 28

Alleviating Premenstrual Syndrome (PMS) Symptoms Using a Natural Factor – Negative Air Ions[#]

Valeria Laza, MD, PhD*
Department of Hygiene, University of Medicine
and Pharmacy, Cluj-Napoca, Romania

Research Summary

There is hardly any other element of the physical environment which has caused so much confusion and controversies as negative air ions (NAI). Despite more than 100 years of study in the field, the knowledge on ion specter is still in an embryonic stage.

However, NAI have found to have good or excellent results, as therapeutic, as well as a prophylactic factor. We used a therapy of moderate doses of negative air ions emitted by a generator, for up to 14-20th days to treat the symptoms of discomfort in Premenstrual Syndrome (PMS). On female students with PMS, the results were very significantly different from the witness group. The premenstrual intense pain decreased from 38% to 9.5% ($p < 0.001$), and generally pain completely disappeared in 45% of cases. Acne decreased from 76% to 43%, and irritability from 76% to 19%.

It is worth mentioning that the premenstrual irritability completely disappeared in 75% of students. Before the experiment 81% of the cases used pain killers, while after the experiment only 24% were still addicted to medication, especially as a preventive measure. Another effect was the regulation of the menstrual cycle, in 89% of the cases with irregular periods. All of these improvements lasted in half of cases up to one year after the treatment (no other known medicine has such a long effect). The items referring to the energetic basis of the neuro-psychic tonus have an ascending trend, except the well-being sensation and self

---

This chapter was previously published in *Advances in Medicine and Biology. Volume 87,* edited by Leon V. Berhardt, New York: Nova Publishers Inc., 2015.

* Corresponding Author: Valeria Laza MD PhD. Associate Professor, Department of Hygiene, University of Medicine and Pharmacy, Cluj-Napoca, Romania. E-mail: v_laza@yahoo.com.

confidence, which were situated from the very beginning at the higher levels of the scale. Negative air ions are not a universal panacea, but they could be considered a physiological factor, very cheap, with no side effects, not addictive, with very few contraindications, and which do not bring any foreign substance inside the organism.

In conclusion, considering the advantages, the artificially ionized air might be a potentially effective biologic factor, which, if properly harnessed, controlled, and utilized, may become a valuable adjunct to other forms of therapy.

In: Medicine Research Summaries. Volume 17
Editors: Zhongwen Liáng and Bibao Zhang

ISBN: 978-1-53612-751-5

Chapter 29

NEUTRALIZATION-ENHANCING RF ANTIBODIES[#]

***Konstantin V. Suslov**[*]*
Institute of Immunology, Moscow, Russia

RESEARCH SUMMARY

Monomeric specific high-affinity IgG antibodies arising during infection process have low avidity to multimeric structures of the pathogen. Moreover, in the case of viruses such antibodies may sometimes enhance FcR-mediated infection of monocytes.

Multistage generation of antibody complexes with high affinity and avidity are important for efficient neutralization of the pathogen. Multimeric IgM or IgA rheumatoid factor (RF) antibodies may specifically bind Fc parts of IgG molecules complexed with pathogen and thus enhance the neutralization activity of pathogen-specific monomeric IgG. Such neutralization-enhancing RF antibodies amplify IgG response via increased aggregation and clearance of antibody-pathogen immune complexes.

Neutralization-enhancing RF antibodies (NeRFa) might be induced via prolonged repeated immunization with protein antigens. Induction of NeRFa would be an important task for creating effective therapeutic and prophylactic vaccines against HIV, malaria, Ebola and other pathogens. Single-administration vaccine technology with pulsatile release of protein antigens from biodegradable polymeric microspheres opens new possibilities to achieve such a goal.

The idea that specific induction of NeRFa can be a universal approach to eradicate any pathogen, including cancer-associated viruses, will be put forward in this review article.

[#] This chapter was previously published in *Advances in Medicine and Biology. Volume 87,* edited by Leon V. Berhardt, New York: Nova Publishers Inc., 2015.

[*] Corresponding Author: Konstantin V. Suslov, Institute of Immunology, 24/2 Kashirskoe Sh., Moscow 115 478, Russia. Telephone: +7 9150661500, e-mail: suslov_kv@mail.ru, Website: http://konstantin.suslov.googlepages.com.

In: Medicine Research Summaries. Volume 17
Editors: Zhongwen Liáng and Bibao Zhang
ISBN: 978-1-53612-751-5

Chapter 30

ADVANCES IN THE DIAGNOSIS, ASSESSMENT, MANAGEMENT AND OUTCOME OF TAKAYASU'S ARTERITIS: A NARRATIVE REVIEW#

Slavica Pavlov-Dolijanovic and Nada Vujasinovic Stupar
School of Medicine University of Belgrade,
Institute of Rheumatology, Serbia

RESEARCH SUMMARY

Takayasu arteritis (TA) is a rare, chronic large-vessel vasculitis (LVV) characterized by granulomatous inflammation of the vessel wall with an unknown etiopathogenesis. TA predominantly affects young females during the 2nd or 3rd decades of life and mainly involves the aortic arch and its major branches, ascending aorta, thoracic descending aorta and abdominal aorta. A physical examination is the first step for disease assessment. Systemic inflammatory response does not always show a positive correlation with inflammatory activity in the vessel wall. Imaging modalities are very important for establishing the diagnosis of TA. Conventional angiography, the gold standard for initial diagnosis, seems to be replaced with the new imaging modalities such as magnetic resonance angiography, ultrasonography, computerized tomography and, 18F-fluorodeoxyglucose positron emission tomography in recent years. Prognosis is possibly getting better with lower mortality in recent years. The most commonly used agents include corticosteroids and conventional immunosuppressive agents such as methotrexate, azathioprine, micophenolate mofetil and leflunomide. However, in resistant and/or intolcrant patients, biologic drugs including anti-TNF agents (mostly infliximab), rituximab and tocilizumab seem to be promising. Antiplatelet treatment may also lower the frequency of ischaemic events in TA. Endovascular interventions (balloon angioplasty or stent graft replacement) or by-pass surgery may be useful for critical arterial occlusions. There is a clear need to develop a validated set of outcome measures in TA, such as measures of disease activity, health-related quality of life and disease-related damage. The OMERACT Vasculitis Working Group has taken on this task and aims to develop a core set of outcomes for LVV.

This chapter was previously published in *Advances in Medicine and Biology. Volume 87,* edited by Leon V. Berhardt, New York: Nova Publishers Inc., 2015.

In: Medicine Research Summaries. Volume 17
Editors: Zhongwen Liáng and Bibao Zhang
ISBN: 978-1-53612-751-5

Chapter 31

MACRONUTRIENTS AND PREMENSTRUAL SYNDROME[#]

Serena C. Houghton and Elizabeth R. Bertone-Johnson
Department of Biostatistics and Epidemiology, University of Massachusetts Amherst, Amherst, MA, US

RESEARCH SUMMARY

Premenstrual syndrome (PMS) has few established risk factors and an unknown etiology. Effective treatment options are limited and most have substantial limitations. It is important to identify modifiable risk factors for PMS including dietary aspects. A number of recommendations concerning macronutrient intake have been made regarding prevention or treatment of PMS. For example, the American Congress of Obstetricians and Gynecologists and the Association of Reproductive Health Professionals recommend consuming regular meals with adequate protein and complex carbohydrates, with reduced fat and sugar intakes to alleviate PMS. However, these recommendations are not evidence-based and largely unsubstantiated.

Potential physiological effects of fats on PMS include inflammation and altered hormonal milieu. Saturated fats act as pro-inflammatory factors and increase estradiol and luteinizing hormone levels, whereas polyunsaturated fats like omega-3s act as anti-inflammatory factors. To date, two cross-sectional studies have examined fat intake and PMS symptom severity, and five small clinical trials have tested whether supplements containing fatty acids are effective at relieving symptoms. Total, saturated, and monounsaturated fats have overall higher symptom scores, particularly pain but total fat intake is related to lower cravings and bloating. The treatment trials show that gamma-linoleic acid supplements reduce symptoms.

Potential effects of carbohydrates include increasing serotonin levels, regulation of blood glucose and insulin sensitivity, and reducing estrogen levels via whole grain fiber. Few studies have directly assessed how carbohydrates impact premenstrual symptoms. These

---

[#] This chapter was previously published in *Advances in Medicine and Biology. Volume 87,* edited by Leon V. Berhardt, New York: Nova Publishers Inc., 2015.

studies have shown inconsistent relationships suggesting that higher carbohydrate intakes are associated with lower symptom experience, particularly for pain and negative affect. Women with PMS show increased intake of total carbohydrates primarily from simple sugars, which are associated with higher symptom severity, whereas whole grains and fiber are not associated, except for breast pain.

Dietary protein may potentially affect premenstrual symptoms through action of the renin-angiotensin-aldosterone system, lowered calcium levels, negation of serotonin increases from carbohydrates, and altered hormonal milieu. Soy protein is related to lower estradiol and progesterone levels, whereas red or processed meats have increased steroid hormones and sex hormone binding globulin. To our knowledge, only three studies have examined the association of protein intake and premenstrual symptoms. It appears that while women with higher intakes of protein have fewer symptoms, there is no difference in severity. Low-fat vegetarian diets show reductions in symptoms and severity, though not related to soy intake.

Several major limitations exist among available literature. All studies have assessed macronutrients as a potential treatment rather than a causal factor of PMS. Among the observational studies, it is unknown whether observed associations are due to reverse causation; specifically, it is unclear whether macronutrient intake contributes to PMS or whether women with PMS have altered their diet to control their symptoms. Lastly, many studies have looked at each macronutrient separately and have not assessed the effects relative to each other, to kilocalorie intake, or to confounding factors. Future research should use prospective designs to determine the temporal relationship between macronutrient intake and PMS controlling for other macronutrients and confounders. This research has the potential to help women prevent PMS via modifiable risk factors or treat symptoms effectively and safely.

In: Medicine Research Summaries. Volume 17
Editors: Zhongwen Liáng and Bibao Zhang
ISBN: 978-1-53612-751-5

Chapter 32

Pressurized Intraperitoneal Aerosol Chemotherapy (PIPAC): Occupational Health and Safety Management#

Loic Reymond[1], Wiebke Solass[2], MD, Clemens Tempfer[3], MD MBA, and Marc A. Reymond[4] MD MBA*

[1]Mechanical Engineering, RWTH Aachen University, Germany
[2]Institute of Pathology, Hanover Medical School, Germany
[3]Department of Gynaecology
[4]Ruhr-University Bochum, Germany

Research Summary

Pressurized IntraPeritoneal Aerosol Chemotherapy (PIPAC) is an innovative drug delivery system applying chemotherapy as a pressurized therapeutic aerosol into the abdominal cavity. PIPAC has superior pharmacological properties and first clinical results concerning efficacy and safety are promising. However, applying chemotherapeutic substances as a toxic aerosol is a challenge for occupational health and safety management. A risk assessment of PIPAC was performed to meet legal requirements. It was not possible to replace chemotherapeutic drugs with other substances since platin based drugs and/or anthracyclines are the drugs of choice in many peritoneal cancers. However the dose of toxic substances could be reduced by 90%. Exposure of health workers to the chemotherapeutic drugs can be cutaneous (liquids) or respiratory (aerosol). Wearing chemotherapy gloves, protective clothing and glasses was effective for preventing cutaneous or ocular exposure,

---

This chapter was previously published in *Advances in Medicine and Biology. Volume 87,* edited by Leon V. Berhardt, New York: Nova Publishers Inc., 2015.

* Corresponding Author: Marc A. Reymond, M.D. M.B.A. Professor and Head, Surgical oncology and Therapy center peritoneal cancer, Marien Hospital Herne, Ruhr-University Bochum, Hölkeskampring 40, 44625 Herne, Germany, Tel.: +49.(0)2323 499-5807, Fax: +49.(0)2323 499-392, E-Mail: marc.reymond@marienhospital-herne.de.

since the drugs applied are not absorbed through the skin. A three-level confinement system was designed to prevent any inhalative exposure of health workers. The first level is the closed abdomen itself, which tightness is controlled before chemotherapy application. The second level is the volume of the operating room together with air exchange through high-flow ventilation. The third confinement is the physical operating room, since the PIPAC procedure is remote-controlled and the team leaves the room during application. At the end of the procedure, the toxic aerosol is exhausted through a Closed Aerosol Waste System (CAWS) over a special line into the external environment, using the same system used for eliminating narcosis gases. Repeated environmental measurements in two different hospitals according to NIOSH protocols at the potential working places of the surgeon and of the anesthesiologist detected no traces of platin in the air. Biological monitoring in the blood of 5 surgeons after 500 procedures showed no traces of platin or doxorubicin. Mathematic modelling of the worst case scenario (immediate release of the toxic aerosol into the working environment) showed a potential respiratory uptake lower than 1/100'000 of a usual systemic chemotherapy dose. Over 650 procedures, to minor incidents related to disconnection in the tubing system were reported in the Critical Incident Reporting System (CIRS). No severe incident, in particular no leakage of the toxic aerosol, was recorded. No pressure- or technology-linked patient complication was noted. Work place measurements remained below the tolerance margin. The safety measures and conditions as defined above are sufficient. PIPAC can be used safely in the clinical setting if the conditions specified above are met. For the drugs tested, PIPAC is in compliance with European Community working safety law and regulations.

In: Medicine Research Summaries. Volume 17
Editors: Zhongwen Liáng and Bibao Zhang

ISBN: 978-1-53612-751-5

Chapter 33

THE CONTROL OF MAO EXPRESSION: A RESOURCE UNDERSCORED BY THE PHARMACOLOGY[#]

Annunziatina Laurino and Laura Raimondi*
Department of NEUFARBA, Section of Pharmacology,
University of Florence, Florence, Italy

RESEARCH SUMMARY

Mitochondrial monoamine oxidases (isoforms A and B; MAO-A and MAO-B respectively) are ubiquitous enzymes located at the outer mitochondria membrane facing toward cytoplasm. This localization results strategic allowing products of enzyme catalysis distributing in cytoplasm as well as into organelles. In this respect, several studies indicate the deleterious role of the hydrogen peroxide produced by MAO catalysis in inducing oxidative damage of structural or mitochondrial proteins (Kaludercic et al., 2010), triggering tissue loss of function and senescence.

Interesting enough, experimental evidence indicate that MAO-A isoform over-activation occurs in degenerative pathologies including heart and kidney failure. These evidence suggested that MAO-A overactivation might be considered as a novel source of free radicals participating to unbalancing the cell redox state, a ground condition for the onset of several diseases.

Accordingly, inhibition of enzyme activity has been proposed as a novel antioxidant strategy to reduce tissue oxidative status. This approach has however, intrinsic limitations including the increase of the the sympathergic tone.

Bach et al., (1988) cloned MAO-A and MAO-B describing interesting differences and similarities between the two isoforms. In this respect they clearly indicated that the promoters of the two isoforms are controlled, as expected, by different regulatory factors. In particular, in addition to sex hormones, they reported that angiotensin-II (AT-II) selectively activates

---

[#] This chapter was previously published in *Advances in Medicine and Biology. Volume 87,* edited by Leon V. Berhardt, New York: Nova Publishers Inc., 2015.

[*] Corresponding Author: Laura Raimondi. Viale G. Pieraccini 6, 50139 Florence, Italy. E-mail: laura.raimondi@unifi.it, phone: ++390552758385.

MAO-A promoter activity. This evidence, which can have clinical implications, has been neglected largely by pharmacologists.

Drugs targeting AT-II and its intracellular cascade are considered gold standard treatments for cardiovascular diseases (CVD). The beneficial effects of such drugs may include the control of MAO-A over-activation, thus working indeed as "indirect antioxidants." This aspect may over-come the use of MAO inhibitors, which *di per se* are endowed of scavenging activity in respect of oxidants, and be considered an added value for drugs rescuing against the cardiovascular risk.

In: Medicine Research Summaries. Volume 17
Editors: Zhongwen Liáng and Bibao Zhang
ISBN: 978-1-53612-751-5

Chapter 34

iMAO: What We Know About[#]

Grzegorz Opielak
Department of Human Anatomy, Medical University of Lublin,
Collegium Anatomicum, Lublin, Poland

Research Summary

MAO inhibitors (MonoAminoOxidase) - iMAO, are a group of antidepressant agents acting through the blocking of the enzymatic pathway of the disintegration of the serotonin - of MAO enzyme decomposing serotonin. One distinguishes two isoenzymes: MAO-A and MAO-B differing in the location and action. Isoenzyme MAO-A is found in a nervous tissue and its action is based on controlling the level of affection, whereas MAO-B is located in non-nervous tissues and with its action it regulates the appropriate blood pressure. Also numerous side effects, which may appear in the course of therapy with MAO, are based on these relations, especially on nonselective ones.

iMAO action was revealed by chance, as these medicines were used in treating tuberculosis, and their influence on the mood was quickly connected with action on neurotransmitters. The entire group of MAO inhibitors are not only drugs used in the treatment of depression, and these are divided in three subgroups. The first, oldest group includes drugs restraining MAO permanently and not selectively. Isoniazid, applied up till today in curing tuberculosis is in this group. The following second group, entails medicines blocking MAO irremediably, but selectively, e.g., Selegiline (MAO-B) - used in therapy of Parkinson's disease. Last, most contemporary group, are selective and reversible medicines, e.g., moklobemid, (MAO-A) that is the most important antidepressant agent being a representative of iMAO entire group.

iMAO group is used universally worldwide, which does not mean that these medicines are deprived of side effects. Above all, an amount of interactions they can enter with other medicines, elevating the serotonin level is quite large. Effects of such combinations are very serious, including serotonin syndrome and death. A wrong diet, containing lots of the tyramine, also decomposed by MAO, has a similar effect. Other adverse effects characteristic of MAO inhibitors are a hepatotoxicity and hypertensive action.

[#] This chapter was previously published in *Advances in Medicine and Biology. Volume 87,* edited by Leon V. Berhardt, New York: Nova Publishers Inc., 2015.

In: Medicine Research Summaries. Volume 17
Editors: Zhongwen Liáng and Bibao Zhang
ISBN: 978-1-53612-751-5

Chapter 35

OVERWEIGHT DURING THE CENTURIES#

Emilia Manzato*
University of Ferrara, Italy National Council Member,
Italian Society for the Study of Eating Disorder (SISDCA), Italy

RESEARCH SUMMARY

There is a growing concern about obesity and overweight worldwide perceived as "epidemic problem".

In this chapter the results of the main surveys regarding the spread of obesity and overweight will be briefly reported.

Most studies have been focused on obesity so far and only recently overweight has gained importance.

Data on overweight give a complex and unclear view: could overweight be considered as a high risk factor to obesity? Or, vice versa, could overweight be the best condition for a longer life expectancy? The results of literature data are contradictory.

In this chapter a broad view about the features of overweight in childhood and adolescence and in women, particularly in the menopausal age will be also given.

Data about health's risks due to overweight condition will be provided in the last part of the chapter.

This chapter was previously published in *The Different Faces of Being Overweight: Risk Factors for the Evolution towards Obesity*, edited by Emilia Manzato, New York: Nova Publishers Inc., 2015.

* Corresponding Author: Emilia Manzato, Psychiatrist; Email: emilia.manzato@gmail.com.

In: Medicine Research Summaries. Volume 17
Editors: Zhongwen Liáng and Bibao Zhang

ISBN: 978-1-53612-751-5

Chapter 36

FOOD ADDICTION: BRAIN AND MIND[#]

Gian Luigi Luxardi[1 2]* and Fiorenza Marchiol[3 4]
[1]Center for Eating Disorders of ASL, "Friuli Occidentale", Italy
[2]Triveneto Section of Italian Society for the Study of Eating Disorders (SISDCA), Italy
[3]Center for Eating Disorders of ASL n.6, "Friuli Occidentale", Italy
[4]Italian Society for the Study of Eating Disorders (SISDCA), Italy

RESEARCH SUMMARY

There have been various attempts to explain why some people chronically overeat and seem unable to restrain their food intake. One explanation relates directly to the markedly "toxic" food environment in recent years. A growing body of clinical and neurobiological evidence has shown how persistent overeating can lead, in vulnerable individuals, to a pattern of compulsive behaviour similar to that seen in addiction disorders. Evidence in scientific literature argues that food reward, not hunger, could be the main driving force behind eating in the modern obesogenic environment. In this chapter, we consider the assumptions related to neural and molecular adaptations in both homeostatic and non-homeostatic appetite regulation that may underlie the formation of an allostatic, non-resilient state, propelling the individual from a basic preference for palatable diets to food craving and compulsive, addiction-like eating behavior. We consider also the interaction of these systems with stress and mood regulation.

This chapter was previously published in *The Different Faces of Being Overweight: Risk Factors for the Evolution towards Obesity*, edited by Emilia Manzato, New York: Nova Publishers Inc., 2015.

* Corresponding Author: Gian Luigi Luxardi, Clinical Psychologist, Chief of Center for Eating Disorders of ASL; President of Triveneto Section of Italian Society for the Study of Eating Disorders; Email: gianluigi.luxardi@ass6.sanita.fvg.it.

In: Medicine Research Summaries. Volume 17
Editors: Zhongwen Liáng and Bibao Zhang ISBN: 978-1-53612-751-5

Chapter 37

DIETARY RESTRAINT AS A RISK FACTOR FOR LOSS OF CONTROL[#]

Nazario Melchionda[12*] and Giulietta Tarrini[3†]
[1]University of Bologna, Italy
[2]Italian Society for the Study of Eating Disorder (SISDCA), Italy
[3]Azienda Ospedaliera di Bologna, Policlinico S.Orsola-Malpighi, Servizio di Malattie del Metabolismo e Dietetica Clinica, Italy

RESEARCH SUMMARY

The subject of the present chapter is extremely topical and it is interesting not only for research purposes but also to find and examine evidence relevant to therapy in clinical practice. This chapter focuses on the risk of loss of control, using definitions for non-experts, recognizing that eating disorders are multi-disciplinary, involving psychological, psychiatric, endocrinological and nutritional disciplines: Binge eating (BE), Binge Eating Disorder (BED), Dietary Restraint (DR), Food Addiction (FA), HSME: Homeostasis System of Metabolism and Energy, HSHR: Homeostasis System of Hedonic Reward, NAc: Nucleus Accumbens, NCAR: Neural Circuitry of Addiction and Reward, VTA: Ventral Tegmental Area. The major sources of historical data are outlined so as to understand the significance of loss of control – in particular, the 1950 Minnesota Study by Angel Keys, in which the characteristic symptoms of eating disorders were activated in volunteer participants by means of caloric restriction; this is followed by observations in Greek literature, the phenomenon of St Anorexics in the Middle Ages and the effect of caloric restriction on a group of Canadian soldiers during World War II. The historical data concludes with the pioneering publication by Stunkard of his case study of a subject with chronic obesity, in which Binge Eating is described for the first time. In addition, there is reference to human and rodent experimental

---

[#] This chapter was previously published in *The Different Faces of Being Overweight: Risk Factors for the Evolution towards Obesity*, edited by Emilia Manzato, New York: Nova Publishers Inc., 2015.

[*] Corresponding Author: Nazario Melchionda, President of Italian Society for the Study of Eating Disorder, Email: melchiondauno@gmail.com.

[†] Corresponding Author: Giulietta Tarrini, Dietista Coordinatrice, Email: gtarrini@gmail.com.

data: in particular regarding the psychological, psychobiological and neurobiological mechanisms related to BED loss of control. Since 2000 considerable research and numerous studies have been carried out employing neuroimaging techniques to determine the effect brain biology has on both normal and pathological behavior. The result is the current recognition that neural systems influence the regulation of normal eating behavior and that they also influence the loss of control that characterizes AN, BN, and BED. The neural systems identified by means of neuroimaging radiological techniques are summarized in the definitions and in the section 'What we can learn from brain biology'. Food Addiction (FA) is the latest chapter in the history of ED research. Three important questions are therefore asked: What are the neurobiological effects of intermittent restriction? What is the level of calorie restriction that results in loss of control? Can we stop eating too much hyper-palatable food? By answering these questions we will be able to make recommendations and suggestions. The final conclusion is that inadequate caloric restriction is not the only risk factor for loss of control but also the cognitive intention to lose weight by means of DR.

In: Medicine Research Summaries. Volume 17
Editors: Zhongwen Liáng and Bibao Zhang
ISBN: 978-1-53612-751-5

Chapter 38

LIFE STAGES AND OVERWEIGHT/OBESITY RISK[#]

Ottavio Bosello[1*], MD, and Angiola Vanzo[2†], MD
[1]Department of Medicine, University of Verona, Italy
[2]Department of Prevention, Food Hygiene and Nutrition Service, ASL 6 Veneto, Italy

RESEARCH SUMMARY

Looking at the natural history of obesity, people tend to accumulate fat during all the life span. In recent years, this phenomenon has modified and the age at highest risk is now the childhood. The prevalence of childhood obesity has increased rapidly to high levels over recent decades, particularly in some communities and states at high economic level but also in developing countries. Given such a high prevalence, is now crucial to identify the risk factors best predicting incident obesity in childhood and what are the contributory characteristics resulting in obesity. The environment is the main accused. Furthermore the children at highest risk must be accurately targeted for early intervention.

As a consequence, in the adulthood the main risk factor for obesity is to have been overweight at the younger age.

The prevalence studies show that the peak of obesity is in the younger elderly (60-65 years). Despite the increase in life expectancy, over the years more advanced obesity is becoming less frequent. The phenomenon is due to the increased risk of morbidity and mortality carried by overweight and obesity, with the finding that at older ages the prevalence of obesity is less common.

Last but not least consideration: nowadays, there is a new tendency to redefine obesogenic environments not as environments that make bodies fat, but as environments that make fat bodies problematic and considering alternative theoretical frameworks in order to avoid the pitfalls of environmental determinism.

[#] This chapter was previously published in *The Different Faces of Being Overweight: Risk Factors for the Evolution towards Obesity*, edited by Emilia Manzato, New York: Nova Publishers Inc., 2015.

[*] Corresponding Author: ottavio.bosello@univr.it. Past president SIO (Italian Society for Obesity) Past president SISDCA (Italian Society for Eating Disorders).

[†] Corresponding Author Email: angiola.vanzo@ulssvicenza.it.

In: Medicine Research Summaries. Volume 17
Editors: Zhongwen Liáng and Bibao Zhang
ISBN: 978-1-53612-751-5

Chapter 39

OVERWEIGHT IN CHILDHOOD AND ADOLESCENCE[#]

Andrea Vania, MD*

ECOG (European Childhood Obesity Group), Belgium
Department of Paediatrics and Paediatric Neuropsychiatry,
"Sapienza" University of Rome, Italy

RESEARCH SUMMARY

About 40% of children with weight troubles (as well as 60% of adolescents in the same conditions) will remain obese during their adult life. With this in mind, it is clear enough that many cases of adulthood's obesity found their roots in paediatric age.

Belonging to a lineage where obesity runs in the family appears as an important risk factor in the development of childhood obesity, but the relationship between parental and offspring obesity is not limited to genetic factors. Actually, environment can play a major role in both generations.

The concept of environment has widened enough, in the recent years, and scientists look at it now as the "envirome", the total complement of environmental characteristics, conditions, and processes required for life form viability and successful adaptation. Genome and environment coexist, and genomic expression can be modified by environment, leading to the idea that genome and envirome can interact through epigenetic modifications, which are active during the individual life-span, but are suspected to have an inter-generational influence as well.

Should epigenomics' hypothesis be confirmed as reliable, then the whole weighing condition, development, and future of an individual would be really decided during the very first periods of his/her life. According to the hypothesis, epigenetic changes start during the gestational period, and – quite possibly – even before it.

We are still trying to understand which external environmental factors can shape the genomic expression, and what impact each factor can have.

[#] This chapter was previously published in *The Different Faces of Being Overweight: Risk Factors for the Evolution towards Obesity*, edited by Emilia Manzato, New York: Nova Publishers Inc., 2015.
* Corresponding Author: Andrea Vania, Former President, ECOG; E-mail: andrea.vania@uniroma1.it.

In: Medicine Research Summaries. Volume 17
Editors: Zhongwen Liáng and Bibao Zhang
ISBN: 978-1-53612-751-5

Chapter 40

EATING DISORDERS AND BIASED EATING BEHAVIORS AS RISK FACTORS FOR OVERWEIGHT[#]

Emilia Manzato*
University of Ferrara, Italy
National Council Member,
Italian Society for the Study of Eating Disorder (SISDCA), Italy

RESEARCH SUMMARY

Eating disorders and biased eating behavior could be risk factors leading to overweight and obesity or encouraging such as status.

In this chapter we deal particularly with binge eating disorder, the most frequent eating disorder in the overweight and obese population, because the presence of binge episodes without compensatory behaviors. Furthermore, the presence lifetime of any eating disorder (anorexia, bulimia or binge eating disorder) represents a risk factor for weight gain. We describe also night eating syndrome, a particular disorder included, for the first time, between the Eating Disorders in DSM5th in the "Other specified feeding or eating disorder" section. These eating disorders, if present, could play an important role in the development of overweight and obesity.

We describe also some other biased eating behavior such as grazing- not included in eating disorders but important because its contribution to the weight gain- and emotional eating.

They are still object of researches programs.

In the last part of the chapter we'll also deal with a particular eating behavior such as "Hyperphagia" as risk factor for overweight and obesity.

[#] This chapter was previously published in *The Different Faces of Being Overweight: Risk Factors for the Evolution towards Obesity*, edited by Emilia Manzato, New York: Nova Publishers Inc., 2015.

* Corresponding Author: Emilia Manzato, Psychiatrist; emilia.manzato@gmail.com.

In: Medicine Research Summaries. Volume 17
Editors: Zhongwen Liáng and Bibao Zhang
ISBN: 978-1-53612-751-5

Chapter 41

NEGATIVE BODY-IMAGE AND BODY DISSATISFACTION IN OVERWEIGHT[#]

Antonia Bolognesi*
Italian Society for the Study of Eating Disorder (SISDCA), Italy

RESEARCH SUMMARY

Body image disorder can be included among the multiple factors, which develop and maintain the overweight condition.

With the term "body image" we refer to the mind representation that an individual has of their body. Although it is structured upon specific individual physical characteristics, it is influenced by psychological, relational and cultural factors. Body image is multifactorial and dynamic construct and it includes- and at the same time overcomes- the physical characteristics.

In such a complex construct, the breaking points may be various: a disturbed body image can be expressed as 'misperception' (body shape is wrongly evaluated), as dissatisfaction (consequence of the gap between perception and a thin ideal) or as excessive evaluation of body shape and weight.

Some authors suggest to give a nosographic validity to body image disorder, placing it in the Diagnostic and Statistics Manual of Mental Disorders5th edition (DSM5). At the moment, body image disorder is not universally recognized as *a* diagnosis, we refer therefore to negative body image to indicate a condition which is more uncomfortable and inhibiting than ordinary body anxiety. Subjects with negative body image can be dissatisfied with their weight and complain that they are too fat, seeing weight loss as a solution strategy.

Sex is an important modulator as far as it concerns the thin ideal, the type of worries and the tendency to express or hide anxiety. In cultures where western influence is more consistent, the ideal of woman beauty is oriented to thinness, while man to muscularity. Since

---

This chapter was previously published in *The Different Faces of Being Overweight: Risk Factors for the Evolution towards Obesity*, edited by Emilia Manzato, New York: Nova Publishers Inc., 2015.

* Corresponding Author: Antonia Bolognesi, Psychologist, Psychotherapist and member of SISDCA; Email: antoniabolognesi@libero.it.

this kind of ideal is almost unreachable for most people, the levels of dissatisfaction in both men and women increase.

Body image is a moderator in the relationship the individual has with eating, physical activity and the consequent evolution of weight and health conditions in life. Literature also stresses how body image mediates the relationship between Body Mass Index (BMI) and psycho-social variables such as self-esteem and life quality.

The sociocultural, individual and relational factors, which play a role in the construction and evolution of body image in overweight people in their lifetime, are numerous.

In a society where the stress on thinness is constant, especially for young women, being overweight or obese is a risk factor FOR the creation and development OF negative body image.

Other factors which cause negative body image are linked to the individual dimension (i.e. low self-esteem and binge eating) as well as relational dimension (family and extra family relationships).

The chapter explores the contributions in literature about body image in overweight people with and without eating disorders, paying particular attention to the factors which play a role in the creation of negative body image and body dissatisfaction among these people.

In: Medicine Research Summaries. Volume 17
Editors: Zhongwen Liáng and Bibao Zhang
ISBN: 978-1-53612-751-5

Chapter 42

LIFESTYLES: SEDENTARY LIFESTYLE AND UNBALANCED DIET[#]

Eleonora Roncarati
Italian Society for the Study of Eating Disorders (SISDCA), Italy

RESEARCH SUMMARY

The epidemic of overweight and obesity are a well-known phenomenon affecting the world population. Mainly, the increase in adipose tissue responsible for weight gain, is related to a gap in the energy balance for which the energy intake (nutrients) are superior than the energy expenditure (Resting Metabolic Rate, thermic effect, physical activity and thermogenesis from other causes). Several studies in the literature suggest that it is more difficult to maintain the energetic balance nowadays than in the past. Urbanization, industrialization and the use of transport have lead to a general decrease in energy expenditure for physical activity that has encouraged the development of "sedentary"; furthermore, there has been an exaggerated use of industrial techniques for processing and food preparation depleting the food from its healthy components, such as fibers vitamins, minerals and enrich it of nutrients that make it hyper palatable and highly caloric (sugar, lipids, especially saturated fats, salt, preservatives and food colourings). So you get a food called "refined and manipulated" very attractive, ready for consumption, low satiety index and high calorie that's easy to "exceed" in the amount of intake and frequency of consumption; the excess that is realized in terms of total energy (calories) and nutrients densely caloric (as lipids and sugars) determines a positive energy balance, which correlates with weight gain. Several studies have also shown that the variations of body weight appear to be more affected by a "combination" of nutrients, rather than by a single nutrient taken in excess. The analysis of dietary patterns therefore provides an opportunity to assess which food styles are more related to the development of overweight and obesity, as well as metabolic diseases, cardiovascular and oncology. The analysis of patter food has led to

[#] This chapter was previously published in *The Different Faces of Being Overweight: Risk Factors for the Evolution towards Obesity*, edited by Emilia Manzato, New York: Nova Publishers Inc., 2015.

identify a “Healthy Patter” that has features common to the "Mediterranean Diet". Various studies have shown that the Mediterranean diet is not related to an increased risk of overweight and obesity and may play a role in the prevention of both. Instead, the food restriction in order to control body weight was unsuccessful in the long term: the imposition of a rigid control promotes the loss of control over food intake resulting in energy and nutrients unscheduled nor manageable.

In: Medicine Research Summaries. Volume 17
Editors: Zhongwen Liáng and Bibao Zhang
ISBN: 978-1-53612-751-5

Chapter 43

OVERWEIGHT AND OBESITY IN INTERNAL MEDICINE[#]

Lorenzo M. Donini*, MD
Experimental Medicine Department, Medical Pathophysiology,
Food Science and Endocrinology Section,
Food Science and Human Nutrition Research Unit,
Sapienza University of Rome, Italy
National Council Member,
Italian Society for the Study of Eating Disorder (SISDCA), Italy

RESEARCH SUMMARY

Obesity may be secondary to other diseases due to genetic or acquired conditions that are characterized by alterations in the control of systems regulating hunger-satiety and / or weight, in the gastrointestinal system and the intestinal microbiota, in endocrine pathways. Secondary obesity may be due to maternal metabolic conditions, to neurobiological and psychological determinants, to sleep debt and smoking cessation, to disability and to various medications.

[#] This chapter was previously published in *The Different Faces of Being Overweight: Risk Factors for the Evolution towards Obesity*, edited by Emilia Manzato, New York: Nova Publishers Inc., 2015.

* Corresponding Author Email: Lorenzomaria.donini@uniroma1.it.

In: Medicine Research Summaries. Volume 17
Editors: Zhongwen Liáng and Bibao Zhang ISBN: 978-1-53612-751-5

Chapter 44

ARTIFICIAL SWEETENERS, GUT MICROBIOTA AND HEALTH[#]

Xiaofa Qin, MD, PhD
GI BiopharmaInc, Westfield, NJ, US

RESEARCH SUMMARY

Most of the currently heavily used artificial sweeteners such as saccharin, sucralose, cyclamate and acesulfame potassium (ace K) are characterized as minimal metabolism by the body and thus believed to be safe. They are very stable and can even keep unchanged for a long time in the environment. However, they have a strong impact on bacteria. For instance, saccharin, the oldest and one of the most widely used artificial sweeteners that has been on the market since 1880s, was used at the very beginning as antiseptic. More and more studies revealed that gut microbiota played a critical role in a wide range of diseases. Recent study demonstrated that the non-caloric high intensity artificial sweeteners like saccharin may induce glucose intolerance and increase the risk of diabetes by altering gut microbiota. Evidence collected by the author suggests that these artificial sweeteners could be important causative factor for inflammatory bowel disease (IBD) through mechanisms such as impaired deactivation of digestive proteases by certain kinds of gut bacteria and the resultant damage of gut tissue. Increased gut permeability has also seen in many other diseases such as irritable bowel syndrome (IBS), food allergy, multiple sclerosis, asthma, atopic dermatitis, cirrhosis, autism, etc. The adverse effect of artificial sweeteners on gut microbiota and health would be worthwhile for further study.

[#] This chapter was previously published in *Advances in Medicine and Biology. Volume 93,* edited by Leon V. Berhardt, New York: Nova Publishers Inc., 2016.

In: Medicine Research Summaries. Volume 17
Editors: Zhongwen Liáng and Bibao Zhang

ISBN: 978-1-53612-751-5

Chapter 45

THALIDOMIDE IN PULMONARY DISEASE[#]

Christine L. Vigeland, MD and Maureen R. Horton, MD
Johns Hopkins University School of Medicine, Baltimore, MD, US

RESEARCH SUMMARY

Originally developed in the mid-1950's as a sedative and anti-emetic the use of thalidomide for those purposes was terminated due to its teratogenic effects [1]. However, more recently, thalidomide has been found to have potent effects modulating immune function, reducing inflammation, and inhibiting angiogenesis [2-5]. These immumomodulatory properties have allowed the re-purposing of this drug to treat a variety of malignancies and autoimmune diseases [4-6]. Within the scope of pulmonary diseases, thalidomide is being investigated for treatment of dysregulated inflammation manifest in such diseases as acute lung injury, idiopathic pulmonary fibrosis, sarcoidosis, COPD, infections and asthma [7-11]. Animal studies have found that the immunomodulatory effects of thalidomide reduce inflammation and injury in animal models of acute lung injury, idiopathic pulmonary fibrosis, and asthma [8, 10, 11]. Human studies investigating the efficacy of thalidomide have demonstrated that it may improve both cutaneous and pulmonary sarcoidosis, as well as decrease cough and improve quality of life in patients with idiopathic pulmonary fibrosis [7, 9]. Thalidomide's immunomodulatory, anti-inflammatory, and anti-angiogenesis effects make it a potentially efficacious therapy for a number of pulmonary diseases characterized by dysregulated inflammation and fibrosis. Current studies in pulmonary diseases show promising effects, and additional studies are needed to fully evaluate the efficacy of thalidomide in treatment of these diseases.

[#] This chapter was previously published in *Advances in Medicine and Biology. Volume 93,* edited by Leon V. Berhardt, New York: Nova Publishers Inc., 2016.

References

[1] Taussig HB (1962) The thalidomide syndrome. *Sci Am* 207: 29-35.

[2] D'Amato RJ, Loughnan MS, Flynn E, Folkman J (1994) Thalidomide is an inhibitor of angiogenesis. *Proc Natl Acad Sci USA* 91: 4082-4085.

[3] Figg WD, Dahut W, Duray P, Hamilton M, Tompkins A, et al. (2001) A randomized phase II trial of thalidomide, an angiogenesis inhibitor, in patients with androgen-independent prostate cancer. *Clin Cancer Res* 7: 1888-1893.

[4] Singhal S, Mehta J, Desikan R, Ayers D, Roberson P, et al. (1999) Antitumor activity of thalidomide in refractory multiple myeloma. *N Engl J Med* 341: 1565-1571.

[5] Eisen T, Boshoff C, Mak I, Sapunar F, Vaughan MM, et al. (2000) Continuous low dose Thalidomide: a phase II study in advanced melanoma, renal cell, ovarian and breast cancer. *Br J Cancer* 82: 812-817.

[6] Lazzerini M, Martelossi S, Magazzu G, Pellegrino S, Lucanto MC, et al. (2013) Effect of thalidomide on clinical remission in children and adolescents with refractory Crohn disease: a randomized clinical trial. *JAMA* 310: 2164-2173.

[7] Fazzi P, Manni E, Cristofani R, Cei G, Piazza S, et al. (2012) Thalidomide for improving cutaneous and pulmonary sarcoidosis in patients resistant or with contraindications to corticosteroids. *Biomed Pharmacother* 66: 300-307.

[8] Asano T, Kume H, Taki F, Ito S, Hasegawa Y (2010) Thalidomide attenuates airway hyper responsiveness and eosinophilic inflammation in a murine model of allergic asthma. *Biol Pharm Bull* 33: 1028-1032.

[9] Horton MR, Santopietro V, Mathew L, Horton KM, Polito AJ, et al. (2012) Thalidomide for the treatment of cough in idiopathic pulmonary fibrosis: a randomized trial. *Ann Intern Med* 157: 398-406.

[10] Tabata C, Tabata R, Kadokawa Y, Hisamori S, Takahashi M, et al. (2007) Thalidomide prevents bleomycin-induced pulmonary fibrosis in mice. *J Immunol* 179: 708-714.

[11] Lv P, Li HY, Ji SS, Li W, Fan LJ (2014) Thalidomide alleviates acute pancreatitis-associated lung injury via down-regulation of NFkappaB induced TNF-alpha. *Pathol Res Pract* 210: 558-564.

In: Medicine Research Summaries. Volume 17
Editors: Zhongwen Liáng and Bibao Zhang

ISBN: 978-1-53612-751-5

Chapter 46

Activation of Thalidomide to Reactive Metabolites by Autoinduced Human Cytochrome P450 3A Enzymes, with Substrate Cooperativity, and Implications for Development of Analogs[#]

Hiroshi Yamazaki[1]*, Goutam Chowdhury[2] and F. Peter Guengerich[3]
[1]Showa Pharmaceutical University, Machida, Tokyo, Japan
[2]Shiv Nadar University, Gautam Buddha Nagar, UP, India
[3]Vanderbilt University School of Medicine, Nashville, TN, US

Research Summary

The teratogen thalidomide has been subsequently approved for the treatment of multiple myeloma, and there is renewed interest in both its toxicity and pharmacological mechanisms. In this review article, the focus is on human metabolic activationof thalidomide and analogs. Pre-treatment with orally administered thalidomide enhanced midazolam clearance in mice with humanized liver due to human cytochromeP450 3A induction, as also evident in *in vitro* studies including enhanced levels of P450 3A4 mRNA, protein expression, and/or oxidation activity in human hepatocytes through the action of the pregnane X receptor (PXR). Homotropic and heterotropic cooperativity of human cytochrome P450 (P450) 3A4/5 by thalidomide was demonstrated using the model substrate midazolam in various *in vitro* systems with human liver microsomes, recombinant P450 enzymes, and hepatocytes *in vivo* models with chimeric mice expressing humanized liver cells. Thalidomide and its human

---

[#] This chapter was previously published in *Advances in Medicine and Biology. Volume 93,* edited by Leon V. Berhardt, New York: Nova Publishers Inc., 2016.

* Corresponding Author: Prof. Hiroshi Yamazaki, PhD, Showa Pharmaceutical University, 3-3165 Higashi-tamagawa Gakuen, Machida, Tokyo 194-8543, Japan, Tel/fax: +81-42-721-1406; E-mail: hyamazak@ac.shoyaku.ac.jp.

primary metabolite 5-hydroxythalidomide were oxidized by human P450 3A enzymes to reactive intermediates involving aromatic ring positions, which were trapped with glutathione conjugates. These findings collectively suggest that thalidomide causes human P450 3A enzyme induction and activation by the same P450 3A enzymes through the human primary metabolite 5-hydroxythalidomide. New thalidomide-related drugs, e.g., pomalidomide and lenalidomide, had limited and no metabolism leading to adducts in the similar systems, respectively. Taken together, screening for avoiding unwanted bioactivation but keeping the immunomodulatory properties is a strategic pathway to new cancer drugs. The possibilities for drug interactions during thalidomide therapy and roles of the reactive metabolites in the efficacy and side effects of thalidomide require further evaluation.

In: Medicine Research Summaries. Volume 17
Editors: Zhongwen Liáng and Bibao Zhang
ISBN: 978-1-53612-751-5

Chapter 47

AUTOMATIC CONTROL OF BRAIN TEMPERATURE BY SURFACE COOLING[#]

Tomohiko Utsuki*, PhD
Department of Biomedical Engineering, School of Engineering,
Tokai University, Shibuya, Tokyo, Japan

RESEARCH SUMMARY

Therapeutic hypothermia is one of the most essential treatments for hypoxic-ischemic encephalopathy after cardiac arrest and also for neonatal asphyxia. However, this treatment requires precise control of brain and/or body temperature because excessive cooling often induces various side effects. Consequently, several automatic brain temperature control systems have been developed for precise control of brain temperature and to minimize the burden on medical staff.

Surface cooling, in particular, is currently the technique most utilized in clinical practice because it is noninvasive and easier to perform than blood cooling, including endovascular cooling. The Arctic Sun® temperature management system is a water-surface cooling apparatus that has a function for automatic control of brain temperature. This apparatus is quite prevalent in clinical practice, because it does not require medical staff to input the patient's parameters such as height, weight, and age. However, its control algorithm cannot be found clearly in academic papers as far as this author checked.

In this study, an automatic water-surface cooling brain temperature control system was developed as a model reference control system with two degrees of freedom. This system has a more flexible algorithm, which is necessary for brain temperature control because the thermal characteristics of a patient are time-variable and in general are much different on an individual basis. The developed system has two selectable types of control algorithms: an

---

[#] This chapter was previously published in *Advances in Medicine and Biology. Volume 93,* edited by Leon V. Berhardt, New York: Nova Publishers Inc., 2016.

* Corresponding Author: Tomohiko Utsuki, PhD: Department of Biomedical Engineering, School of Engineering, Tokai University, 143 Shimo-Kasuya Isehara-shi Kanagawa-ken 259-1193, Japan. Phone: +81-463-1121, Email: tom.utsuki@tokai-u.jp.

optimal-adaptive control algorithm and a model reference fuzzy control algorithm. The results of application of the system in clinical practice on three patients with cerebral venous infarction showed that the control errors of the system were kept within ± 0.20°C on average, with root mean square approximately 0.06°C.

Thus, the control performance of the developed system was confirmed as being of sufficiently high quality, despite much time variations in the thermal characteristics.

An automatic air-surface cooling brain temperature control system was also developed using the model reference control algorithm with two degrees of freedom, as with the water-cooling system. An air-cooling system can conserve electric power, reduce the degree of compression of the cooling blankets/pads, and reduce the risk of contamination caused by leakage from a control apparatus, because air has a lower specific heat capacity and lower density than water. Thus, it represents the next stage in the development of a high performance clinically usable system.

In: Medicine Research Summaries. Volume 17
Editors: Zhongwen Liáng and Bibao Zhang
ISBN: 978-1-53612-751-5

Chapter 48

SWIMMING ANOMALIES IN ANIMALS WITH CEREBELLAR LESIONS[#]

Robert Lalonde[1,*] and Catherine Strazielle[2,†]
[1]Université de Rouen, Département de Psychologie,
Laboratoire ICONES EA 4699, Mont-Saint-Aignan Cedex, France
[2]Université de Lorraine, Laboratoire "Stress, Immunité, Pathogènes" EA 7300,
and Service de Microscopie, Faculté de Médecine and CHU de Nancy,
Vandoeuvre-les-Nancy, France

RESEARCH SUMMARY

The evaluation of anti-ataxic substances usually comprises motor coordination in rotorod, stationary beam, or bar-suspension assays as well as the control of gait in footprint analyses. But other measures may be used to evaluate the effects of cerebellar lesions, notably those requiring swimming movements. Unlike animals with vestibular damage, often unable to keep their head above water, those with damage to the cerebellum are able to swim efficiently. But when placed into a small basin with no possibility of escape, normal mice quickly float on the water, making only those movements necessary to keep their head above the surface, while cerebellar-damaged animals have great difficulty in maintaining the floating posture and continue to swim around the basin. Likewise, cerebellar-lesioned fish are unable to maintain a steady position. In addition, whereas normal fish swim straight, cerebellar-lesioned fish undulate their body. Unlike deactivation occurring in several brain regions during forced swimming, brain metabolism measured by fluorodeoxyglucose uptake in normal rats indicates increased activity in the cerebellum and striatum. Examples are given as to the feasibility of rapid evaluations of swimming in rodents and fish as a supplement to motor coordination tests.

[#] This chapter was previously published in *Advances in Medicine and Biology. Volume 93,* edited by Leon V. Berhardt, New York: Nova Publishers Inc., 2016.

[*] Corresponding Author: Université de Rouen, Département de Psychologie, Laboratoire ICONES EA 4699, 76821 Mont-Saint-Aignan Cedex, France, E-mail: robert.lalonde@univ-rouen.fr.

[†] Corresponding Author: Université de Lorraine, Laboratoire "Stress, Immunité, Pathogènes" EA 7300, and Service de Microscopie, Faculté de Médecine and CHU de Nancy, 54500 Vandoeuvre-les-Nancy, France, Email: catherine.strazielle@univ-lorraine.fr.

In: Medicine Research Summaries. Volume 17
Editors: Zhongwen Liáng and Bibao Zhang
ISBN: 978-1-53612-751-5

Chapter 49

NUCLEIC ACID DRUGS TO PREVENT CORONARY RESTENOSIS AFTER STENT IMPLANTATION[#]

Jun-ichi Suzuki*
Department of Advanced Clinical Science and Therapeutics,
The University of Tokyo, Tokyo, Japan

RESEARCH SUMMARY

Nuclear factor-kappa B (NF-kB) plays a pivotal role in restenosis after stent implantation. To evaluate the effectiveness of an NF-kB decoy oligodeoxynucleotide (ODN), we performed experimental studies and clinical trials. Firstly, murine femoral arteries were injured using flexible wires and we performed *in vivo* NF-kB decoy ODN transfection in the injured arteries. Pathologically, the NF-kB decoy ODN transfection group showed smaller neointima per media area ratios than those in the control groups. Immunohistochemistry revealed that enhanced expression of inflammatory factors was observed in non-treated injured arteries, while the NF-kB decoy ODN suppressed the expression. Based on these experimental results, we initiated an open label phase I/IIa clinical trial to evaluate the safety and effectiveness of NF-kB decoy ODN. Seventeen patients, who were suffering from angina, were treated with NF-kB decoy ODN after bare metal stent implantation. Three days after stent implantation, serum MCP-1 levels were significantly suppressed in NF-kB decoy ODN treated patients compared to the non-treated patients. Six months after stent implantation and decoy ODN transfection, significant restenosis was found in only 1 of the 17 patients, and the average restenosis rate was less than 40%. In-stent thrombosis was not found and no significant systemic adverse effect occurred in any of the patients in the six-months observation period. One of the 17 cases has been regularly examined for eight years after ODN transfection. We revealed that decoy ODN treatment suppressed neointimal formation in comparison to the stent lesion without ODN transfection in the same artery. Thus, we showed the safety and long-term usefulness of NF-kB decoy ODN transfer after coronary stent implantation.

[#] This chapter was previously published in *Advances in Medicine and Biology. Volume 93,* edited by Leon V. Berhardt, New York: Nova Publishers Inc., 2016.

* Corresponding Author: Jun-ichi Suzuki, Department of Advanced Clinical Science and Therapeutics, Graduate School of Medicine, The University of Tokyo, 7-3-1 Hongo, Bunkyo, Tokyo 113-8655, Japan; phone 81-3-5800-9116, fax 81-3-5800-9182, e-mail junichisuzuki-circ@umin.ac.jp.

In: Medicine Research Summaries. Volume 17
Editors: Zhongwen Liáng and Bibao Zhang
ISBN: 978-1-53612-751-5

Chapter 50

DOES ANOSOGNOSIA AFFECT THE SHORT-TERM GOALS ACHIEVEMENT IN MEDICAL REHABILITATION FOR PATIENTS WITH ACUTE ISCHEMIC STROKE?[#]

V. N. Grigoryeva and T. A. Sorokina
Nizhniy Novgorod State Medical Academy, Nizhny Novgorod Oblast, Russia

RESEARCH SUMMARY

Insufficiency of self-awareness for neurological deficits may negatively affect the functional outcomes in medical rehabilitation due to the decreased engagement of the patients in the rehabilitation process [1-4]. However, its relationships with rehabilitation goals attainment in the patients with acute ischemic stroke (IS) have not yet been clarified.

References

[1] Prigatano G.P. Anosognosia: clinical and ethical considerations. *Curr. Opin. Neurol.* 2009 Dec; 22(6): 606-11.
[2] Kortte K.B., Hillis A.E. Recent trends in rehabilitation interventions for visual neglect and anosognosia for hemiplegia following right hemisphere stroke. *Future Neurol.* 2011 Jan; 6(1): 33–43.
[3] Vossel S., Weiss P.H., Eschenbeck P., Fink G.R. Anosognosia, neglect, extinction and lesion site predict impairment of daily living after right-hemispheric stroke. *Cortex* 2013 Jul-Aug; 49(7): 1782-9 [PubMed].
[4] Wang Y.C., Kapellusch J., Garg A. Important factors influencing the return to work after stroke. *Work.* 2014;47(4):553-9 [PubMed].

[#] This chapter was previously published in *Advances in Medicine and Biology. Volume 93,* edited by Leon V. Berhardt, New York: Nova Publishers Inc., 2016.

In: Medicine Research Summaries. Volume 17
Editors: Zhongwen Liáng and Bibao Zhang

ISBN: 978-1-53612-751-5

Chapter 51

ELECTRO-ACUPUNCTURE FOR LOWER URINARY TRACT DYSFUNCTION[#]

Ran Pang*[*], *Xinyao Zhou and Zhishun Liu
Guang An Men Hospital,
China Academy of Chinese Medical Sciences, Beijing, China

RESEARCH SUMMARY

Electro-acupuncture, as a component of acupuncture, has been used for various urological diseases and has gained acceptance in urologists. In this chapter, we will present the evidence about electro-acupuncture's effectiveness, as well as its potential mechanism, on lower urinary tract (LUT) dysfunction, a most common urological disorder. Because LUT function is basically divided into two parts, storage and voiding function, we will discuss the effect of electro-acupuncture on the two kinds of LUT functions, respectively. In terms of storage LUT dysfunction, overactive bladder and each type of urinary incontinence will be discussed respectively. For voiding LUT dysfunction, two common diseases including benign prostatic hyperplasia and bladder dysfunction secondary to anesthesia will be involved. In addition, the limitation of current electro-acupuncture study will also be discussed.

[#] This chapter was previously published in *Advances in Medicine and Biology. Volume 93,* edited by Leon V. Berhardt, New York: Nova Publishers Inc., 2016.

[*] Corresponding Author: Ran Pang, M.D., Division of Urology, Guang An Men Hospital, China Academy of Chinese Medical Sciences. No. 5 Bei Xian Ge Street, Xi Cheng District, Beijing, China, 100053, FAX: +8610-63014195, Telephone: +8610-88001040, e-mail: pangran2002@gmail.com or pangran2002@sina.com.

In: Medicine Research Summaries. Volume 17
Editors: Zhongwen Liáng and Bibao Zhang

ISBN: 978-1-53612-751-5

Chapter 52

PERIORBITAL NECROTIZING FASCIITIS: A CAUSE OF TOXIC SHOCK SYNDROME#

Shantha Amrith, FRCS (Edin)
Department of Ophthalmology,
National University Hospital, Singapore

RESEARCH SUMMARY

Toxic Shock resulting from periorbital necrotizing fasciitis (NF) is uncommon due to the excellent blood supply to that area; nevertheless, it can sometimes result in death. The aim of this paper is to present a systematic review and analyze factors associated with death.

We carried out a systematic literature review of all cases of periorbital NF published in the English language over the past twenty years and present the predisposing conditions, triggering factors, organisms causing NF, presence or absence of toxic shock and the prognosis. The significance of various risk factors leading to death was analysed.

We traced a total of 94 patients with periorbital NF from 61 reports. There were no triggering incidents in 25 cases (26.6%). In 48 cases (51.1%) the organism responsible for NF was *Group A beta hemolytic Streptococcus* (*GABHS*). Toxic shock occurred in 29 (30.9%) cases and loss of vision in 13 (13.8%). Surgical debridement was done in 80 (85.1%) cases. There were 8 cases (8.5%) of death. This seems to be less than previously reported figures. Toxic shock syndrome ($p < 0.001$), type 1 infections ($p = 0.018$), facial involvement ($p = 0.032$) and blindness due to periorbital NF ($p = 0.035$) were significantly associated with mortality.

Mortality due to NF arising from the periorbital area seems to be on the decline. However, it is important to recognize it early and institute treatment to avoid toxic shock that leads to death. Major morbidity is loss of vision followed by soft tissue defects affecting function and cosmesis.

This chapter was previously published in *Advances in Medicine and Biology. Volume 93,* edited by Leon V. Berhardt, New York: Nova Publishers Inc., 2016.

In: Medicine Research Summaries. Volume 17
Editors: Zhongwen Liáng and Bibao Zhang
ISBN: 978-1-53612-751-5

Chapter 53

ETIOPATHOGENESIS OF ROTATORS CUFF TEARS[#]

Antonio Gigante, MD, Carlo Bottegoni*, MD and Mario Marinelli, MD
Department of Clinical and Molecular Sciences,
Polytechnic University of Marche, Ancona, Italy

RESEARCH SUMMARY

Rotator cuff tears are the most common cause of shoulder pain, leading to considerable disability. Despite their frequency, etiology and pathogenesis are still debated. Rather than being a process that is purely intrinsic or extrinsic to the tendons themselves, the origin of rotator cuff disease is likely multifactorial, including age-related degeneration, fatigue damage accumulation from repetitive use, microtrauma and macrotrauma. Smoking, hypercholesterolemia, and genetics have all been shown to influence the development of rotator cuff tearing. Extrinsic factors are anatomic variables, such as acromial morphologic characteristics, os acromiale, and acromial spurs that compress the rotator cuff by bony impingement or direct pressure from the surrounding soft tissue. Intrinsic factors arise from the tendon itself, because of tensile overload, microvascular supply, traumatisms, or degeneration.

An attempt to unify intrinsic and extrinsic theories regards the formation of fibrous cartilage in rotator cuff tendons induced by repeated stimulation in compression, probably through the reduction of partial oxygen tension. By inhibiting the angiogenesis, cartilage glycosaminoglycans give rise to a poorly vascular tissue, predisposing themselves the formation of fibrous cartilage. The consequent alteration of matrix synthesis and the remodeling of the existing matrix result in a tendon less resistant to traction and more susceptible to tears. Little information is available from a cellular and molecular point of

---

[#] This chapter was previously published in *Advances in Medicine and Biology. Volume 93,* edited by Leon V. Berhardt, New York: Nova Publishers Inc., 2016.

* Corresponding Author: Carlo Bottegoni, MD, Department of Clinical and Molecular Sciences, Polytechnic University of Marche, Via Tronto 10/A, 60020 Ancona, Italy. Tel.: +39 3343427530 (mobile). Fax: +39 071 220 6066. E-mail address: bottegonicarlo@gmail.com.

view. The tissue in the ruptured area undergoes marked rearrangement at molecular levels, involving the activity of MMP 1, 2 and 3. Seemingly intact parts of the injured tendons can present tendinopathic features, with altered cellular metabolism. These changes could be pathogenic precursors of subsequent tear, with extension to the portion medial to the rupture site. Understanding the etiopathogenesis of rotator cuff tears would facilitate the rationale for therapeutic interventions, thus guiding and improving treatment strategies such as preventive measures, biologic modulation and surgical techniques.

In: Medicine Research Summaries. Volume 17
Editors: Zhongwen Liáng and Bibao Zhang
ISBN: 978-1-53612-751-5

Chapter 54

REHABILITATION APPROACHES OF ROTATOR CUFF INJURIES[#]

Raoul Saggini [1], Simona Maria Carmignano[2] and Rosa Grazia Bellomo[3]
[1]PRM, Department of Medical Sciences,
Oral and Biotechnology, "G. d'Annunzio" University, Chieti, Italy
[2]School of Specialties in PRM, "G. d'Annunzio" University, Chieti, Italy
[3]PRM, Department of Medicine and Science of Aging,
"G. d'Annunzio" University, Chieti, Italy
Carmignano Carmela Giovanna for the english translation/correction/amend
Degree Interpreters and Translators
"G. d'Annunzio" University, Chieti, Italy"

RESEARCH SUMMARY

Rotator cuff injury is one of the most common disorders of the shoulder. The spectrum of injuries includes tendinosis, partial thickness tear, and complete tear. It is a common reasons for a high number of patients with shoulder pain for visiting a general practice. It also causes work absenteeism and claims for sick leaves. Both extrinsic and intrinsic factors of the cuff tendon are thought to be involved in the pathogenesis, leading to a spectrum of conditions ranging from sub-acromial bursitis to mechanical failure of the cuff tendon itself. The degenerations in the tendons is based on the structure of the tendon collagen fibers and the feature of the tendon fibroblasts. Inside these degenerate tendons, the expression of the matrix metalloproteinase (MMP) enzymes (produced by the tenocytes to mediate the matrix turnover) is altered compared to normal tendons, showing that the tendons degeneration is an active, cell-mediated process. Evidences of the tendon degeneration have been found mostly thanks to the detection of highly sulphated glucosaminoglycans (GAGs) in the inflamed supraspinatus tendon.

[#] This chapter was previously published in *Advances in Medicine and Biology. Volume 93,* edited by Leon V. Berhardt, New York: Nova Publishers Inc., 2016.

The sometimes associated calcification is a cell-mediated calcification resembling an incomplete endochondral ossification. Rehabilitation is always difficult in the shoulder, whose complex function involves not only local anatomic and biomechanical integrity, but also biomechanical and physiologic contributions from distant body segments.

Numerous studies support conservative therapy as the mainstay of the treatments for the mildest forms of the rotator cuff pathologies. Several treatments are recognized and utilized to reduce pain and improve a range-of-motion faster than the natural course of the disease. The treatment for rotator cuff injuries with symptoms less than 1 year and tears less than 1 cm is, fundamentally, conservative: FANS, cortisone-based infiltration or hyaluronic acid injections, Platelet-Rich Plasma (PRP) with ice to alleviate the pain, manual therapy and therapies using physical energy such as ultrasound, lasers, hyperthermia, electro-analgesia and shock waves to restore the compromised mobility of the joint.

Eccentric exercises have been proposed to promote collagen fiber cross-linkage within the tendon, enhancing the remodeling process.

The therapeutic exercise, i.e., the muscular selective reinforcement and the increasing development of the force in the different patterns of movement, together with the proprioceptive recovery, allow a good recovery of the motor control.

In the last few years, as per our clinical experience and research, ESWT (Extracorporeal Shock Wave Therapy) has been proposed as an elective therapy in the first phase of treatment, later integrated with a progressive increase of the work load carried out with complete strengthening of the shoulder muscles and the proprioceptive re-education, using also hyaluronic acid injections in the shoulder. The proprioceptive re-education is performed through the Multi Joint System, which is a system for the evaluation and rehabilitation of the shoulder consisting of an anthropomorphous arm which, guided by the patient, can move freely in a three dimensional space to recuperate the mobility and muscle strength of the shoulder. With the purpose to improve the body and shoulder posture, a postural rebalancing in microgravity environment with Dynamic Antigravitational Postural System (SPAD) and hydrokinesitherapy has been used.

Patients with symptomatic full thickness rotator cuff tears failing to improve with conservative management, often require an operative treatment. In these kind of patients, the applied rehabilitation plays an important role in the improvement of the surgery results both before and after the surgery itself.

In: Medicine Research Summaries. Volume 17
Editors: Zhongwen Liáng and Bibao Zhang
ISBN: 978-1-53612-751-5

Chapter 55

The Story Behind the Naming of HELLP Syndrome[#]

Louis Weinstein, MD, FACOG[*]
Department of Obstetrics and Gynecology, Thomas Jefferson University
Philadelphia, Pennsylvania, US

Research Summary

Robert Hooke (1635-1703) the great philosopher, scientist and Renaissance man of the 17th century, wrote in Micrographia in 1665 that "the truth is, the science of nature has been already too long made only a work of the brain and the fancy. It is now high time that it should return to the plainness and soundness of observations on material and obvious things."

Currently with the stated importance of randomized control trials, meta-analyses and evidence-based medicine, the powers of observation by a physician often have been relegated to only a historical role. An example of the importance of observation was demonstrated by Sir Norman McAllister Gregg, an Australian ophthalmologist who in 1941 made the observation that congenital cataracts were related to fetal exposure to rubella in utero. This astute observation lead to Gregg's description of congenital rubella syndrome. Gregg published two papers which summarized and supported his findings. His work was initially discredited by the prestigious journal Lancet which wrote that he 'failed to adequately prove his case'. This is reflective of my experience with my original observations on HELLP syndrome. The initial manuscript describing the first 29 patients with HELLP syndrome was rejected by a prestigious Ob/Gyn journal secondary to the reviewers stating there was minimal scientific basis for the entity of HELLP syndrome.

An appreciation of the importance of observation, the good fortune to be in the right place at the right time, and perseverance to try to answer a perplexing clinical question lead to

---

[#] This chapter was previously published in *The 2015 Compendium for HELLP Syndrome: From Bench to Bedside*, edited by James N. Martin, Jr., New York: Nova Publishers Inc., 2015.

[*] Corresponding Author Email: Louis.weinstein@jefferson.edu.

my discovery of the variant of severe preeclampsia that included hemolysis, elevated liver enzymes and low platelets called HELLP syndrome [1].

Reference

[1]. Weinstein, L. Syndrome of hemolysis, elevated liver enzymes, and low platelet count: a severe consequence of hypertension in pregnancy. *Am J Obstet Gynecol*, 1982,142, 159-67.

In: Medicine Research Summaries. Volume 17
Editors: Zhongwen Liáng and Bibao Zhang
ISBN: 978-1-53612-751-5

Chapter 56

THE PATHOGENESIS OF HELLP SYNDROME: SIMILARITIES AND DIFFERENCES WITH PREECLAMPSIA[#]

Babbette LaMarca, PhD*
Department of Pharmacology and
Maternal-Fetal Medicine Fellowship Program

RESEARCH SUMMARY

Even though HELLP syndrome is considered a distinct type of preeclampsia that has been known to us for more than three decades, there is much that remains unknown about its pathogenesis and pathophysiology. What is known will be summarized in the review to follow with the intention of delineating the differences between preeclampsia and HELLP syndrome. Many studies have been performed particularly during the last decade to address the gaps in our knowledge. There are a number of promising new directions that research will take us over the coming years to more fully clarify the important features of HELLP syndrome, a disorder which greatly impacts maternal and perinatal morbidity and mortality on a global scale.

[#] This chapter was previously published in *The 2015 Compendium for HELLP Syndrome: From Bench to Bedside*, edited by James N. Martin, Jr., New York: Nova Publishers Inc., 2015.

* Corresponding Author: Babbette LaMarca, Professor, Dept. of Pharmacology and Thesis Director, Maternal-Fetal Medicine Fellowship Program; Email: bblamarca@umc.edu.

In: Medicine Research Summaries. Volume 17
Editors: Zhongwen Liáng and Bibao Zhang

ISBN: 978-1-53612-751-5

Chapter 57

HELLP SYNDROME: CLINICAL AND LABORATORY DIAGNOSIS[#]

Nana-Ama E. Ankumah, MD[*]
and Baha M. Sibai, MD, FACOG
University of Texas Health Science Center at Houston
Houston, Texas, US

RESEARCH SUMMARY

In the setting of preeclampsia with severe features and eclampsia, cases with concurrent thrombocytopenia, microangiopathic anemia, and abnormal liver function have been described in the literature since the mid-1950s [1-5]. This entity was later named HELLP syndrome (*h*emolysis, *e*levated *l*iver enzymes, *l*ow *p*latelets) by Weinstein in 1982 following his series of 29 women with severe preeclampsia and eclampsia who exhibited abnormal peripheral blood smears, elevated liver enzymes, and thrombocytopenia [6]. HELLP syndrome has since been substantiated in several subsequent case studies [7-9]; however, there has been variation in the laboratory diagnosis of HELLP syndrome, as original studies did not quantify laboratory findings needed to establish the diagnosis [5]. Here, we will detail common clinical findings and laboratory criteria in complete HELLP syndrome as well as a differential diagnosis for other conditions that mimic HELLP syndrome.

References

[1] Pritchard, JA; Weisman, Jr. R; Ratnoff, OD; Vosburgh, GJ. Intravascular hemolysis, thrombocytopenia and other hematologic abnormalities associated with severe toxemia of pregnancy. *N Engl J Med*, 1954, 250(3), 89-98.

[#] This chapter was previously published in *The 2015 Compendium for HELLP Syndrome: From Bench to Bedside*, edited by James N. Martin, Jr., New York: Nova Publishers Inc., 2015.

[*] Corresponding Author Email: Nana.ama.e.ankumah@uth.tmc.edu.

[2] McKay, DG. Hematologic evidence of disseminated intravascular coagulation in eclampsia. *Obstet Gynecol Surv*, 1972, 27(6), 399-417.
[3] Killam, AP; Dillard, SH; Patton, PC; Pederson, PR. Pregnancy-induced hypertension complicated by acute liver disease and disseminated intravascular coagulation. Five case reports. *Am J Obstet Gynecol*, 1975, 123(8), 823-828.
[4] López-Llera, M; de la Luz Espinosa, M; Diaz de León, MD; Linares, GR. Abnormal coagulation and fibrinolysis in eclampsia: a clinical and laboratory correlation study. *Am J Obstet Gynecol*, 1976, 124(7), 681-687.
[5] Sibai, BM. Diagnosis, Controversies, and Management of the Syndrome of Hemolysis, Elevated Liver Enzymes, and Low Platelet Count. *Obstet Gynecol*, 2004, 103(5), 981-991.
[6] Weinstein, L. Syndrome of hemolysis, elevated liver enzymes, and low platelet count: a severe consequence of hypertension in pregnancy. *Am J Obstet Gynecol*, 1982, 142(2), 159-167.
[7] Sibai, BM; Taslimi, MM; el-Nazer, A; Amon, E; Mabie, BC; Ryan, GM. Maternal-perinatal outcome associated with the syndrome of hemolysis, elevated liver enzymes, and low platelets in severe preeclampsia-eclampsia. *Am J Obstet Gynecol*, 1986, 155(3), 501-509.
[8] Sibai, BM; Ramadan, MK; Usta, I; Salama, M; Mercer, BM; Friedman, SA. Maternal morbidity and mortality in 442 pregnancies with hemolysis, elevated liver enzymes, and low platelets (HELLP syndrome). *Am J Obstet Gynecol*, 1993, 169(4), 1000-1006.
[9] Martin, Jr. JN; Blake, PG; Perry, Jr. KG; McCaul, JF; Hess, LW; Martin, RW. The natural history of HELLP syndrome: patterns of disease progression and regression. *Am J Obstet Gynecol*, 1991, 164(6 Pt 1), 1500-1509.

In: Medicine Research Summaries. Volume 17
Editors: Zhongwen Liáng and Bibao Zhang
ISBN: 978-1-53612-751-5

Chapter 58

CLASSIFICATION AND CATEGORIZATION OF HELLP SYNDROME[#]

James N. Martin, Jr., MD*
Department of Obstetrics and Gynecology,
The University of Mississippi Medical Center
Jackson, Mississippi, US

RESEARCH SUMMARY

The essential considerations for correctly diagnosing HELLP syndrome in pregnant and postpartum patients have been presented in a preceding chapter. Recognition that very dangerous forms of preeclampsia-eclampsia exist has been evident since case reports first appeared in the late nineteenth [1] and early twentieth century [2-5]. Between 1950-1980, several case series were published that related patient case histories and poor obstetric outcomes to clinical and laboratory findings that currently we recognize as consistent with the diagnosis of probable HELLP syndrome [6-17]. Dr. Louis Weinstein, soon after completion of his fellowship in maternal-fetal medicine, gets the credit for formally consolidating the concept and creating the acronym of HELLP [H=hemolysis, EL=elevated liver enzymes and LP=low platelets] in 1982 based on observations within a group of 29 pregnant patients he considered to have a distinct subset of severe preeclampsia/eclampsia [18]. All patients exhibited findings reflective of microangiopathic hemolytic anemia with moderate to severe thrombocytopenia, abnormally shaped red cells on peripheral smear, and abnormal liver function tests. Usually this was encountered in patients that had symptoms of nausea, vomiting, epigastric/right upper quadrant pain and occasional, inconsistent signs of hypertension and proteinuria.

[#] This chapter was previously published in *The 2015 Compendium for HELLP Syndrome: From Bench to Bedside*, edited by James N. Martin, Jr., New York: Nova Publishers Inc., 2015.

* Corresponding Author Email: Jmartin6@comcast.net.

References

[1] Schmorl, G. Pathologisch-anatomische Untersuchungen uber Puerperal-Eklampsie., *Leipzig, FCW Vogel*, 1893.

[2] Dienst, A. Experimentaelle Studien uber die Aetiologische Bedeutung des Fibrinsferments und Fibrinogens fur die Schwangerschaftsniere und die Eklampsie. *Arch Gynaekol*, 1912, 96,43-170.

[3] Denecke, G. Blut and Lymphe. In Hinselman H (ed) Die Eklampsie. Bonn, *Cohen*, 1924, 293-360. (Cited in Chesley.)

[4] Chesley, LC. Disseminated intravascular coagulation. In: *Hypertensive Disorders in Pregnancy*. 1978: Appleton-Century-Crofts, New York, 88-118.

[5] Dieckmann, WJ. Toxemias of Pregnancy, ed 3. St. Louis, Mosby,1952, 362-69.

[6] Pritchard, JA; Weisman, R; Jr. Ratnoff, OD; Vosburgh, GJ. Intravascular hemolysis, thrombocytopenia and other hematologic abnormalities associated with severe toxemia of pregnancy. *New Engl J Med*, 1954, 250, 89-98.

[7] Pritchard, JA; Cunningham, FG; Mason, RA. Coagulation changes in eclampsia: their frequency and pathogenesis. *Am J Obstet Gynecol*, 1976, 124, 855-64.

[8] Brain, MC; Kuah, KB; Dixon, HG. Heparin treatment of haemolysis and thrombocytopenia in pre-eclampsia. *J Obstet Gynaecol Br Commonw,* 1967, 74, 702-11.

[9] Scott, R; Gordon, S; Schatz, A; Casella, S. Acute hemolysis and thrombocytopenia in eclampsia. *Obstet Gynecol*, 1970, 36, 128-31.

[10] McKay, DG. Hematologic evidence of disseminated intravascular coagulation in eclampsia. *Obstet Gynecol Surv*, 1972, 27,399-407.

[11] Kitzmiller, JL; Lang, JF; Yellenosky, PF; Lucas, WE. Hematologic assays in pre-eclampsia. *Am J Obstet Gynecol*, 1974,118, 362-7.

[12] Vardi, J; Fields, GA. Microangiopathic hemolytic anemia in severe pre-eclampsia. *Am J Obstet Gynecol*, 1974, 119, 617-22.

[13] Killam, AP; Dillard, SH; Jr. Patton, RC; Pederson, PR. Pregnancy-induced hypertension complicated by acute liver disease and disseminated intravascular coagulation. *Am J Obstet Gynecol*, 1975, 123, 823-8.

[14] Lopez-Llera, M; de la Luz Espinosa, M; Diaz de Leon, M; Linares, GR. Abnormal coagulation and fibrinolysis in eclampsia. A clinical and laboratory correlation study. *Am J Obstet Gynecol*, 1976, 128, 681-92.

[15] Schwartz, ML; Brenner, WE. The obfuscation of eclampsia by thrombotic thrombocytopenic purpura. *Am J Obstet Gynecol*, 1978, 131, 18-24.

[16] Goodlin, RC. Severe pre-eclampsia: another great imitator. *Am J Obstet Gynecol*, 1976, 126, 855-64.

[17] Goodlin, RC; Cotton, DB; Haesslein, HC. Severe EPH gestosis. *Am J Obstet Gynecol*, 1978, 132, 595-8.

[18] Weinstein, L. Syndrome of hemolysis, elevated liver enzymes, and low platelet count: a severe consequence of hypertension in pregnancy. *Am J Obstet Gynecol*, 1982, 142, 159-167.

In: Medicine Research Summaries. Volume 17
Editors: Zhongwen Liáng and Bibao Zhang

ISBN: 978-1-53612-751-5

Chapter 59

CORE CONCEPTS AND COMPONENTS OF BEST MANAGEMENT FOR PATIENTS WITH HELLP SYNDROME#

James N. Martin, Jr., MD*
Department of Obstetrics and Gynecology,
The University of Mississippi, Medical Center,
Jackson, Mississippi, US

RESEARCH SUMMARY

The 2012 Howard Taylor Lecture presented to the XX FIGO World Congress of Gynecology and Obstetrics in Rome, Italy was delivered by the author with the title "Milestones in the Quest for Best Management of Patients with HELLP Syndrome" [1]. For the purposes of this chapter, we will not review all of the milestones covered in the 2012 Taylor Lecture but will instead focus on best management for patients with HELLP syndrome based on available evidence in the scientific literature and professional experience acquired during 40+ years of clinical care of complicated obstetric patients, approximately 1500 of which had this variant severe form of preeclampsia. This will be integrated within the five goals of HELLP therapy—the different gestational periods will be discussed in relation to core management principles. We must consider the differences between HELLP management with regard to the antepartum versus postpartum patient as well as how management transitions once the HELLP patient moves from antepartum to postpartum status. How cervical ripening, labor and delivery decisions are impacted by HELLP management will be addressed. Four basic clinical scenarios will be summarized to help focus the management discussion about this dangerous pregnancy complication which contributes greatly and globally to preterm birth, perinatal morbidity/mortality and severe maternal morbidity and mortality.

This chapter was previously published in *The 2015 Compendium for HELLP Syndrome: From Bench to Bedside*, edited by James N. Martin, Jr., New York: Nova Publishers Inc., 2015.

*Corresponding Author: ACOG Past President 2011-2012; Jmartin6@comcast.net.

In: Medicine Research Summaries. Volume 17
Editors: Zhongwen Liáng and Bibao Zhang

ISBN: 978-1-53612-751-5

Chapter 60

HELLP SYNDROME: CONTROVERSY OVER CORTICOSTEROIDS[#]

John R. Barton, MD[*]
Maternal-Fetal Medicine, Baptist Health Lexington
Lexington, Kentucky, US

RESEARCH SUMMARY

It is well established that antenatal glucocorticoid therapy reduces neonatal complications and neonatal mortality in women with severe preeclampsia at 34 weeks or less gestation. Observational, retrospective and prospective studies have found that different regimens of corticosteroids in combination with magnesium sulfate therapy and control of severe hypertension have been associated with a severe maternal morbidity-related decrease in HELLP syndrome. Reported benefits from corticosteroid use in patients with HELLP syndrome have included an increase in platelet count, a decrease in transaminase levels, a decrease in LDH levels and a reduction in blood pressure. Further, retrospective studies have shown that administration of dexamethasone increases the rate of regional anesthesia use in women with antepartum HELLP syndrome, particularly in those who achieved a latency of 24 hours before delivery. Corticosteroids also appear to have a potential to restore the imbalance among antiangiogenic and inflammatory factors known to be significantly elevated in women with HELLP syndrome.

Although corticosteroids have been shown to significantly improve laboratory parameters of HELLP syndrome, thereby leading to a longer diagnosis to delivery interval, they have not been shown to improve maternal or perinatal outcome in large prospective randomized, double-blind, placebo-controlled trials. These studies, however, have been criticized for study design, particularly for the use of duration of hospitalization as a primary outcome and for the presence of severe morbidities at the time of enrollment confusing the issue of whether

[#] This chapter was previously published in *The 2015 Compendium for HELLP Syndrome: From Bench to Bedside*, edited by James N. Martin, Jr., New York: Nova Publishers Inc., 2015.

[*] Corresponding Author Email: jbarton@bhsi.com.

corticosteroids can improve outcome with advanced disease. Subgroup analysis from randomized studies however has suggested that among patients with the most severe HELLP syndrome (Class 1 HELLP with a platelet count less than 50,000/mm^3); there is a shorter average platelet count recovery and less duration of hospitalization in those receiving corticosteroids.

Potential maternal risks with corticosteroid therapy in HELLP syndrome can include rebound thrombocytopenia (once the effect of corticosteroids wane), masking of potential complications or other disease processes, hyperglycemia, infection and adrenal suppression. Admitting the limitations in sample size and study design of previous studies, corticosteroids should be provided to patients with HELLP syndrome identified at less than 34 weeks' gestation and considered in those at a more advanced gestation in which an improvement in platelet count is considered useful. There remains, however, a definite need in both antepartum and postpartum HELLP syndrome patients for a well-designed, adequately powered, randomized, placebo-controlled trial regarding dosage and timing of corticosteroids.

In: Medicine Research Summaries. Volume 17
Editors: Zhongwen Liáng and Bibao Zhang

ISBN: 978-1-53612-751-5

Chapter 61

HELLP Syndrome: Severe Maternal Morbidity#

James N. Martin, Jr., MD, and Jamil Elfarra, MD
Department of Obstetrics and Gynecology
The University of Mississippi Medical Center
Jackson, Mississippi, US

Research Summary

The development of HELLP syndrome as a severe form of preeclampsia/eclampsia in the pregnant patient places her at significant risk for severe maternal morbidity and death, especially if diagnosis is delayed and/or management is suboptimal [1-6]. At the present time, in the absence of a single drug or drug(s) to target the arrest and reversal of the course of HELLP syndrome or to prevent its development altogether, one of the major decisions facing any physician caring for a patient with HELLP syndrome today is whether or not to supplement early delivery, control of severe hypertension and intravenously infused magnesium sulfate with the early initiation of potent glucocorticoids as a standard component of management that is undertaken regardless of gestational age. Uniform early initiation of what is termed the "Mississippi Protocol" or MP (intravenous dexamethasone, intravenous magnesium sulfate, and tight control of maternal blood pressure to minimize or prevent severe systolic hypertension) in 190 sequentially treated patients with HELLP syndrome between 2000-2007 resulted in no maternal death, stroke or liver rupture [6]. Moreover, early initiation of MP also inhibits HELLP syndrome disease progression and severity, decreasing the number of patients who develop the most advanced form of the disease (class 1 HELLP syndrome) and decreasing severe maternal morbidity for patients with class 1 HELLP syndrome who are first encountered with already advanced disease [6]. Since the MP became increasingly used in patients treated at the University of Mississippi Medical Center, severe maternal morbidity and mortality with HELLP syndrome has progressively decreased [6, 8-

This chapter was previously published in *The 2015 Compendium for HELLP Syndrome: From Bench to Bedside*, edited by James N. Martin, Jr., New York: Nova Publishers Inc., 2015.

11]. Thus whether or not a HELLP patient receives corticosteroids either primarily for fetal lung maturity purposes or primarily for maternal treatment likely impacts the patient's risk for severe maternal morbidity and possibly maternal mortality [1-3, 6-8].

References

[1] Isler, CM; Rinehart, BK; Terrone, DA; Martin, RW; Magann, EF; Martin, JN; Jr. Maternal mortality associated with HELLP syndrome. *Am J Obstet Gynecol*, 1999, 181, 924-8.

[2] Martin, JN; Jr. Rose, CH; Briery, CM. Understanding and managing HELLP syndrome: the integral role of aggressive glucocorticoids for mother and child. *Am J Obstet Gynecol*, 2006, 195, 914-34.

[3] Martin, JN; Jr. Milestones in the quest for best management of patients with HELLP syndrome (microangiopathic hemolytic anemia, hepatic dysfunction, thrombocytopenia): the 2012 FIGO Howard Taylor Lecture. *Int J Gyn Obstet*, 2013, 121, 202-207.

[4] Sibai, BM. Diagnosis, controversies, and management of the syndrome of hemolysis, elevated liver enzymes, and low platelet count. *Obstet Gynecol*, 2004, 103, 981-91.

[5] Sibai, BM; Ramadan, MK; Usta, I; Salama, M; Mercer, BM; Friedman, SA. Maternal morbidity and mortality in 442 pregnancies with HELLP syndrome. *Am J Obstet Gynecol*, 1993, 169, 1000-6.

[6] Martin, JN; Jr. Owens, MY; Keiser, SD; Parrish, MR; Tam Tam, KB; Brewer, JM; Cushman, JL; May, WL. Standardized Mississippi Protocol treatment of 190 patients with HELLP syndrome: slowing disease progression and preventing new major maternal morbidity. *Hyperten Preg*, 2012, 31, 79-90.

[7] O'Brien, JM; Milligan, DA; Barton, JR. Impact of high dose corticosteroid therapy for patients with HELLP syndrome. *Am J Obstet Gynecol*, 2000, 183, 921-4.

[8] Martin, JN; Jr. Thigpen, BD; Rose, CH; Cushman, J; Moore, A; May, WL. Maternal benefit of high-dose intravenous corticosteroid therapy for HELLP syndrome. *Obstet Gynecol*, 2003, 189, 830-4.

In: Medicine Research Summaries. Volume 17
Editors: Zhongwen Liáng and Bibao Zhang
ISBN: 978-1-53612-751-5

Chapter 62

HELLP Syndrome: Maternal Mortality[#]

Charlene H. Collier, MD, MPH, MHS, FACOG[*]
and Ashley M. Johnson, MD
Department of Obstetric and Gynecology,
The University of Mississippi Medical Center
Jackson, Mississippi, US

Research Summary

Maternal mortality is defined as the death of a woman while pregnant or within 42 days of delivery or termination of pregnancy, from any cause related to, or aggravated by pregnancy or its management, but excluding deaths from incidental or accidental causes and is presented as a ratio of deaths per 100,000 live births [1]. Maternal mortality remains a significant public health problem worldwide despite advances in intensive care, blood banking capacities and high-risk obstetric medicine. In 2013 there were 289,000 maternal deaths contributing to a global maternal mortality ratio (MMR) of 210 maternal deaths per 100,000 live births [2]. The vast majority of these deaths occur within developing regions (MMR: 230) led by Sub-Saharan Africa (MMR: 510). While this represents an overall decline in maternal deaths of 45% since 1990, certain populations including the United States have seen little improvement and worsening of maternal death rates over the past twenty years [2]. The most recent world Health Organization 2014 data showing global maternal mortality ratios (MMR), number and percent of maternal deaths for the year 2013 is contained within the following Table 1.

[#] This chapter was previously published in *The 2015 Compendium for HELLP Syndrome: From Bench to Bedside*, edited by James N. Martin, Jr., New York: Nova Publishers Inc., 2015.

[*] Corresponding Author Email: Ccollier2@umc.edu.

Table 1. WHO 2013 data for global maternal mortality ratios (MMR), number and percent of maternal deaths

Region	MMR*	Maternal Deaths	Percent of Maternal Deaths
World	210	289,000	-
Developed regions**	16	2300	0.8%
Developing regions	230	286,000	99.2%
Sub-Saharan Africa	510	179,000	62%
Southern Asia	190	69,000	23.9%
Caribbean	190	1400	0.5%
Oceania	190	510	0.2%
South-eastern Asia	140	16,000	5.5%
Latin America	77	7900	2.7%
Western Asia	74	3600	1.2%
Northern Africa	69	2700	0.9%
Caucasus and Central Asia	39	690	0.2%
Eastern Asia	33	6400	2.2%

* The MMR have been rounded according to the following scheme: <100, no rounding; 100–999, rounded to nearest 10; and >1000, rounded to nearest 100. The numbers of maternal deaths have been rounded as follows: <100, no rounding; 100–999, rounded to nearest 10; 1000–9999, rounded to nearest 100; and >10 000, rounded to nearest 1000.

** Albania, Australia, Austria, Belarus, Belgium, Bosnia and Herzegovina, Bulgaria, Canada, Croatia, Cyprus, Czech Republic, Denmark, Estonia, Finland, France, Germany, Greece, Hungary, Iceland, Ireland, Israel, Italy, Japan, Latvia, Lithuania, Luxembourg, Malta, Montenegro, The Netherlands, New Zealand, Norway, Poland, Portugal, Republic of Moldova, Romania, Russian Federation, Serbia, Slovakia, Slovenia, Spain, Sweden, Switzerland, The former Yugoslav Republic of Macedonia, Ukraine, United Kingdom of Great Britain and Northern Ireland, United States of America.

Source: World Health Organization, 2014.

References

[1] *International Classification of Diseases and Related Health Problems*. Geneva: World Health Organization, 1992.

[2] *Trends in maternal mortality: 1990 to 2013*. Estimates by WHO, UNICEF, UNFPA, The World Bank and the United Nations Population Division. World Health Organization, 2014. Accessed online: 3/12/2015http://apps.who.int/iris/bitstream/10665/112682/2/9789241507226_eng.pdf?ua=.

In: Medicine Research Summaries. Volume 17
Editors: Zhongwen Liáng and Bibao Zhang

ISBN: 978-1-53612-751-5

Chapter 63

The Central Nervous System in HELLP Syndrome: Evidence for Impairment[#]

Kedra Wallace*[1,*]*, PhD, and Marilyn Cipolla*[2]*, PhD

[1]Departments of Obstetrics and Gynecology and Department of Neurobiology and Anatomical Sciences, The University of Mississippi Medical Center, Jackson, Mississippi, US

[2]Departments of Neurological Sciences, Obstetrics, Gynecology and Reproductive Sciences, and Pharmacology, University of Vermont, Burlington, Vermont, US

Research Summary

In response to the increase in hormones and circulating factors that occurs during normal human gestation, the pregnant woman's central nervous system (CNS) undergoes a variety of changes such as cerebral artery and venous remodeling and increased neuronal excitability [1-3]. During pregnancy there is diminished cerebrovascular resistance and hyper-permeability in the maternal brain, which increases the risk of neurological complications and brain edema. Both of these are exacerbated during acute hypertension, as seen in patients with HELLP [4, 5]. HELLP syndrome is associated with CNS and visual complications, such as stroke, cerebral edema, headaches unrelieved with acetaminophen, vision loss, somnolence, cerebral vasospasm and hypertensive encephalopathy [6-8]. Several investigators have reported a high mortality rate among women with severe hypertension who developed HELLP syndrome in association with preeclampsia [9, 10]. Intracerebral hemorrhage has been reported to be the primary cause of death in women with HELLP syndrome, ranging from 27-45% [11, 12], with 25.4% of these cases being accompanied by hemorrhagic stroke in the postpartum period. Immediately following delivery, the puerperal woman with HELLP syndrome appears to be most vulnerable to CNS injury [13-15]. However, despite the growing number of case reports which describe various abnormalities in women with HELLP syndrome, there is very

---

[#] This chapter was previously published in *The 2015 Compendium for HELLP Syndrome: From Bench to Bedside*, edited by James N. Martin, Jr., New York: Nova Publishers Inc., 2015.

[*] Corresponding Author Email: Kwallace2@umc.edu.

little the information about the events that led up to changes in the CNS. This chapter will provide a brief overview of the most commonly reported case reports involving CNS injury in HELLP patients.

References

[1] Cipolla, M; Pusic, A; Grinberg, Y; Chapman, A; Poynter, M; Kraig, R. Pregnant serum induces neuroinflammation and seizure activity via TNFalpha. *Experimental Neurology*, 2012, 234, 398-404.

[2] Chapman, A; Chan, S; Cipolla, M. An enhanced myogenic vasodilatory response to hypotension in posterior cerebral arteries of pregnant rats is nitric oxide dependent. *Reprod Sci*, 2012,19,175A.

[3] Cipolla, M. The adaptation of the cerebral circulation to pregnancy: mechanisms and consequences. *Journal of Cerebral Blood Flow and Metabolism*, 2013, 33, 465-78.

[4] Duvekot, J; Peeters, L. Maternal cardiovascular hemodynamic adaptation to pregnancy. *Obstet Gynecol*, 1994, 49, S1-S14.

[5] Cipolla, M; Sweet, J; Chan, S. Cerebral vascular adaptation to pregnancy and its role in the neurological complications of eclampsia. *Journal of Applied Physiology*, 2011, 110, 329-39.

[6] Sibai, B. Diagnosis, controversies, and management of the syndrome of hemolysis, elevated liver enzymes and low platelet count. *Obstetrics and Gynecology*, 2004, 103, 981-91.

[7] Haram, K; Svendsen, E; Abildgaard, U. The HELLP syndrome: Clinical issues and management. A Review. *BMC Pregnancy and Childbirth*, 2009, 9.

[8] Harscher, S; Witte, O; Moller, U; Bloos, G; Pfleiderer, S; Terborg, C. Cerebral vasospasms with hemodynamic infarctions as a complication of HELLP syndrome. *Nervenarzt*, 2003, 74, 1122-26.

[9] Vigil-de Gracia, P; Garcia-Caceres, E. Thrombocytopenia, hypertension and seizures in eclampsia. *International Journal of Gynaecology and Obstetrics*, 1998, 61, 15-20.

[10]Martin, JJ; Thigpen, B; Moore, R; Cushman, J; May, W. Stroke and severe preeclampsia and eclampsia: A paradigm shift focusing on systolic blood pressure. *Obstet Gynecol*, 2005, 105, 246-54.

[11]Isler, C; Rinehart, B; Terrone, D; Martin, R; Magann, E; Martin, Jr. J. Maternal mortality associated with HELLP syndrome. *American Journal of Obstetrics and Gynecology*, 1999, 181, 924-28.

[12]Vigil-de Gracia, P. Maternal deaths due to eclampsia and HELLP syndrome. *International Journal of Gynaecology and Obstetrics*, 2009, 104, 90-94.

[13]James, A; Bushnell, C; Jamison, M; Myers, E. Incidence and risk factors for stroke in pregnancy and the puerperium. *Obstet Gynecol*, 2005, 106, 509-16.

[14]Kamel, H; Navi, B; Sriram, N; Hovsepian, D; Devereux, R; Elkind, M. Risk of a thrombotic event after the 6-week postpartum period. *N Eng J Med*, 2014, 370, 1307-15.

[15]Hovsepian, D; Sriram, N; Kamel, H; Fink, M; Navi, B. Acute cerebrovascular disease occurring after hospital discharge for labor and delivery. *Stroke*, 2014, 45, 1947-50.

In: Medicine Research Summaries. Volume 17
Editors: Zhongwen Liáng and Bibao Zhang

ISBN: 978-1-53612-751-5

Chapter 64

CARDIOPULMONARY MORBIDITY COMPLICATING HELLP SYNDROME[#]

Marc Parrish, DO, FACOG [*]
Division of Maternal-Fetal Medicine, Kansas University Medical Center,
University of Kansas School of Medicine
Kansas City, Kansas, US

RESEARCH SUMMARY

Although the pathogenesis of HELLP syndrome remains to be fully elucidated, the disorder likely has its origins from aberrant placental development and function. With preeclampsia, it is believed that abnormal placental invasion results in dysregulation of a variety of pathways that affect maternal endothelial and immunologic function. Previous models of preeclampsia have demonstrated that in the presence of placental dysfunction there is widespread activation of the maternal vascular endothelium resulting in up-regulation of vasoconstrictive and oxidative analytes in addition to enhancement of vascular sensitivity, down regulation of vasodilators and an imbalance in angiogenic and anti-angiogenic factors [1-3]. In a similar manner, it has been proposed that HELLP syndrome also results from a placental derived, liver-targeted, acute inflammatory condition [4-6]. This placenta-instigated attack on the maternal system results in endothelial abnormalities, which in turn, leads to hypertension and global endothelial dysfunction [3, 7-9]. These endothelial effects ultimately yield a clinical state that is similar to the systemic inflammatory response syndrome (SIRS) resulting in multi-organ dysfunction. The similarity between HELLP syndrome and SIRS has been demonstrated in multiple investigations [10-12]. Therefore, it is not surprising that significant cardio-pulmonary morbidity is observed in these patients with HELLP syndrome. In fact, morbidity involving the cardiopulmonary system has been shown to be second in frequency only to hematologic/coagulation dysfunction in patients with HELLP syndrome

---

[#] This chapter was previously published in *The 2015 Compendium for HELLP Syndrome: From Bench to Bedside*, edited by James N. Martin, Jr., New York: Nova Publishers Inc., 2015.

[*] Corresponding Author: Assistant Professor, University of Kansas School of Medicine; Email: mparrish@kumc.edu.

[13]. Additionally, the mortality associated with cardio-pulmonary complications is second only to the central nervous system in patients with HELLP syndrome [14].

References

[1] Young, BC; Levine, RJ; Karumanchi, SA. *Pathogenesis of preeclampsia. Annual Review of Pathology*, 5 (2010), 173–192.

[2] James, JL; Whitley, GS; Cartwright, JE. Pre-eclampsia: fitting together the placental, immune and cardiovascular pieces. *Journal of Pathology,* 221(2010), 363–378.

[3] Gilbert, JS; Michael, J. R; LaMarca, BB; Sedeek, M; Murphy, SR; Granger, JP. Pathophysiology of hypertension during preeclampsia: linking placental ischemia with endothelial dysfunction. *American Journal of Physiology - Heart and Circulatory Physiology*, Feb 2008, 294(2) H541-H550.

[4] Martin, JN; Jr. Magann, EF; Isler, CM. HELLP Syndrome: the scope of disease and treatment. M.A. Belfort, S. Thornton, G.R. Saade (Eds.), Hypertension in pregnancy. *Chap 7*, *Marcel Dekker, Oxford*, (2003), 141–188.

[5] Landi, B; Tranquilli, AL. HELLP syndrome and placental inflammatory pathology. *Minerva Ginecologica*, 60 (2008), 389–398.

[6] Venkatesha, S; Toporsian, M; Lam, C; et al. Soluble endoglin contributes to the pathogenesis of preeclampsia. *Nature Medicine*, 12 (2006), 642–649.

[7] Abildgaard, U; Heimdal, K. Pathogenesis of the syndrome of hemolysis, elevated liver enzymes, and low platelet count (HELLP): a review. *Eur J Obstet Gynecol Reprod Biol*, 2013, 166, 117.

[8] Benedetto, C; Marozio, L; Tancredi, A; et al. Biochemistry of HELLP syndrome. *Adv Clin Chem*, 2011, 53, 85.

[9] Jebbink, J; Wolters, A; Fernando, F; et al. Molecular genetics of preeclampsia and HELLP syndrome - a review. *Biochim Biophys Acta,* 2012, 1822, 1960.

[10] Bone, RC. Immunologic dissonance: a continuing evolution in our understanding of the systemic inflammatory response syndrome (SIRS) and the multiple organ dysfunction syndrome (MODS). *Ann Intern Med*, 125(1996), 680–687.

[11] Balderas-Pena, LM; Canales-Munoz, JL; Angulo-Vazqule, J; Anaya-Prado, R; Gonzalez Ojeda, A. The HELLP syndrome: evidence of a possible systemic inflammatory response in preeclampsia? *Ginecol Obstet Mex*, 70 (2002), 328–337.

[12] Redman, CWG; Sargent, IL. Preeclampsia and the systemic inflammatory response. *Semin Nephrol*, *24* (2004), 565–570.

[13] Martin, JN; Jr. Magann, EF; Blake, PG; Terrone, DA; Rinehart, BK; May, WL. Early risk assessment of severe preeclampsia: admission battery of symptoms and laboratory tests to predict likelihood of subsequent significant maternal morbidity. *Am J Obstet Gynecol*, 1999, 180, 1407–14.

[14] Isler, CM; Rinehart, BK; Terrone, DA; Martin, RW; Magann, EF; Martin, JN Jr. Maternal mortality associated with HELLP syndrome. *Am J Obstet Gynecol*, 181 (1999), 924–928.

In: Medicine Research Summaries. Volume 17
Editors: Zhongwen Liáng and Bibao Zhang
ISBN: 978-1-53612-751-5

Chapter 65

HELLP Syndrome and the Liver: Hepatic Pathology, Hemorrhage, Rupture and Failure[#]

Jamil Elfarra[1,*], MD, Marie M. Darby[2], MD, MS, FACOG and Richard R. Viscarello[3], MD, FACOG

[1]Maternal-Fetal Medicine
Department of Obstetrics and Gynecology
The University of Mississippi Medical Center
Jackson, Mississippi, US
[2]Hattiesburg Clinic and Forrest General Hospital
Hattiesburg, Mississippi, US
[3]Maternal Fetal Care P.C.
Stamford, Connecticut, US

Research Summary

The liver plays a critical role in the evolution of HELLP Syndrome, exhibiting a wide spectrum of clinical presentations which range from mild to life-threatening. In the absence of widespread use of a single drug or drug(s) to target the arrest and reversal of the course of HELLP syndrome or to prevent its development altogether, such as the administration of potent glucocorticoids to patients early in the disease process [1, 2], obstetricians will continue to infrequently encounter these potentially catastrophic situations. Vigilant surveillance leading to early recognition of the associated signs and symptoms is necessary to ensure patient safety. A multidisciplinary approach in a tertiary center with adequate resources to manage such complicated clinical scenarios is critically important in order to decrease the associated maternal-perinatal morbidity and mortality.

This chapter was previously published in *The 2015 Compendium for HELLP Syndrome: From Bench to Bedside*, edited by James N. Martin, Jr., New York: Nova Publishers Inc., 2015.

* Corresponding Author Email: jelfarra@umc.edu.

Most of the complications of HELLP Syndrome, including those of the liver, (Table 1) usually resolve in the first 48-96 hours following delivery [3, 4]. However, it is prudent to acknowledge that until resolution of the disease spectrum is complete, the potential for severe maternal morbidity and mortality exists. The rarity of the most severe complications of HELLP syndrome makes it difficult to conduct optimal clinical trials or high quality randomized controlled trials of sufficient size to detect differences between management protocols. Most of the available information about liver-related severe maternal morbidity in patients with HELLP syndrome is based on Level III evidence contained in case reports, small series, or expert opinion which renders recommendations for treatment somewhat controversial in many instances.

In the absence of direct maternal liver trauma, hepatic hemorrhage and rupture are rare and are encountered almost exclusively (98%) as a complication of HELLP syndrome [5, 6]. Although hepatic hemorrhage and rupture occur in less than 5% of patients with HELLP Syndrome, the consequences are profound, with reported mortality in the range of 18 to 86 percent [5-7].

Table 1. Liver complications associated with HELLP syndrome

LIVER COMPLICATIONS ASSOCIATED WITH HELLP SYNDROME
Potential complications of the liver in the setting of HELLP Syndrome include: Elevation in liver enzymes (classic presentation) Liver capsular hematoma and rupture Liver ischemia, necrosis, and failure Disseminated intravascular coagulation disorder (DIC)

References

[1] Martin JN Jr, Owens MY, Keiser SD, Parrish MR, Tam Tam KB, Brewer JM, Cushman JL, May WL. Standardized Mississippi Protocol treatment of 190 patients with HELLP syndrome: slowing disease progression and preventing new major maternal morbidity. Hyp*erten Preg.* 2012;31:79-90.

[2] Martin JN Jr, Brewer JM, Wallace K, Sunesara I, Canizaro A, Blake PG, LaMarca B, Owens MY. HELLP syndrome and composite major maternal morbidity: importance of Mississippi classification system. *J. Mat-Fet Neo Med.* 2013;26:1201-6.

[3] Martin JN Jr, Blake PG, Perry KG Jr, McCaul JF, Hess LW, Martin RW. The natural history of HELLP syndrome: patterns of disease progression and regression. *Am. J. Obstet. Gynecol.*1991;164:1500-9

[4] Martin JN Jr, Blake PG, Lowry SL, Perry KG Jr, Files JC, Morrison JC. Pregnancy complicated by preeclampsia-eclampsia with the syndrome of hemolysis, elevated liver enzymes, and low platelet count: how rapid is postpartum recovery? *Obstet. Gynecol.* 1990;76:737-41.

[5] Rinehart BK, Terrone DA, Magann EF, Martin RW, May WL, Martin JN Jr. Preeclampsia-associated hepatic hemorrhage and rupture: mode of management related to maternal and perinatal outcome. *Obstet. Gynecol* Surv 1990; 54:196-202.

[6] Zarinpar A, Farmer DG, Ghobrial RM, Lishutz GS, GU Y, Hiatt JR, et al. Liver transplantation for HELLP syndrome. *Am. Surg.* 2007;73(10):1013-6.
[7] Kinthala S, Fakoory M, Greaves T, Kandamaran L, Thomas H, Moe S. Karateke A, et al. HELLP syndrome complicated by subcapsular Hematoma of liver. *Int. J. Obstet. Anesth.* 2012; 21(3):276-9.

In: Medicine Research Summaries. Volume 17
Editors: Zhongwen Liáng and Bibao Zhang
ISBN: 978-1-53612-751-5

Chapter 66

THE KIDNEY AND ACUTE KIDNEY INJURY IN HELLP SYNDROME[#]

Sarah Novotny*, MD, MS, FACOG
and Nicole M. Lee, MD, MPH, MS
Division of Maternal-Fetal Medicine
Department of Obstetrics and Gynecology
The University of Mississippi Medical Center
Jackson, Mississippi, US

RESEARCH SUMMARY

Acute kidney injury (AKI), previously termed acute renal failure, is defined the abrupt loss of kidney function that can range from transient depression of renal function to irreversible renal disease and death. Over the last five decades, rates of AKI in pregnancy have decreased dramatically due largely to decreased rates of septic abortion and improvements in obstetric care [1-4]. Today HELLP syndrome and severe forms of preeclampsia account for approximately 40% of all cases of AKI in pregnancy [2]. However, despite the recent overall decrease in pregnancy-associated AKI, its occurrence in patients with HELLP syndrome has continued to range between 3-15% over multiple decades where renal injury in such patients can have a complex and lasting effect [4-7]. Some investigators have reported that 30-50% of patients with acute renal failure (ARF) and HELLP syndrome require dialysis, and when patients develop AKI in HELLP syndrome, the perinatal mortality rate reaches 26% [2, 5, 7]. Patients with pre-existing renal disease that develop HELLP syndrome have an even higher risk of perinatal mortality. Due to these risks, understanding renal injury in the setting of HELLP syndrome is of clinical importance for acute patient management as well as the prevention of long term morbidity.

[#] This chapter was previously published in *The 2015 Compendium for HELLP Syndrome: From Bench to Bedside*, edited by James N. Martin, Jr., New York: Nova Publishers Inc., 2015.

* Corresponding Author Email: Assistant Professor, snovotny@umc.edu.

References

[1] Prakash J, Vohra R, Wani IA, Murthy AS, Srivastva PK, Tripathi K, et al. Decreasing incidence of renal cortical necrosis in patients with acute renal failure in developing countries: a single-centre experience of 22 years from Eastern India. *Nephro Dial Transplant* 2007: 22: 1213-7.

[2] Prakash J. The kidney in pregnancy: A journey of three decades. *Indian Journal of Nephro* 2012; 22: 159-167.

[3] Martin JN Jr, Blake PG, Perry KG Jr, McCaul JF, Hess LW, Martin RW. The natural history of HELLP syndrome: patterns of disease progression and regression. *Am. J. Obstet. Gynecol.* 1991; 164; 1500-13

[4] Stratta P, Besso L, Canavesce C, Grill A, Todros T, Benedetto C, et al. Is pregnancy-related acute renal failure a disappearing entity? *Ren Fail* 1996; 18:575-84.

[5] Gul A, Aslan H, Cebeci A, Polat I, Ulusoy S, Ceylan Y. Maternal and fetal outcomes in HELLP complicated with acute renal failure. *Ren Fail* 2004; 26:557-62.

[6] Hadded B, Barton JR, Livingston JC, Chahing R, Sibai BM. Risk factors for adverse maternal outcomes among women with HELLP syndrome. *Am. J. Obstet. Gynecol.* 2000; 183: 444-8.

[7] Sibai BM, Ramadan MK, Usta I., Salama M, Mercer BM, Friedman SA. Maternal morbidity in 442 pregnancies with hemolysis, elevated liver enzymes, and low platelets (HELLP syndrome). *Am. J. Obstet. Gynecol.* 1993; 169: 1000-6.

In: Medicine Research Summaries. Volume 17
Editors: Zhongwen Liáng and Bibao Zhang
ISBN: 978-1-53612-751-5

Chapter 67

COMPOUNDED COMPLEXITY: WHEN HELLP SYNDROME AND ECLAMPSIA ARE CONCURRENT[#]

Rose Gasnier*[*]*, MD, MSc
Hospital de Clínicas de Porto Alegre
Universidade Federal do Rio Grande do Sul, Brazil
Wolfson Medical Center, Holon
Sackler University, Tel Aviv, Israel

RESEARCH SUMMARY

Hypertensive disorders are among the most common medical complications of pregnancy, affecting about 7- 10% of all pregnant women. These disorders are a major cause of maternal and perinatal morbidity worldwide [1, 2]. It is considered the second cause of maternal mortality in Africa after postpartum hemorrhage and the leading cause in Latin America [3]. In the United States, it is the second cause of mortality, after pulmonary embolism [4]. It can occur at any time during the second half of pregnancy, intrapartum or in the first few weeks postpartum.

Preeclampsia is classically recognized as hypertension that begins after week 20 of pregnancy with significant proteinuria that disappears until 12 weeks after the labor. The Australasian Society for the Study of Hypertension in Pregnancy (ASSHP) already had suggested that proteinuria not be included as a diagnostic criterion for preeclampsia [5]. It is well known that preeclampsia and even eclampsia can develop in the absence of either hypertension or proteinuria. According to The American Congress of OBGYN Task Force on Hypertension in Pregnancy, proteinuria was eliminated as a requirement for the diagnosis of preeclampsia. Preeclampsia is no longer classified as mild and severe, but rather by having evidence of hypertensive pathology, and its severe form is defined by having severe features, since a mild case can progress to a more severe presentation [6].

[#] This chapter was previously published in *The 2015 Compendium for HELLP Syndrome: From Bench to Bedside*, edited by James N. Martin, Jr., New York: Nova Publishers Inc., 2015.

[*] Corresponding Author Email: Gasnier.rose@gmail.com

Hypertension is considered to be the hallmark for the diagnosis of preeclampsia. HELLP syndrome represents a severe form of preeclampsia-eclampsia, currently regarded as a variant of severe preeclampsia or a complication of the disease, and is characterized by hemolysis, elevated liver enzymes and low platelets. It occurs in 0.5-0.9% of all pregnancies and in 10-20% of cases with severe preeclampsia [7]. Diagnosis can be difficult, as blood pressure (BP) values may be only slightly elevated. HELLP/Eclampsia or Eclampsia/HELLP is defined as the presence of eclampsia and HELLP syndrome in the same women. Patients with HELLP syndrome with or without eclampsia represent an important complication because it is associated with severe maternal morbidity and mortality in women with preeclampsia-eclampsia. Both presentations – HELLP syndrome and eclampsia – can cause significant morbidity and mortality for the fetus and the woman. In the past it was postulated that eclampsia is the final expression of preeclampsia in a linear progression and that it represents the worst prognosis for the patient, but this is not the case. Similarly, a patient with HELLP syndrome can present with as much morbidity as a patient with eclampsia, and the two occurring together can be especially dangerous.

References

[1] Lindheimer MD, Umans JG. Explaining and predicting preeclampsia. *N. Engl. J. Med.* 2006; 335 (10): 1056-8.

[2] Sibai B, Dekker G, Kupferminc M. Pre-eclampsia. *Lancet* 2005; 365 (9461): 785-99.

[3] Trends in maternal mortality: 1990 to 2008 Estimates developed by WHO, UNICEF, UNFPA and The World Bank http://www.int//reproductivehealth/publications /monitoring/9789241500265/en/index.htlm (2011)

[4] Creanga AA, Berg CJ, Syverson C, et al. Pregnancy-related mortality in the Unites States, 2006-2010. *Obstet. Gynecol.* 2015; 125:5.

[5] Brown MA, Hague WM, Higgins J, et al. The detection, investigation and management of hypertension in pregnancy. *Aust. N. Z. J. Obstet. Gynaecol.* 2000; 40: 133-55.

[6] Moussa HN, Arian SE, Sibai BM. Management of hypertensive disorders in pregnancy. *Women's Wealth* 2014; 10(4): 385-404.

[7] Haram K. The HELLP syndrome: clinical issues and management. A review. *BMC Pregnancy Childbirth* 2009; 9(1):8.

In: Medicine Research Summaries. Volume 17
Editors: Zhongwen Liáng and Bibao Zhang
ISBN: 978-1-53612-751-5

Chapter 68

WHEN HELLP MIGHT BE SOMETHING ELSE: THE DIFFERENTIAL DIAGNOSIS OF HELLP SYNDROME#

Rachael Morris*, MD, MS and
James N. Martin, Jr., MD, FACOG, FRCOG ad eundem
Department of Obstetrics and Gynecology
Division of Maternal-Fetal Medicine
The University of Mississippi Medical Center
Jackson, Mississippi, US

RESEARCH SUMMARY

The pregnant patient presenting in the latter half of gestation or postpartum with laboratory evidence of hemolysis, elevated liver function tests, and moderate to severe thrombocytopenia (platelets <100,000/uL) likely has HELLP syndrome. This is especially likely in the presence of other evidence suggestive of preeclampsia such as hypertension, proteinuria and symptoms of epigastric pain, nausea, and vomiting. Sometimes other disease entities masquerade as complete or incomplete/partial HELLP syndrome or HELLP can occur concurrently with them. Considering the possibility of HELLP-like disease entities with timely consultation usually to an experienced hematologist, extended laboratory testing and the initiation of alternative therapy such as plasma exchange can be critical to patient survival. This chapter is focused on the differential diagnosis of HELLP-like disorders. There are other chapters of this book which are very relevant including the ones on HELLP classification, HELLP management and TPE (therapeutic plasma exchange) for complicated HELLP.

This chapter was previously published in *The 2015 Compendium for HELLP Syndrome: From Bench to Bedside*, edited by James N. Martin, Jr., New York: Nova Publishers Inc., 2015.

* Corresponding Author Email: Assistant Professor; rmorris@umc.edu.

In: Medicine Research Summaries. Volume 17
Editors: Zhongwen Liáng and Bibao Zhang
ISBN: 978-1-53612-751-5

Chapter 69

THERAPEUTIC PLASMA EXCHANGE USE IN PATIENTS WITH HELLP SYNDROME AND HELLP-LIKE DISORDERS[#]

Michelle Y. Owens*, MD, MS, FACOG and Cynthia Bean, MD, FACOG
Department of Obstetrics and Gynecology
Division of Maternal-Fetal Medicine
The University of Mississippi Medical Center
Jackson, Mississippi, US

RESEARCH SUMMARY

HELLP (hemolysis, elevated liver enzymes and low platelets) syndrome is a rare and serious complication of pregnancy. If the diagnosis of HELLP syndrome is made early and managed appropriately, the majority of patients improve within 24-48 hours [1, 2]. On rare occasion, patients will develop a HELLP syndrome-like picture with progressively worsening clinical and laboratory parameters with features of a complex thrombotic microangiopathy or consumptive coagulopathy with or without single or multiple organ injury. The disease process is often difficult to define and does not respond to traditional medical therapies. In these specific situations, postpartum therapeutic plasma exchange has been used.

[#] This chapter was previously published in *The 2015 Compendium for HELLP Syndrome: From Bench to Bedside*, edited by James N. Martin, Jr., New York: Nova Publishers Inc., 2015.

* Corresponding Author Email: Associate Professor; myowens@umc.edu.

In: Medicine Research Summaries. Volume 17
Editors: Zhongwen Liáng and Bibao Zhang
ISBN: 978-1-53612-751-5

Chapter 70

ANESTHESIA CONSIDERATIONS WITH HELLP SYNDROME#

Arthur Calimaran*, MD, and Nicole M. Lee†, MD, MPH, MS
[1]Education Residency Program Director
Obstetric Anesthesiology
Department of Anesthesiology
The University of Mississippi Medical Center,
Jackson, Mississippi, US
[2]Maternal Fetal Medicine
Department of Obstetrics and Gynecology
The University of Mississippi Medical Center,
Jackson, Mississippi, US

RESEARCH SUMMARY

In the past, due to the risk of spinal-epidural hematoma with regional anesthesia, general anesthesia with endotracheal intubation was thought to be the anesthetic of choice in the setting of HELLP syndrome, regardless of the platelet count [1]. This concept has been challenged in several different clinical scenarios by a number of investigators. Regional anesthesia such as epidural and spinal anesthesia for labor and delivery should no longer be considered contraindicated in HELLP patients, provided there is no severe clotting abnormality [2]. Several factors confound the management of anesthesia for vaginal and cesarean deliveries in the setting of HELLP syndrome. In this chapter, we will review the literature and report issues with management and considerations when choosing a mode of anesthesia for delivery.

This chapter was previously published in *The 2015 Compendium for HELLP Syndrome: From Bench to Bedside*, edited by James N. Martin, Jr., New York: Nova Publishers Inc., 2015.

* Corresponding Author: Associate Professor and Vice Chair for Education Residency Program Director, Chief of Obstetric Anesthesiology; Email: acalimaran@umc.edu.

† Corresponding Author: Fellow, Maternal Fetal Medicine; Email: nmlee@umc.edu.

References

[1] Crosby E. Obstetrical anaesthesia for patients with the syndrome of Haemolysis, Elevated Liver Enzymes and Low Platelets. *Obstet and Gynecol Survey. 1991*; 46:11, 744-746.

[2] Hogg B, Hauth JC, Caritis SN, Sibai BM, Lindheimer M, Van Dorsten JP, et al. Safety of labor epidural anesthesia for women with severe hypertensive disease. National Institute of Child Health and Human Development Maternal-Fetal Medicine Units Network. *Am J Obstet Gynecol* 1999;181:1096-101.

In: Medicine Research Summaries. Volume 17
Editors: Zhongwen Liáng and Bibao Zhang
ISBN: 978-1-53612-751-5

Chapter 71

HELLP SYNDROME: ANESTHESIA CONSIDERATIONS WHEN OTHER DISEASES COMPLICATE[#]

***Monica del-Rio-Vellosillo*[1,*], *MD*,**
and Jose Javier Garcia-Medina*[2,†], *MD

[1]Department of Anesthesia
University Hospital Virgen de la Arrixaca, El Palmar,
Murcia, Spain
[2]Department of Ophthalmology,
University Hospital Reina Sofia
University School of Medicine,
University of Murcia, Murcia, Spain

RESEARCH SUMMARY

The HELLP syndrome (hemolysis, high liver enzymes and low platelets syndrome) is a severe, life-threatening pregnancy disorder that is usually resolved with delivery without sequelae [1]. In the absence of other concurrent conditions, laboratory disturbances associated with the HELLP syndrome include evidence of hemolysis, thrombocytopenia, and characteristic histological abnormalities [2, 3]. Although the causative factor(s) for the development of HELLP syndrome remain elusive, the clinical and laboratory manifestations are well described and include activation of the coagulation system [4, 5].

When other disorder(s) occur concomitant with HELLP syndrome, they challenge the health care provider to not only make the correct diagnoses but also to make sometimes difficult decisions regarding the specific needs of the patient to have each disorder managed

---

[#] This chapter was previously published in *The 2015 Compendium for HELLP Syndrome: From Bench to Bedside*, edited by James N. Martin, Jr., New York: Nova Publishers Inc., 2015.

[*] Corresponding Author Email: Senior Conusltant Anesthetist; Email: monicadelriov@hotmail.com.

[†] Corresponding Author Email: Senior Consultant; Email: josegarciam@yahoo.com.

well in order to minimize severe maternal morbidity and maximize the patient's chance for intact survival. A number of pregnancy disorders can complicate the care of patients with HELLP syndrome including certain thrombophilic diseases such as antiphospholipid syndrome, systemic lupus erythematosus, and resistance to activated protein C (mutation R506Q, Leiden V factor) [6-10]. Other diseases which have been reported to complicate HELLP syndrome management include idiopathic thrombocytopenic purpura and diabetes insipidus. In these circumstances when minor or major surgery is required it can be particularly challenging for the anesthesiologist to devise a plan of management which takes into account all of the special issues to consider in such a rarely encountered situation. In addition, anesthesiologists must consider the potential for these HELLP-related conditions to complicate anesthesia care for patients with HELLP syndrome and render anesthetic management difficult. Some of the most important considerations relative to these issues are reviewed in light of published literature and experience.

References

[1] Weinstein L. Syndrome of hemolysis, elevated liver enzymes, and low platelet count: a severe consequence of hypertension in pregnancy. *Am J Obstet Gynecol.* 1982;142:159-67.

[2] van Pampus MG, Wolf H, Mayruhu G, Treffers PE, Bleker OP. Long-term follow-up in patients with a history of HELLP syndrome. *Hypertens Pregnancy.* 2001;20:15-23.

[3] Soltesz P, Szekanecz Z, Vegh J, Lakos G, Toth L, Szakall S. Catastrophic antiphospholipid antibody syndrome in cancer. *Haematologia.* 2000;30:303-11.

[4] Krauss T, Augustin HG, Osmers R, Meden H, Unterhalt M, Kuhn W. Activated protein C resistance and factor V Leiden in patients with hemolysis, elevated liver enzymes, low platelets syndrome. *Obstet Gynecol.* 1998;92:457-60.

[5] de Boer K, Büller HR, Ten Cate JW, Treffers PE. Coagulation studies in the syndrome of hemolysis, elevated liver enzymes and low platelets. *Br J Obstet Gynaecol.* 1991;98:42-7.

[6] Kupferminc MJ, Eldor A, Steinman N, Many A, Bar-Am A, Jaffa A, Fait G, Lessing JB. Increased frequency of genetic thrombophilia in women with complications of pregnancy. *N Engl J Med.* 1999;340:9-13.

[7] Yasuda M, Takakuwa K, Tokunaga A, Tanaka K. Prospective studies of the association between anticardiolipin antibody and outcome of pregnancy. *Obstet Gynecol.* 1995;86:555-9.

[8] Grandone E, Margaglione M, Colaizzo D, Cappucci G, Sciannamé N, Montanaro S, Paladini D, Martinelli P, Di Minno G. Prothrombotic genetic risk factors and the occurrence of gestational hypertension with or without proteinuria. *Thromb Haemost.* 1999;81:349-52.

[9] Middeldorp S. Thrombophilia and pregnancy complications: cause or association? *J Thromb Haemost.* 2007;5:276-82.

[10] Robertson L, Wu O, Langhorne P, Twaddle S, Clark P, Lowe GD, Walker ID, Greaves M, Brenkel I, Regan L, Greer IA; Thrombosis: Risk and Economic Assessment of Thrombophilia Screening (TREATS) Study. Thrombophilia in pregnancy: a systematic review. *Br J Haematol.* 2006;132:171-96.

In: Medicine Research Summaries. Volume 17
Editors: Zhongwen Liáng and Bibao Zhang
ISBN: 978-1-53612-751-5

Chapter 72

Reduced Pseudocholinesterase Activity in Patients with HELLP Syndrome[#]

Samuel Lurie*, MD
Department of Obstetrics and Gynecology
Edith Wolfson Medical Center, Holon
Sackler School of Medicine
Tel Aviv University, Tel Aviv, Israel

Research Summary

The prevalence of reduced pseudocholinesterase activity in patients with HELLP syndrome is significantly increased. Its deficiency results in abnormally slow metabolic degradation of exogenous choline-ester drugs such as succinylcholine, a condition that is usually recognized clinically when paralysis of the respiratory and other skeletal muscles fails to spontaneously recover following the administration of choline-ester drugs during general anesthesia. Pseudocholinesterase is a plasma enzyme that was first identified in 1932 but it has no known apparent physiologic function [1, 2]. Deficiency of the enzyme is either inherited or acquired by a variety of pathologic conditions or diseases such as HELLP syndrome or revealed when certain medications are employed. In view of its increased prevalence in patients who develop HELLP syndrome, the potentially reduced pseudocholinesterase activity becomes particularly important when choosing general anesthesia for obstetric indications such as cesarean delivery or revision of uterine cavity in women with antepartum HELLP syndrome. Regional anesthesia for cesarean delivery may be indicated in the presence of pseudocholinesterase deficiency in women with HELLP syndrome.

[#] This chapter was previously published in *The 2015 Compendium for HELLP Syndrome: From Bench to Bedside*, edited by James N. Martin, Jr., New York: Nova Publishers Inc., 2015.

* Corresponding Author: Professor; Email: drslurie@hotmail.com.

References

[1] Stedman E, Stedman E, Easson LH. Choln-esterase. An enzyme present in the blood-serum of the horse. *Biochem J* 1932;26:2056-66.

[2] Whittaker M. Cholinesterase. *Karger, Basel.* 1986. pp.1-7, 68-9.

In: Medicine Research Summaries. Volume 17
Editors: Zhongwen Liáng and Bibao Zhang

ISBN: 978-1-53612-751-5

Chapter 73

PERINATAL AND NEONATAL ASPECTS OF HELLP SYNDROME[#]

Carl H. Rose*, MD, MS, FACOG
Division of Maternal-Fetal Medicine,
Department of Obstetrics and Gynecology,
Mayo Clinic, Rochester, Minnesota, US

RESEARCH SUMMARY

Marked progress in management of the preterm infant over the past two decades has contributed to a substantial reduction in both immediate mortality and longstanding morbidity. However, the primary determinants of neonatal outcome remain gestational age at delivery and birth weight [1]. Given the median gestational age at diagnosis of 34.5 weeks, HELLP syndrome commonly mandates preterm delivery for maternal indication [2] Although minimal data directly addresses long-term outcomes in this specific subpopulation, most investigators have described neonatal outcomes similar to those of patients with severe preeclampsia [3, 4]. This chapter will review the existing evidence and potential fetal and neonatal implications of maternal diagnosis of HELLP syndrome.

References

[1] Mathews TJ, MacDorman MF. Infant mortality statistics from the 2010 period linked birth/infant death data set. *Natl Vital Stat Rep.* 2013 Dec 18;62(8):1-26.
[2] Fitzpatrick KE, Hinshaw K, Kurinczuk JJ, Knight M. Risk factors, management, and outcomes of hemolysis, elevated liver enzymes, and low platelets syndrome and

---

[#] This chapter was previously published in *The 2015 Compendium for HELLP Syndrome: From Bench to Bedside*, edited by James N. Martin, Jr., New York: Nova Publishers Inc., 2015.

* Corresponding Author: Associate Professor; Email: rose.carl@mayo.edu.

elevated liver enzymes, low platelets syndrome. *Obstet Gynecol.* 2014 Mar;123(3):618-27.

[3] Magann EF, Graves GR, Roberts WE, Blake PG, Morrison JC, Martin JN Jr. Corticosteroids for enhanced fetal lung maturation in patients with HELLP syndrome: impact on neonates. *Aust N Z J Obstet Gynaecol.* 1993 May; 33(2):131-5.

[4] Abramovici D, Friedman SA, Mercer BM, Audibert F, Kao L, Sibai BM. Neonatal outcome in severe preeclampsia at 24 to 36 weeks' gestation: does the HELLP (hemolysis, elevated liver enzymes, and low platelet count) syndrome matter? *Am J Obstet Gynecol.* 1999 Jan;180(1 Pt 1):221-5.

In: Medicine Research Summaries. Volume 17
Editors: Zhongwen Liáng and Bibao Zhang
ISBN: 978-1-53612-751-5

Chapter 74

INFECTION AND ANTIBIOTIC CONSIDERATIONS IN PATIENTS WITH HELLP SYNDROME[#]

Ana Martínez Aspas*[*]*, MD,
and Mª José Esquembre Gratacós*[†]*, MD
Department of Obstetrics and Gynecology
Hospital Clínico Universitario de Valencia, Valencia, Spain

RESEARCH SUMMARY

HELLP syndrome is associated with a high risk of infection for at least three reasons. The first reason is the high likelihood of transfusion which develops in proportion to the severity of HELLP with microangiopathic hemolytic anemia, an increased risk for blood loss at delivery, possibly a need for platelets to undergo cesarean delivery, and sometimes the need to mitigate the consequences of disseminated intravascular coagulation (DIC), surely one of the most feared complications of this serious pregnancy disorder. A second reason is the possibility of massive bleeding that these patients can incur when there is cerebral hemorrhage, formation of a subcapsular liver hematoma, or the rupture of a liver hematoma. A third reason for increased risk for infection is patient exposure to nosocomial infections secondary to the likelihood of invasive procedures to which these patients are subjected in intensive care units.

Despite these potential risk factors for infection with HELLP, antibiotic prophylaxis in these patients is not indicated. In fact, preventive antibiotic treatment is not routinely used or recommended for patients with HELLP. These patients usually receive only one dose of prophylactic antibiotic when a cesarean section is performed, the method of delivery most commonly employed to end these complicated pregnancies. Antibiotic prophylaxis for

---

[#] This chapter was previously published in *The 2015 Compendium for HELLP Syndrome: From Bench to Bedside*, edited by James N. Martin, Jr., New York: Nova Publishers Inc., 2015.
[*] Corresponding Author Email: amaras82@hotmail.com.
[†] Corresponding Author Email:mp.esquembre@gmail.com.

cesarean delivery is utilized due to the risk of infection associated with laparotomy rather than one associated with HELLP syndrome itself.

Thrombocytopenia is defined variably as a platelet count below 130,000 to 150,000/ul according to the country and laboratory systems in place. Thrombocytopenia becomes clinically significant below a threshold of 100,000/ul, developing either due to a lack of production by the bone marrow or an increased destruction or consumption which occurs with HELLP syndrome due in large part to pathological platelet-endothelial inflammatory interaction that can develop into a vicious cycle of platelet recruitment, endothelial damage and fibrin deposition [1-5].

If the patient has a superimposed septic process, platelet destruction is greater. There is an inverse relationship between the severity of the septic process and the mother's platelet count. It is important to emphasize that thrombocytopenia per se is not an independent risk factor for infection. Instead it is infection itself which can cause a decrease in platelets to merit a diagnosis of thrombocytopenia consequent to bone marrow damage.

After this brief introduction, we will discuss each of the above mentioned scenarios that may contribute to the development of a greater number of infections in patients with HELLP.

In: Medicine Research Summaries. Volume 17
Editors: Zhongwen Liáng and Bibao Zhang

ISBN: 978-1-53612-751-5

Chapter 75

HELLP Syndrome: Epidemiology and Recurrence Risk[#]

Pavan Parikh*[1,*]*, MD,
and Imran Sunesara*[2,†]*, MBBS MPH
[1]Obstetrics and Gynecology
Department of Obstetrics and Gynecology
The University of Mississippi Medical Center,
Jackson, Mississippi, US
[2]Department of Medicine
Biostatistician in Center of Biostatistics and Bioinformatics
The University of Mississippi Medical Center,
Jackson, Mississippi, US

Research Summary

Among the more than 2000 citations in the obstetric literature that reflect our current knowledge about HELLP syndrome, there is a growing amount of information regarding the epidemiology of the disorder, its demographics and the rates of recurrence for the various categories of complete or incomplete/partial HELLP syndrome. In this chapter we consider the state of our knowledge regarding these issues.

[#] This chapter was previously published in *The 2015 Compendium for HELLP Syndrome: From Bench to Bedside*, edited by James N. Martin, Jr., New York: Nova Publishers Inc., 2015.

[*] Corresponding Author: Pavan Parikh, Resident in Obstetrics and Gynecology; Email: pparikh@umc.edu.
[†] Corresponding Author: Imran Sunesara, Instructor, Dept. of Medicine; Email: isunesara@umc.edu.

In: Medicine Research Summaries. Volume 17
Editors: Zhongwen Liáng and Bibao Zhang
ISBN: 978-1-53612-751-5

Chapter 76

RISK FACTORS FOR HELLP SYNDROME[#]

Llanos Belmonte Andujar[1,*], MD,
María Teresa Gómez García[2,3], PhD,
Ana María Fuentes Rozalén, MD,
Carolina Serrano Diana[2], MD,
and Esther López del Cerro[2], MD
[1]Obstetrics and Gynecology Department Hospital of Almansa, Albacete, Spain
[2]Obstetrics and Gynecology Department, University and Hospital of Albacete, Spain
[3]Medical Science Department, School Of Medicine of Albacete,
Universidad de Castilla-La Mancha, Spain

RESEARCH SUMMARY

HELLP syndrome is one of the most severe complications that can occur during pregnancy. It is considered a multisystem and multifactorial condition. Although its physiopathology is not exactly known, many likely factors related to its development have been studied. HELLP syndrome has historically been supposed to be more frequent in multiparous, older, obese or Caucasian women, but actually there is no conclusive consensus research about its risk factors.

HELLP syndrome has been considered as a severe manifestation of preeclampsia, with a common physiopathology. However, the risk factors associated with each are slightly different, for example race. HELLP syndrome occurs more frequently in White women than in African-Americans or Hispanics, while Black race is regarded as a risk factor of preeclampsia. Despite these differences in risk, many published studies related to risk factors of preeclampsia and HELLP syndrome do not make a distinction between the two conditions, analyzing the different possible risk factors as if both were the same clinical entity.

[#] This chapter was previously published in *The 2015 Compendium for HELLP Syndrome: From Bench to Bedside*, edited by James N. Martin, Jr., New York: Nova Publishers Inc., 2015.
[*] Corresponding Author Email: belmonte.llanos@gmail.com.

There is great variability in the incidence of preeclampsia and HELLP syndrome worldwide, with preeclampsia ranging from 1.5% in Sweden, to 3.8% in the United States, to 7.5% in Brazil [1, 2] Preeclampsia estimated general incidence is 2.16% to 4.6% [3, 4], with HELLP syndrome ranging from 1-8 per 1,000 pregnancies and from 8 to 24% of pregnancies complicated with preeclampsia or eclampsia [5].

This chapter serves as a bibliographic review of HELLP and preeclampsia in order to establish the main risk factors of HELLP syndrome and those which differ from preeclampsia. Knowledge of the different risk factors associated with these complex diseases will allow for the development of appropriate preventive strategies for the future and reduce adverse fetal and maternal outcomes experienced worldwide.

References

[1] Saftlas AF, Olson DR, Franks AL, Atrash HK, Pokras R. Epidemiology of preeclampsia and eclampsia in the United States, 1979-1986. *Am J Obstet Gynecol.* 1990 Aug;163(2):460–5.

[2] Gaio DS, Schmidt MI, Duncan BB, Nucci LB, Matos MC, Branchtein L. Hypertensive disorders in pregnancy: frequency and associated factors in a cohort of Brazilian women. *Hypertens Pregnancy.* 2001;20(3):269–81.

[3] Abalos E, Cuesta C, Carroli G, Qureshi Z, Widmer M, Vogel JP, et al. Pre-eclampsia, eclampsia and adverse maternal and perinatal outcomes: a secondary analysis of the World Health Organization Multicountry Survey on Maternal and Newborn Health. *BJOG Int J Obstet Gynaecol.* 2014 Mar;121 Suppl 1:14–24.

[4] Abalos E, Cuesta C, Grosso AL, Chou D, Say L. Global and regional estimates of preeclampsia and eclampsia: a systematic review. *Eur J Obstet Gynecol Reprod Biol.* 2013 Sep;170(1):1–7.

[5] Sibai BM. *HELLP syndrome..* In: UpToDate, Charles J Lockwood, Keith D Lindor (Ed), UpToDate. Accessed on March 25, 2015.

In: Medicine Research Summaries. Volume 17
Editors: Zhongwen Liáng and Bibao Zhang
ISBN: 978-1-53612-751-5

Chapter 77

BEYOND HELLP SYNDROME: PROGNOSIS, RECOVERY AND IMPACT ON FUTURE MATERNAL HEALTH[#]

Michelle Y. Owens[1,*], MD, MS, FACOG, and Eleni Z. Tsigas[2,†]

[1]Department of Obstetrics and Gynecology
Division of Maternal-Fetal Medicine
The University of Mississippi Medical Center,
Jackson, Mississippi, US
[2]Preeclampsia Foundation, Melbourne, Florida, US

RESEARCH SUMMARY

HELLP syndrome represents one of the most serious variants in the spectrum of hypertensive disorders of pregnancy. It is associated with complications for both the mother and neonate. Significant perinatal and maternal morbidity and mortality can occur. Upon recovery from HELLP syndrome, attention must also be given to the long-term effects of HELLP syndrome for both mother and child.

[#] This chapter was previously published in *The 2015 Compendium for HELLP Syndrome: From Bench to Bedside*, edited by James N. Martin, Jr., New York: Nova Publishers Inc., 2015.

[*] Corresponding Author: Michelle Y. Owens, Associate Professor, Department of Obstetrics and Gynecology; Email: myowens@umc.edu.

[†] Corresponding Author: Eleni Z. Tsigas, Executive Director, Preeclampsia Foundation; Email: eleni.tsigas@preeclampsia.org.

In: Medicine Research Summaries. Volume 17
Editors: Zhongwen Liáng and Bibao Zhang ISBN: 978-1-53612-751-5

Chapter 78

HELLP SYNDROME: THE PATIENT PERSPECTIVE#

Laney Poye[1], MA, Melissa Wilson[2], MPH, PhD and Eleni Z. Tsigas[1,*], BA
[1]Preeclampsia Foundation, Melbourne FL, US
[2]University of Southern California, Los Angeles, California, US

RESEARCH SUMMARY

From the patient's perspective, the experience of having HELLP syndrome lasts longer than the pregnancy, labor and delivery, or the days that immediately follow. While physicians continue to wrestle with issues of timely diagnosis and effective management to lessen or eliminate severe maternal morbidity and mortality for the mother and child, patients must deal with the physical and emotional after-effects from their experiences for the remainder of their lives. There is much to learn from the patient perspective with regard to HELLP syndrome. It may not seem important to physicians as to whether HELLP is a unique disorder or closely related to preeclampsia, but it might matter to patients processing their experience. Since HELLP can be so insidious in onset, how does this affect patient education about the most frequently experienced symptoms that patients might or might not report to their physicians? What is the extent of unmet mental health needs consequent to patient experiences with HELLP syndrome encounters? In this chapter we address some of these concerns and summarize what has been learned so far in the realm of living with the after-effects of a HELLP pregnancy.

This chapter was previously published in *The 2015 Compendium for HELLP Syndrome: From Bench to Bedside*, edited by James N. Martin, Jr., New York: Nova Publishers Inc., 2015.

* Corresponding Author Email: eleni.tsigas@preeclampsia.org.

In: Medicine Research Summaries. Volume 17
Editors: Zhongwen Liáng and Bibao Zhang

ISBN: 978-1-53612-751-5

Chapter 79

FALLS IN OLDER PEOPLE: PREVALENCE, RISK FACTORS, ASSESSMENT AND INTERVENTION STRATEGIES#

Juliana Hotta Ansai[1,*], Thais Rabiatti Aurichio[1] and Larissa Pires de Andrade[2]

[1]Postgraduate Program of Physiotherapy, Federal University of São Carlos, São Carlos, Brazil

[2]Physiotherapy Department, Federal University of São Carlos, São Carlos, Brazil

RESEARCH SUMMARY

Falls are considered as one of the accidents that take more loss of functionality, mainly in older adults. This chapter describes the prevalence of falls among different populations, the most used definitions and classifications for falls and their physical, social and psychological consequences. Health professional and society need to know the main risk factors for falls in order to screen older adults at greater risk and draw correct prevention strategies. The authors talked about the importance of identifying the combination of risk factors presented in each person. Since the prevalence of falls increases to 60% among older people with cognitive impairment and their consequences tend to be more serious, a brief text was inserted in this chapter. A large amount of sensitive methods has been described to assess falls and screen susceptible people for this event. This chapter helps health professionals to select the most appropriate tools to each patient or target population. Finally, prevention and rehabilitation strategies were mentioned, thinking about the complex interaction between environment, individual and task. To reduce the public health burden and fall-related injuries, it is imperative that effective preventive strategies are put in place.

This chapter was previously published in *Accidental Falls: Risk Factors, Prevention Strategies and Long-Term Outcomes*, edited by Brenda Evans, New York: Nova Publishers Inc., 2015.

* Corresponding Author Email: julianaansai@gmail.com.

In: Medicine Research Summaries. Volume 17
Editors: Zhongwen Liáng and Bibao Zhang
ISBN: 978-1-53612-751-5

Chapter 80

DETERMINANTS OF ACCIDENTAL FALLS AND FALL-RELATED INJURIES: RECOMMENDATIONS FOR FALLS AND FALL-RELATED INJURIES PREVENTION SET ON THE ANALYSIS OF A THEORETICAL DYNAMIC SYSTEM INVOLVING THE OLDER ADULT, THE ENVIRONMENT, AND THE TASK PERFORMANCE#

Catarina Lino Neto Pereira**
and Ana Isabel Carvalho Cruz-Ferreira
Departamento de Desporto e Saúde; Escola de Ciências e Tecnologia;
Universidade de Évora; Research Center in Sports Sciences,
Health and Human Development (CIDESD); Évora, Portugal

RESEARCH SUMMARY

This work aims to provide easy and practical recommendations for falls and fall-related injuries prevention set on the analysis of a theoretical dynamic system involving the subject (older adult), the environment, and the task performance.

In accordance with this system, accidental falls occur while performing physical activities/tasks. In the absence of movement the probability of falling will be almost zero. However, immobility decreases the subject´s ability of performance. The fall usually occurs when the demands of a given task exceed the subject's ability. The demands of a task are determined by its difficulty and by environmental conditions. In a hostile environment, the demands of a given task increase. As result, the task demands may exceed the subject's ability causing a fall.

This chapter was previously published in *Accidental Falls: Risk Factors, Prevention Strategies and Long-Term Outcomes*, edited by Brenda Evans, New York: Nova Publishers Inc., 2015.

* Corresponding Author Email: clnp@uevora.pt.

The ability to perform daily tasks without falling tends to decline with age due to associated frailty (notably the increased morbidities and the diminished physical, sensorial, and neural fitness). However, falls may also be a problem before the age of 60 years. The main immediate consequence of a fall is injury, which may be fatal. Another possible short-term consequence is an increased fear of falling that often conducts to a loss of independence while performing daily tasks and, consequently, leads to a decline in the subject's ability.

It was observed that the determinant factor for the rupture of this system balance (resulting in falls and fall-related injuries) in older adults is the subject, namely his/her condition of frailty. As the subject becomes more fragile and as the risk of intrinsic factors increases, their susceptibility to extrinsic factors rises, especially with regard to environmental hazards. Thereafter, the subject's likelihood of falling and injuring increases. However, a good level of physical fitness can also increase the threat of falling and injuring, because fitter people are more confidence in performing more demanding tasks and in more hazardous environments. Thereby, they expose themselves to more dangerous situations.

Given the above and reporting recent research findings, the primary recommendations for fall and fall-related injuries prevention are the following:

- A healthy lifestyle, in order to avoid co-morbidities or, at least, to minimize its effects.
- The reduction of environmental hazards, principally when fitness decreases and frailty increases, and the restraint of difficult tasks in hazardous environments.
- The practice at least 1,150 MET-min.wk^{-1} of physical activity, with no more than 500 MET-min.wk^{-1} (~60 min. wk^{-1}) of vigorous physical activity (due to associated hazards). For example a combination of 1 hour of walking, 2 hours of moderate physical activity (such as carrying light loads or bicycling at a regular pace) and 20 minutes of vigorous physical activity (such as heavy lifting, digging, aerobics, or fast bicycling) per week, what computes ~1,150 MET-min.wk^{-1}.
- The implementation of exercise programs to prevent physical fitness loss, especially balance. Further, muscle strength and gait exercises may be particularly relevant for less fit and frail people.
- The performance of functional exercises that mimic everyday life tasks and promote self-confidence.
- Regarding women, special attention must be taken because they tend to be more fragile. Regarding men, special attention must be taken because they tend to expose themselves to more hazardous situations.

In: Medicine Research Summaries. Volume 17
Editors: Zhongwen Liáng and Bibao Zhang

ISBN: 978-1-53612-751-5

Chapter 81

FALL PREVENTION IN A PERSON WITH PARKINSON'S DISEASE: A CASE STUDY REPORT[#]

Lynne M. Chapman*[*], *MS, OTR/L, LICDC
Department of Occupational Therapy
The University of Toledo, Toledo, OH, US

RESEARCH SUMMARY

A sensorimotor approach that included the use of repetitive, fast, and gross movement patterns was chosen for as the theoretical foundation for this case study. This approach is intended for use across disciplines and the principles of this approach have been correlated with fall prevention in persons who have a diagnosis of Parkinson's disease. It was hypothesized that there would be a significant decrease in the reported number of falls following successful completion of intervention that consisted of the use of the sensorimotor approach to intervention. The intervention included preparatory, purposeful, and occupation-based interventions using fast, repetitive gross motor patterns of movement. The goal of this sensorimotor approach was to teach the participant a new way of moving that would now be required in order to safety engage in everyday occupations. The process of learning and using new ways of moving by altering the effort required and type of movement required for task completion is a phenomenon referred to in the literature as "recalibration." Upon completion of the intervention, the participant had achieved success in gaining a new awareness of the effort required to internally regulate the movements required for safe and successful completion of occupations of daily living. The average rate of reported falls prior to the participant's participation in the study was one per month and at six month follow-up from the initiation of his participation in the study, patient had no falls to report.

[#] This chapter was previously published in *Accidental Falls: Risk Factors, Prevention Strategies and Long-Term Outcomes*, edited by Brenda Evans, New York: Nova Publishers Inc., 2015.

[*] Corresponding Author Email: Lynne M. Chapman, Clinical Assistant Professor/Coordinator of Professional Development/Senior Clinician; Email: Lynne.Chapman@utoledo.edu.

In: Medicine Research Summaries. Volume 17
Editors: Zhongwen Liáng and Bibao Zhang
ISBN: 978-1-53612-751-5

Chapter 82

SELF-PERCEIVED HEALTH AND THE RISK OF FALLING IN A BRAZILIAN COMMUNITY SAMPLE[#]

Patricia Morsch*
Institute of Geriatrics and Gerontology,
Pontifical Catholic University of Rio Grande do Sul,
Porto Alegre, Brazil

RESEARCH SUMMARY

In Brazil and in the United States, the prevalence of falls is approximately 30%. A lot of measures have been adopted trying to reduce this rate; however, the number of older adults who fall is still rising. Falling is associated with increased disability rates, as well as hospital and nursing home admissions. Research has identified many risk factors for falling, including physical and environmental hazards. In addition, as many chronic diseases older adults present, higher is the risk of falling. Self-perceived health has been used in research as a good indicator of individuals' actual health. Using a secondary dataset the relationship between self-perceived health and falls was tested in community dwelling older adults from the state of Rio Grande do Sul, Brazil. The data were used to test whether self-perceived health is associated with falling, controlling for sociodemographic variables (age, gender and monthly household income). Analysis was conducted using bivariate cross tabulation and noting of chi-square values. To sum up, self-perceived health has a relationship with falls and this is an important finding since inquiring self-perceived health is a simple and fast measure that might be useful in identifying older adults at risk of falling.

[#] This chapter was previously published in *Accidental Falls: Risk Factors, Prevention Strategies and Long-Term Outcomes*, edited by Brenda Evans, New York: Nova Publishers Inc., 2015.

[*] Corresponding Author Email: patriciamorsch@hotmail.com.

In: Medicine Research Summaries. Volume 17
Editors: Zhongwen Liáng and Bibao Zhang
ISBN: 978-1-53612-751-5

Chapter 83

PRACTICAL DESIGN SEARCH FOR OPTIMAL FLOOR SURFACE FINISHES TO PREVENT FALL INCIDENTS[#]

In-Ju Kim*
Department of Industrial Engineering,
College of Engineering King Saud University,
Riyadh, Saudi Arabia

RESEARCH SUMMARY

Increasing traction properties of the floor surface would be desirable as a general rule, but a very high level of slip-resistance may impede safe and comfortable ambulation. There is lack of evidences whether traction properties are linearly correlated with surface features of the floor or what levels of floor surface finishes are required to effective control of slipperiness. It is also scarce to find studies and/or guidelines on the operational ranges of floor surface roughness required for optimal slip-resistance performance. The objectives of this chapter are to investigate the effects of floor surface finishes on slip-resistance performance under different environmental and shoe-type conditions, and identify operational ranges of floor surface roughness as practical design information for the prevention of fall incidents. A theory model of three operative zones was suggested to characterize functional levels of floor surface roughness on slip-resistance performance. To test the theory model, dynamic friction tests were conducted using 3 shoes and 9 floor specimens under 2 lubricated environments: wet and soapy conditions. The test results showed that significant effects of floor-type on dynamic friction coefficient (DFC) were found in both lubricated conditions. As compared to the floor-type effects, shoe-type effects were relatively small. Slip-resistance performance was significantly affected by and well correlated with the floor surface roughness under the soapy environment. Polynomial regression analyses amongst the floor surface roughness, DFCs and environments allowed to estimating operational ranges for

[#] This chapter was previously published in *Accidental Falls: Risk Factors, Prevention Strategies and Long-Term Outcomes*, edited by Brenda Evans, New York: Nova Publishers Inc., 2015.

* Corresponding Author Email: slipsafety@gmail.com.

optimal slip-resistance performance. Under the soapy environment, floor surfaces with 17 and 52 μm in *Ra* roughness parameter most likely represented the lower and upper bounds of the operational ranges. The test result also identified that the soapsuds-covered soapy floors required rougher surface finishes than the wet ones in their lower boundary roughness range. However, there were lack of correlations between the surface roughness and slip-resistance properties under the wet surface condition. The current study suggests that designs for the floor surface finishes would require different levels of surface roughness for different types of environmental conditions to effectively control slippery walking environments.

In: Medicine Research Summaries. Volume 17
Editors: Zhongwen Liáng and Bibao Zhang

ISBN: 978-1-53612-751-5

Chapter 84

SLIP-RESISTANCE MEASUREMENTS FOR ASSESSING PEDESTRIAN FALL INCIDENTS: FACTS AND FALLACIES[#]

In-Ju Kim*
Department of Industrial Engineering,
College of Engineering King Saud University,
Riyadh, Saudi Arabia

RESEARCH SUMMARY

Pedestrian falls resulting from slips and/or trips are one of the leading categories of non-traffic incidents in terms of serious injuries and fatalities. They are a primary cause of industry injuries, as well as one of the leading causes of injury-related deaths for the elderly aged 65 and over. Fall incidents involve multi-factors, but have been commonly assessed by slip-resistance measurements as a simplified format of coefficient of friction (COF) quantity amongst shoes, floors and environments. However, slip-resistance properties have unique and specific features to any combination of the shoe, floor and environment. Notwithstanding such complex characteristics, COFs consistently change because slip-resistance properties are inherently noisy and geometric dimensions between the shoes and floors are largely modified during repetitive measurements. Whilst controversies on the friction measurements for the evaluation of slipperiness remain, slip-resistance properties are still commonly measured by COF readings in many studies and practices for slip and fall safety assessments. To enhance the validity and reliability of friction measurements, therefore, it is necessary to improve our understanding on the slip-resistance mechanics, mechanisms, and related tribo-physical characteristics of the sliding interface amongst the shoes, floors and environments. Because surface topographies of the shoes and floors are largely modified throughout the course of ambulation, this may considerably affect friction and wear behaviours and be one of the most

---

[#] This chapter was previously published in *Accidental Falls: Risk Factors, Prevention Strategies and Long-Term Outcomes*, edited by Brenda Evans, New York: Nova Publishers Inc., 2015.

* Corresponding Author Email: slipsafety@gmail.com.

important factors on the slip-resistance properties. Furthermore, surface features significantly affect the degree of slip-resistance performance and have a direct correlation to the ease of cleaning. A high profile surface finish is hard to clean and eventually loses its texture due to inability to remove dirt and physical erosions of the floor surface. This will also increase the risk of slipperiness. However, these issues are hardly investigated in the literature. This study explores the current knowledge gaps and misinterpretations on slip-resistance measurements that are mainly caused by oversimplified perceptions on friction phenomena between the shoes and floors and suggests a new paradigm on slip-resistance assessments for future researches on pedestrian fall incidents.

In: Medicine Research Summaries. Volume 17
Editors: Zhongwen Liáng and Bibao Zhang
ISBN: 978-1-53612-751-5

Chapter 85

QUALITY OF LIFE UNDER THE PERSPECTIVE OF COMPLEXITY[#]

Guanis de Barros Vilela Júnior*[1], *DSc
***Gustavo Celestino Martins*[2], *MS*, *Erika da Silva Maciel*[3],**
***Jaqueline Girnos Sonati*[4] *and Roberto Vilarta*[5]**
[1]Faculty of Physical Education, University Methodist of Piracicaba (UNIMEP), Piracicaba, São Paulo, Brazil
[2]Faculty Euclides da Cunha (FEUC), Brasil
[3]University and Lutheran Center of Palmas (CEULP-ULBRA), Palmas, Tocantins, Brazil
[4]Nursing School, State University of Campinas (UNICAMP). Campinas, São Paulo, Brazil
[5]Faculty of Physical Education, State University of Campinas (UNICAMP), Campinas, São Paulo, Brazil

RESEARCH SUMMARY

Promoting *Health* and *Quality of Life* is not a one-off challenge for the scientific community and professionals in this field. Currently, it is a consensus that this challenge is a transdisciplinary and complex struggle that permeates the dynamic perception of individuals about their lives as physical, social and political beings that interact with the environment (of which they are part), changing and being changed by it. However, methodological strategies in scientific research, education and public policies are at the same time arrogant and ingenuous. Arrogant because many argue that human supremacy and science will solve all the evils plaguing the planet. Ingenuous because they simplify, reduce and face difficulties to "think outside the box". The objective of this chapter is to reflect on promoting *Health* and *Quality of Life* under the paradigm of complexity, the limitations of hegemonic

[#] This chapter was previously published in *Quality of Life and Public Health: Assessment and Intervention*, edited by Erika da Silva Maciel and Jaqueline Girnos Sonati, New York: Nova Publishers Inc., 2015.

methodologies and the trans-phenomenal proposals to think about human's role in the sustainability of the planet and maintenance of civilization as we know it in the so-called Anthropocene period, in which a thousand years ago, we began to interfere with the climate of the planet.

In: Medicine Research Summaries. Volume 17
Editors: Zhongwen Liáng and Bibao Zhang
ISBN: 978-1-53612-751-5

Chapter 86

QUALITY OF LIFE AND PHYSICAL ACTIVITY#

Dênis Marcelo Modeneze[1], DSc, Erika da Silva Maciel[2], Jaqueline Girnos Sonati[3] and Fernando Rodrigues Peixoto Quaresma[4]

[1] State University of Campinas (UNICAMP) Campinas, São Paulo, Brazil
[2]University of São Paulo, University and Lutheran Center of Palmas (CEULP-ULBRA) Palmas, Tocantins, Brazil
[3]Nursing School, State University of Campinas (UNICAMP) Campinas, São Paulo, Brazil
[4]Nursing School, University Federal of Tocantins (UFT) Palmas, Tocantins, Brazil
ABC Medical Foundation (FMABC). Laboratory of Epidemiology and Data Analysis, Santo André, São Paulo, Brazil
University and Lutheran Center of Palmas (CEULP-ULBRA). Palmas, Tocantins, Brazil

RESEARCH SUMMARY

In recent decades, physical activity performed in an organized manner within the physical limits of each person has been considered a scientifically proven remedy for the prevention and control of various diseases such as obesity, diabetes, hypertension and musculoskeletal disorders. Recent research shows that active lifestyle, at least three times a week of moderate exercise, can provide better quality of life to individuals as listed by the World Health Organization through its group called the WHOQOL-group. Among the listed domains, "physical" and "psychological" are mostly affected by a sedentary lifestyle. A healthy and physically fit body can withstand more setbacks in life and contribute to a better quality of life. Physical fitness provides individuals good aerobic capacity, muscular strength, endurance, flexibility, healthy body composition with adequate levels of fat percentage, lean mass and bone weight. In combination with a balanced diet, it helps control levels of cholesterol, triglycerides and glucose in the blood. In this chapter, we propose to list many benefits that physical exercise provide to a better quality of life proposed by the WHO.

This chapter was previously published in *Quality of Life and Public Health: Assessment and Intervention*, edited by Erika da Silva Maciel and Jaqueline Girnos Sonati, New York: Nova Publishers Inc., 2015.

In: Medicine Research Summaries. Volume 17
Editors: Zhongwen Liáng and Bibao Zhang

ISBN: 978-1-53612-751-5

Chapter 87

Quality of Life and Food Consumption[#]

Anne Cristine Rumiato, Rosana Evangelista Poderoso and Inês Monteiro
University of Campinas (UNICAMP), Campinas, Brazil

Research Summary

Food consumption may affect the quality of life of the population, since one's diet can be associated with chronic diseases. The adoption of eating guidelines provides strategies for disseminating scientific knowledge about the health nutrition of the population. Countries with greater access to processed foods have a higher tendency to an increase in the obesity of the population. To assess the population's diet, indexes have been proposed and applied in population studies showing a portrait of the health of various population segments. In this scenario, this chapter aims to address the conditions of the availability of food and its relationship with consumption in the global context. Objectives: To identify the importance of eating healthy food for the world population; to describe the consumption of processed foods and the risk of obesity; to correlate food advertisements with encouraging healthy eating habits; to describe the evaluation indexes of diet quality utilized by the population. A systematic review was performed with the search strategy applied to the most relevant databases with the terms: Food Habit, Quality of life e Health food. No other filters have been assigned to the search, making it possible to identify all the relevant studies.

[#] This chapter was previously published in *Quality of Life and Public Health: Assessment and Intervention*, edited by Erika da Silva Maciel and Jaqueline Girnos Sonati, New York: Nova Publishers Inc., 2015.

In: Medicine Research Summaries. Volume 17
Editors: Zhongwen Liáng and Bibao Zhang
ISBN: 978-1-53612-751-5

Chapter 88

QUALITY OF LIFE AND THE IMPACT OF CHANGES ON SLEEP[#]

Milva Maria Figueiredo De Martino
Nursing School, State University of Campinas (UNICAMP), Campinas, São Paulo, Brazil

RESEARCH SUMMARY

In this chapter, the concept of quality of life proposed by the World Health Organization is discussed, which encompasses areas of physical health, social relationships, degree of independence, environment, psychological and spiritual variables and the impact of changes on sleep. Generally, people that show changes of sleep patterns often shows impaired quality of life. The consequences of sleep disorders are strongly related to quality of life. The schedules of work shifts are among the factors that affect sleep in modern societies. Changes of habits related to light-dark cycles affect the biological clock, altering the circadian system resulting in sleep disorders. An internal pacemaker in the suprachiasmatic nucleus (SCN) in the hypothalamus regulates the sleep-wake cycle. It consists of a brain structure located immediately above the optic chiasm, where the nerves cross. It has very specific functions related to cognition called suprachiasmatic nucleus (SCN) whose main function is to regulate the biological clock. Sleep disorders cause adverse consequences in people's lives by reducing their daily functions, leading to psychiatric disorders, cognitive deficits, and aggravation of health problems, as well as other issues regarding risks of traffic accidents, work absenteeism, compromising quality of life. Work shifts and unemployment risks can affect the quality of sleep and life of an individual because the need for work in these situations increases sleep latency and awakenings.

[#] This chapter was previously published in *Quality of Life and Public Health: Assessment and Intervention*, edited by Erika da Silva Maciel and Jaqueline Girnos Sonati, New York: Nova Publishers Inc., 2015.

In: Medicine Research Summaries. Volume 17
Editors: Zhongwen Liáng and Bibao Zhang

ISBN: 978-1-53612-751-5

Chapter 89

RELATED TO STAGE OF CHANGE IN EXERCISE BEHAVIOR AND QUALITY OF LIFE OF BRAZILIAN ADMINISTRATIVE WORKERS[#]

Cynara Cristina Domingues Alves Pereira[1] and Ana Lúcia Rodrigues Maretti[2]

[1]Institute of Physical Education, State University of Campinas (UNICAMP), Campinas, São Paulo, Brazil
[2]Health Sciences, University of São Paulo (USP), São Paulo, Brazil

RESEARCH SUMMARY

Sedentary people are subject to increased risks to their quality of life. The objective of this study was to describe the quality of life and the stage of change in the physical exercise behavior of Brazilian administrative workers. A cross-sectional study was conducted with 54 administrative workers (ADM); mostly women (73.9%) aged between 17 and 29 years old (63.6%), of a private company in the city of Salt, State of São Paulo, Brazil. The stage of change to exercise (transtheoretical model - TTM), as well as the domains and facets of quality of life (QoL) (WHOQOL-BREF), were the variables collected through an electronic form. The TTM reported a higher percentage for the contemplation stage (37.0%), followed by a tie between preparation and maintenance (20.4%), action (14.8%) and pre-contemplation (7.4%). The total QoL (83.2 ± 12.0), as well as the social physical domains (81.3 ± 10.0) and (83.0 ± 10.3) were classified as excellent, while the overall QoL (76.9 ± 14.6), the psychological fields (78.4 ± 5.0), and environmental field (68.7 ± 9.2) were classified as intermediate and good, with the lowest rate described for the environmental domain. The results described showed expressive values related to TTM and QoL. Although we cannot say that these data are directly related to each other, there is a positive positioning of Brazilian ADM workers when it comes to physical activity and quality of life.

[#] This chapter was previously published in *Quality of Life and Public Health: Assessment and Intervention*, edited by Erika da Silva Maciel and Jaqueline Girnos Sonati, New York: Nova Publishers Inc., 2015.

In: Medicine Research Summaries. Volume 17
Editors: Zhongwen Liáng and Bibao Zhang

ISBN: 978-1-53612-751-5

Chapter 90

Quality of Life at Work, Absenteeism and Job Satisfaction: A Case Study in Manufacturing Industry[#]

Telma Silva, DSc and Inês Monteiro
Nursing School, State University of Campinas (UNICAMP)
Campinas, São Paulo, Brazil

Research Summary

Scientific evaluation of causes for absenteeism in organizations demonstrated a scenario of multiple causes, involving socio-demographic characteristics, quality of life domains, and job satisfaction aspects. This case study had an objective to identify the socio-demographic variables, quality of life and job satisfaction perception associated with absenteeism among electronic manufacturing workers. A cross-sectional epidemiological study was made of employees from an electronics manufacturing company in Brazil, based on the numbers of absences in the last twelve months. Self-administered questionnaires were used: The Job Satisfaction Scale from Occupational Stress Indicator (OSI) and WHOQOL Bref. The associations between variables were analyzed by analysis of variance and covariance. Models of simple and multiple logistic regressions were also used. Being absent more days at work was associated with the female gender ($p = 0.0006$) along with having a second job ($p = 0.0041$), working a night shift ($p = 0.0001$) and psychological ($p = 0.0005$), physical ($p = 0.0001$), and environmental ($p = 0.0025$) domains of quality of life.

The employees' perception regarding job satisfaction and quality of life was related to absenteeism, which is associated with multi-causal factors that suggest a worker's coping strategy. The analysis of these variables depends on scientific methods and a consistent theoretical basis in order to achieve improvements to the quality of life at work.

[#] This chapter was previously published in *Quality of Life and Public Health: Assessment and Intervention*, edited by Erika da Silva Maciel and Jaqueline Girnos Sonati, New York: Nova Publishers Inc., 2015.

In: Medicine Research Summaries. Volume 17
Editors: Zhongwen Liáng and Bibao Zhang
ISBN: 978-1-53612-751-5

Chapter 91

SOCIO-DEMOGRAPHICS, LIFESTYLE, HEALTH AND WORK ASPECTS RELATED TO QUALITY OF LIFE AMONG PHARMACEUTICAL INDUSTRY WORKERS*,#

Inês Monteiro[1,†], Eloisa Petruci Hodge[2] and Aparecida Mari Iguti[3]
[1]Faculty of Nursing, University of Campinas (UNICAMP) Brazil
[2]Clinical Nurse at Occupational Health Center,
Centre de Sante' et de Services Sociaux de la Montagne
[3]Faculty of Medical Sciences
University of Campinas (UNICAMP), Brazil

RESEARCH SUMMARY

Aspects of quality of life are important and often undervalued in studies about industrial workers. The objective of this study was to correlate the socio-demographics, lifestyle, health and work aspects with the quality of life among workers in the pharmaceutical industry. A cross-sectional study was conducted in two plants of a pharmaceutical industry, in Campinas, with a sample of 357 workers, of which 293 were performing activities in the production of drugs for oral administration and, 64, in the injectable products factory. A questionnaire about socio-demographics, lifestyle and work and a question on current work ability was used. Data analysis was performed through statistical modelling including socio-demographic variables (gender, age, marital status, children and school education); relating to work (demand, function, perception if the work is tiresome/fatigue); health (self-reported health) and lifestyle (physical activity, smoking and alcohol intake).

---

* Data from Eloisa Petruci Hodge Master Dissertation and Research Productivity scholarship – CNPq of Inês Monteiro.

This chapter was previously published in *Quality of Life and Public Health: Assessment and Intervention*, edited by Erika da Silva Maciel and Jaqueline Girnos Sonati, New York: Nova Publishers Inc., 2015.

† Corresponding Author: Inês Monteiro, Associate Professor; Email: inesmon@unicamp.br.

In: Medicine Research Summaries. Volume 17
Editors: Zhongwen Liáng and Bibao Zhang
ISBN: 978-1-53612-751-5

Chapter 92

PERCEPTION OF PAIN AND QUALITY OF LIFE AT WORK OF TRUCK DRIVERS IN CITIES OF SÃO PAULO STATE[#]

Luciane Manzatto[1], Guanis de Barros Vilela Junior[2], Antonio Jose Grande[3], Erika da Silva Maciel[4], Gustavo Celestino Martins[5], Tulio Brandão Xavier Rocha[6] and Jaqueline Girnos Sonati[7]

[1,2,3,5]Faculty of Physiotherapy, University Methodist of Piracicaba (UNIMEP)
Piracicaba, São Paulo, Brazil
[4]University and Lutheran Center of Palmas
(CEULP-ULBRA) Palmas, Tocantins, Brazil
[6]Faculty of Physiotherapy, Integrated College Pythagoras
Montes Claros, Minas Gerais, Brazil
[7]Nursing School, State University of Campinas (UNICAMP)
Campinas, São Paulo, Brazil

RESEARCH SUMMARY

The aim of this study was to analyze the perception of truck drivers regarding quality of life and pain. The study was descriptive and cross-sectional, using 38 male volunteers at an average age of 43 years. The instruments of quality of life at work and health (QVS-80) as well as the Corlett diagram were used. Drivers perceive good health and quality of life in their activities, even those that reported suffering pain. Regarding discomforts, the lumbar spine region was reported with greater pain incidence, followed by the right shoulder. Aspects related to improving health conditions, such as exercise programs, are needed for these professionals.

[#] This chapter was previously published in *Quality of Life and Public Health: Assessment and Intervention*, edited by Erika da Silva Maciel and Jaqueline Girnos Sonati, New York: Nova Publishers Inc., 2015.

In: Medicine Research Summaries. Volume 17
Editors: Zhongwen Liáng and Bibao Zhang

ISBN: 978-1-53612-751-5

Chapter 93

QUALITY OF LIFE X QUANTITY OF LIFE: THE RIGHT TO DIE WITH DIGNITY PROTECTED BY THE ADVANCED DIRECTIVES INSTITUTES[#]

Bruna Sitta Deserti[1], Hélio Veiga Júnior[1], Patrícia Borba Marchetto[1,2], Roberto Brocanelli Corona[1] and Thiago Soares Lamenha Gomes[3]

[1]Faculty of Humanities and Social Sciences, State University Paulista (UNESP), Franca, São Paulo, Brazil

[2]Faculty of Science, Arts and Humanities, State University Paulista (UNESP), Araraquara, São Paulo, Brazil

[3]Family Medicine of the Regional Center of Family Medicine Community, University of São Paulo (USP), RibeirãoPreto, São Paulo, Brazil

RESEARCH SUMMARY

In the last century we have witnessed a great development in medicine. New drugs and sophisticated surgical interventions present the proposal for a long life, almost as a product available on the market. Facing death as a natural process is increasingly distant from people's lives nowadays. Quantity of life does not mean quality of life. In cases of incurable diseases, the best treatment is to accept the condition and offer palliative cares to ensure the quality of life that still remains. It cannot be forgotten that behind all the medical techniques in development there are human beings who ought to be at the center of the medical-patient relation and have their dignity and autonomy respected. There is a juridical mechanism called "Advanced Directives," popularly known as "Living Will," which is a public document to register all the medical directions regarding health care treatments and procedures that the patients do not wish to be submitted to, that can be used to ensure that the patient's wishes concerning his life will be respected when he may not be able to express his will. The advanced directives defend the dignity of every human being and the palliative cares rather than the pursuit of a cure.

[#] This chapter was previously published in *Quality of Life and Public Health: Assessment and Intervention*, edited by Erika da Silva Maciel and Jaqueline Girnos Sonati, New York: Nova Publishers Inc., 2015.

In: Medicine Research Summaries. Volume 17
Editors: Zhongwen Liáng and Bibao Zhang

ISBN: 978-1-53612-751-5

Chapter 94

QUALITY OF LIFE OF CAREGIVERS OF PEOPLE WITH DISABILITIES[#]

Fernando Rodrigues Peixoto Quaresma[1], Airton Tetelbon Stein[2], Erika da Silva Maciel[3] and Fernando Adami[4]

[1]Nursing School, University Federal of Tocantins (UFT), Palmas, Tocantins, Brazil
Medicine School, ABC Medical Foundation (FMABC),
Laboratory of Epidemiology and Data Analysis, Santo André, São Paulo, Brazil
University and Lutheran Center of Palmas
(CEULP-ULBRA), Palmas, Tocantins, Brazil
[2]UFCSPA, ULBRA Canoas and Coordinator of HTA of Grupo Hospitalar Conceição,
Rio Grande do Sul, Brazil
[3]University of São Paulo,
University and Lutheran Center of Palmas
(CEULP-ULBRA), Palmas, Tocantins, Brazil
[4]Medicine School, ABC Medical Foundation (FMABC),
Laboratory of Epidemiology and Data Analysis, Santo André, São Paulo, Brazil
UNESC - Extreme South in Santa Catarina, Brazil
IBESPA - Brazilian Institute for Applied Research

RESEARCH SUMMARY

The different conceptions and relationships involving people with disabilities (PwD) have been notably marked by contempt, social segregation and care dependence. In the long term, this dependence causes significant impacts on family relationships and on physical and mental health, affecting quality of life (QOL) of caregivers. Caregivers, usually a family member of PwD or teachers in nursing institutions for people with special needs, often have their QOL affected; thus, they need attention regarding their physical and mental health. In this sense, monitoring health conditions and developing preventive actions to promote health should be considered for caregivers of PwD.

[#] This chapter was previously published in *Quality of Life and Public Health: Assessment and Intervention*, edited by Erika da Silva Maciel and Jaqueline Girnos Sonati, New York: Nova Publishers Inc., 2015.

In: Medicine Research Summaries. Volume 17
Editors: Zhongwen Liáng and Bibao Zhang
ISBN: 978-1-53612-751-5

Chapter 95

MANAGEMENT OF OBSTRUCTIVE AND CENTRAL SLEEP APNEA[#]

Seckin O. Ulualp*
Department of Otolaryngology: Head and Neck Surgery,
University of Texas Southwestern Medical Center,
Dallas, TX, US

RESEARCH SUMMARY

The spectrum of sleep-disordered breathing ranges from primary snoring at one end to obstructive sleep apnea and central sleep apnea at the other end. Obstructive sleep apnea and central sleep apnea have an impact on sleep quality and overall health. Repeated episodes of cessation or decrease in airflow and arousals from sleep occur during obstructive and central sleep apnea events. These episodes may lead to day time manifestations including, but not limited to, unrefreshed sleep, sleepiness, poor attention, hyperactivity, and fatigue. Unrecognized obstructive sleep apnea and central sleep apnea may cause cardiovascular, pulmonary, neurologic, metabolic, and neurocognitive morbidities. Better understanding the underlying pathophysiology of obstructive sleep apnea and central sleep apnea, and early diagnosis of sleep apnea and its consequences potentially prevent adverse effects on the individual. This article will provide current state of knowledge about the mechanisms of obstructive sleep apnea and central sleep apnea and review emerging therapies for these disorders.

[#] This chapter was previously published in *Obstructive and Central Sleep Apnea*, edited by Joan McCormick, New York: Nova Publishers Inc., 2015.

* Corresponding Author: Seckin O. Ulualp, MD, Department of Otolaryngology-Head and Neck Surgery, University of Texas Southwestern Medical Center, 5323 Harry Hines Blvd, Dallas, Texas, 75390-9035. Phone: (214) 456-2905. Fax: (214) 648-9122. E-mail: seckin.ulualp@ utsouthwestern.edu.

In: Medicine Research Summaries. Volume 17
Editors: Zhongwen Liáng and Bibao Zhang

ISBN: 978-1-53612-751-5

Chapter 96

SPECIFIC NEUROLOGICAL DISORDERS AND SLEEP DISTURBANCES#

***K. A. Norremose*[1] *and M. F. Oliveira*[2,*]**
[1]Neurology Service, Santa Paula Hospital, São Paulo, Brazil
[2]Department of Neurosurgery, Hospital do Servidor Público Estadual de São Paulo, São Paulo, Brazil

RESEARCH SUMMARY

Sleep apnea, characterized by repetitive cessation of breathing during sleep, has been reported to be prevalent in up to 30% of the general population and may be of obstructive or central origin. It has usually multifatorial causes and affects multiple organic systems resulting in increased cardiovascular morbidity, disturbing sleep quality, metabolic balance, glucose and cholesterol levels, arterial hypertension and thus increasing cardiopulmonary and vascular morbidity. Such complexity is generally assessed by several professionals, like clinical physicians, cardiologists, nutritionists, physical therapists, otorhinolaryngologists, pneumologists, endocrinologists and neurologists. Many neurological disorders, like epilepsy, dementia, neuromuscular affections, headache, multiple sclerosis and stroke may manifest or be characterized by specific sleep patterns, including sleep apnea. We summarize the main findings in literature and perform a brief and concise differential diagnosis.

This chapter was previously published in *Obstructive and Central Sleep Apnea*, edited by Joan McCormick, New York: Nova Publishers Inc., 2015.

* Corresponding Author: Matheus Fernandes de Oliveira. Av. Pedro de Toledo, 1800 – Vila Clementino, São Paulo – São Paulo – Brazil. E-mail: mafernoliv@yahoo.com.br.

In: Medicine Research Summaries. Volume 17
Editors: Zhongwen Liáng and Bibao Zhang

ISBN: 978-1-53612-751-5

Chapter 97

NEUROSURGICAL TOPICS AND SLEEP APNEA[#]

M. F. Oliveira[1,], K. A. Norremose[2] and F. C. G. Pinto[3]*
[1]Department of Neurosurgery, Hospital do Servidor Público Estadual de São Paulo, São Paulo, Brazil
[2]Neurology Service, Santa Paula Hospital, São Paulo, Brazil
[3]Division of Functional Neurosurgery of the Institute of Psychiatry, Hospital das Clínicas, Universidade de São Paulo, São Paulo, Brazil

RESEARCH SUMMARY

Sleep apnea, characterized by repetitive cessation of breathing during sleep, has been reported to be prevalent in up to 30% of the general population and may be of obstructive or central origin. It has usually multifactorial causes and affects multiple organic systems like cardiovascular, sleep quality, metabolic balance, glucose and cholesterol levels, arterial hypertension and thus increasing cardiopulmonary and vascular morbidity. Such complexity is generally assessed by several professionals, like clinical physicians, cardiologists, nutritionists, physical therapists, otorhinolaryngologists, pneumologists, endocrinologists and neurologists. Nevertheless, increasing evidence points to the association of neurosurgical pathologies with sleep apnea, with potential reversibility after proper treatment. In this scenario, we expose and discuss current evidence of neurosurgical conditions and their role in the genesis and progression of sleep apnea. Additionally, we emphasize the adequate treatment and future perspectives.

[#] This chapter was previously published in *Obstructive and Central Sleep Apnea*, edited by Joan McCormick, New York: Nova Publishers Inc., 2015.

[*] Corresponding Author: Matheus Fernandes de Oliveira. Av. Pedro de Toledo, 1800 – Vila Clementino, São Paulo – São Paulo – Brazil. E-mail: mafernoliv@yahoo.com.br.

In: Medicine Research Summaries. Volume 17
Editors: Zhongwen Liáng and Bibao Zhang
ISBN: 978-1-53612-751-5

Chapter 98

CHANGES IN THE EYE RELATED TO OBSTRUCTIVE SLEEP APNEA SYNDROME#

Blanca Ferrandez[1], MD, Pilar Calvo[1], MD, PhD, and Antonio Ferreras[1,2], MD, PhD

[1] Department of Ophtalmology. Miguel Servet University Hospital. Aragon Health Research Institute, IIS Aragón, Zaragoza, Spain
[2]University of Zaragoza, Spain

RESEARCH SUMMARY

Obstructive sleep apnea syndrome (OSAS) is defined by partial (hypopnea) or complete (apnea) intermittent episodes of upper airway collapse during sleep. The hypoxia resulting from these repetitive episodes leads to oxidative stress, sympathetic activation, endothelial dysfunction, systemic inflammation, and metabolic abnormalities. These pathophysiologic mechanisms are the source of many systemic diseases, such as blood and pulmonary hypertension, insulin resistance, metabolic syndrome, arrhythmia, myocardial infarction, congestive heart failure, and stroke. OSAS affects approximately 24% of men and 9% of women in the general population, and its prevalence increases with age. Different ophthalmologic disorders are also associated with OSAS: floppy eyelid syndrome, retinal vein occlusion, primary open angle glaucoma, normal-tension glaucoma, papilledema, non-ischemic anterior optic neuropathy, and central serous retinopathy. Changes in the optic nerve head (ONH) and retinal nerve fiber layer (RNFL) thickness in patients with OSAS have been a topic of controversy in recent years. Some studies have hypothesized that the hypoxia resulting from apnea-hypopnea episodes could compromise ONH vascularization. This condition may produce retinal ganglion cell damage and, consequently, reduce RFNL thickness. Some investigators report that OSAS and its severity could be related to decreased RNFL thickness or reduced retinal sensitivity measured with standard automated perimetry. On the other hand, other studies found no evidence of a correlation between OSAS and RFNL

This chapter was previously published in *Obstructive and Central Sleep Apnea*, edited by Joan McCormick, New York: Nova Publishers Inc., 2015.

thickness loss. Different study designs, methodology, inclusion and exclusion criteria, age, and level of OSAS make it difficult to compare the results among several studies.

Thus, the structural and functional changes in the retina and optic disc due to OSAS remain unclear. Further prospective longitudinal studies are needed to elucidate the effect of OSAS on the eye.

In: Medicine Research Summaries. Volume 17
Editors: Zhongwen Liáng and Bibao Zhang

ISBN: 978-1-53612-751-5

Chapter 99

QT DISPERSION IN PATIENTS WITH OBSTRUCTIVE SLEEP APNEA[#]

Igor A. Kelmanson*
Institute of Special Education and Special Psychology of the Raoul Wallenberg International University for Family and Child, St. Petersburg, Russia

RESEARCH SUMMARY

Exaggerated dispersion of repolarization is likely to play a role in both the initiation and the maintenance of malignant ventricular arrhythmias. Inter-lead QT interval differences within a 12-lead ECG termed "QT dispersion" may reflect regional differences in myocardial refractoriness. QT dispersion is simply defined as the difference between the longest (QTmax) and the shortest (QTmin) QT intervals within a 12-lead ECG. Since the QT interval on its own may vary according to the heart rate, it may be corrected using Bazett's formula ($QT/\sqrt{RR}$) to give rise to QTc intervals, and the difference between QTcmax and QTcmin is the QTc dispersion (heart rate-corrected QT dispersion, QTcd). It has been supposed that one of the causes of the disturbed repolarization might be linked with autonomic imbalance, in that a decreased parasympathetic innervation exposes the heart to unopposed stimulation by sympathetic nerves. This assuming, abnormal QT dispersion may be related to obstructive sleep apnea syndrome (OSAS). A meta-analysis encompassing 222 patients with diagnosed OSAS and 182 control subjects found higher values of QT dispersion in OSAS patients. Another finding was more prominent increase in QT dispersion in the female OSAS patients. The reasons may be significantly longer values of QTd and QTcd found in healthy men. These normally higher values may explain why the OSAS in male patients resulted in less effect compared with women. Increased QT dispersion in OSAS patients may reflect disturbed myocardial repolarization and predispose to cardiac arrhythmias.

[#] This chapter was previously published in *Obstructive and Central Sleep Apnea*, edited by Joan McCormick, New York: Nova Publishers Inc., 2015.

* Corresponding Author Email: iakelmanson@hotmail.com.

In: Medicine Research Summaries. Volume 17
Editors: Zhongwen Liáng and Bibao Zhang
ISBN: 978-1-53612-751-5

Chapter 100

Update in Management of Paget's Disease of The Breast and Review of Literature: Case Report[#]

Victoria Marcos González, Cristina del Valle Rubido and Maria Concepción Sánchez Martínez
Ramon y Cajal Hospital, Spain

Research Summary

Paget´s Disease of the breast is characterized by the association of cutaneous symptoms of the areola – nipple complex and the appearance of a malignant breast carcinoma in a mean time between 6 months and two years.

Traditionally, treatment has been based on mastectomy, even in those cases where there was no evidence of breast neoplasia. However, posterior research has proven that conservative surgery with supplementary radiotherapy is acceptable from an oncologic point of view in patients with early- stage carcinoma, and even in patients in which malignant pathology has not yet been demonstrated.

Patients with cutaneous symptoms and histological confirmation of the disease, but no imaging tests that confirm a malignant breast carcinoma, arouse concern among the clinicians. Although scientific evidence defends conservative surgery in these cases, there is no consensus in literature on the long- term management of these patients.

In this chapter we will perform a comprehensive revision of the management of this entity. We will focus on the cases that present clinical symptoms and histopathological examination of Paget disease with no evidence of underlying tumors in the imaging techniques, as the diagnosis of these cases is more complex. This exposition will be illustrated with a case report of Paget´s disease of the breast that was diagnosed and treated in our hospital.

[#] This chapter was previously published in *Advances in Medicine and Biology. Volume 88,* edited by Leon V. Berhardt, New York: Nova Publishers Inc., 2015.

In: Medicine Research Summaries. Volume 17
Editors: Zhongwen Liáng and Bibao Zhang

ISBN: 978-1-53612-751-5

Chapter 101

The Importance of an Extended Gastric Myotomy for Achalasia[#]

Allison Porter*[*]*, MD, and Brant Oelschlager, MD
University of Washington Department of Surgery, Seattle, WA, US

Research Summary

Over the past 25 years, laparoscopic Heller myotomy with partial fundoplication has become the gold standard the treatment of achalasia. Historically, it was assumed that the lower esophageal sphincter was primarily made up of the musculature of the distal esophagus. As a result, the preferred approach was the left chest, first via thoracotomy and eventually thoracoscopy. When an abdominal approach was adopted via laparoscopy, a standard myotomy was performed which included the division of muscular fibers of the esophagus with extension onto the stomach for a distance of 1-2 cm beyond the gastroesophageal junction. As the approaches evolved, there became a greater appreciation of the gastric sling fiber contribution onto the LES. In 2001, research suggested that an extended gastric myotomy, including > 3 cm of length onto the stomach, resulted in less postoperative dysphagia and a reduced need for reintervention. Postoperative reflux did not increase with the extended myotomy when combined with Toupet fundoplication. These findings were confirmed in 2007, and the extended gastric myotomy has provided the best results for the treatment of achalasia. The extended myotomy is thought to include complete division of the sling fibers of the gastroesophageal junction extending onto the gastric cardia, which may contribute to postoperative dysphagia in patients who have failed after standard myotomy.

[#] This chapter was previously published in *Advances in Medicine and Biology. Volume 88,* edited by Leon V. Berhardt, New York: Nova Publishers Inc., 2015.

[*] Corresponding Author Email: allison4@uw.edu.

In: Medicine Research Summaries. Volume 17
Editors: Zhongwen Liáng and Bibao Zhang

ISBN: 978-1-53612-751-5

Chapter 102

BISPHOSPHONATE TREATMENT IN PAGET'S DISEASE OF BONE[#]

Winnie Zee Man Wat[*]
Department of Medicine, Pamela Youde Nethersole Eastern Hospital, Hong Kong

RESEARCH SUMMARY

Paget's disease of bone (PDB) is a chronic metabolic bone disease with focal increase in bone turnover. It is caused by accelerated bone resorption with subsequent compensatory chaotic bone formation, which results in bone pain, deformity and pathological fracture. Bisphosphonate is the mainstay of treatment for Paget's disease of bone. Bisphosphonates are analogs of inorganic pyrophosphate that bind avidly to the calcium/phosphate inorganic mineral phase of bone and are not hydrolyzed which lead to their sustained effects on reducing bone resorption. While symptom is the main indication for bisphosphonate treatment, the benefits to treat asymptomatic patients remain controversial and lack supporting evidence, and hence decision to treat should be based on individual risk and benefit profile. Different types and regimes of bisphosphonates have been used to treat Paget's disease of bone. Zoledronate has been shown to achieve high rates of biochemical remission and sustain long duration of suppression more than six years by a single intravenous dose. Vitamin D and calcium supplement should be given to patients at risk of vitamin D insufficiency especially when given zoledronate, as symptomatic hypocalcemia may develop. Atypical femoral fracture and osteonecrosis of the jaw are reported possibly related to the use of bisphosphonates. The risks of developing these two possible side effects in patients with Paget's disease of bone remains unknown, but are likely to be very low as the dose used are lower than the reported cases.

[#] This chapter was previously published in *Advances in Medicine and Biology. Volume 88,* edited by Leon V. Berhardt, New York: Nova Publishers Inc., 2015.

[*] Corresponding Author Email: watzm@ha.org.hk.

In: Medicine Research Summaries. Volume 17
Editors: Zhongwen Liáng and Bibao Zhang

ISBN: 978-1-53612-751-5

Chapter 103

Revealing Secrets of Hernial Sac with Advancement in Medicine#

Kumar Jayant[1,2], MD, MS, MRCS, Swati Agrawal[3], Santosh Kumar[2], MS, Mch, FRCS, S. K. Singh[2], MS, Mch, Palkesh Agrawal[4] MS, R. K. Agrawal[5], MS, K. G. Dayama[5], MS, and Rajesh Roat[2], MS

[1]Royal College of Surgeons, Edinburgh, UK
[2]Department of Urology, Postgraduate Institute of Medical Education and Research, Chandigarh, India
[3]Department of Maternal and Fetal Medicine, University of Chicago, US
[4]All India Institute of Medical sciences, New Delhi, India
[5]Sudha Hospital and Medical Research Center, Kota Rajasthan India

Research Summary

As advancement in surgery took place, we started exploring hernial sac, which showed various unexpected pathological entities of significant values. A hernia is the protrusion of abdominal contents (usually parietal peritoneum and viscera such as fat, gut or omentum) through an opening in the wall of abdomen that is designed to allow a normal structure to enter or exit. For example, inguinal hernia is hernia occurring alongside the spermatic cord, or the femoral hernia through femoral canal where hernia is seen along the lymphatics. [1, 2] Approximately 90% of abdominal hernias are in the inguinal region. The two main types are indirect inguinal hernias (~75%) and direct inguinal hernias (~25%).

This chapter was previously published in *Advances in Medicine and Biology. Volume 88,* edited by Leon V. Berhardt, New York: Nova Publishers Inc., 2015.

In: Medicine Research Summaries. Volume 17
Editors: Zhongwen Liáng and Bibao Zhang
ISBN: 978-1-53612-751-5

Chapter 104

THERMOLUMINESCENCE DETECTION OF Γ-RAY IRRADIATED HERBS[#]

Baskaran Purushothaman and Joon Myong Song*
College of Pharmacy, Seoul National University, Seoul, South Korea

RESEARCH SUMMARY

In this study, thermoluminescence detection methods like pulsed photo-stimulated luminescence (PPSL) and thermoluminescence (TL) were investigated to identify the gamma-ray irradiated medicinal herbs. Different parts as well as whole plants of the nineteen dried herb verities were irradiated using 60Co irradiator at 0-50kGy. Out of 19 non-irradiated control samples fifteen had photon counts(PCs) less than the lower threshold values(700 counts/60 s). The PCs of four other control samples (roots of osterici, angelica gigas, liriope, and whole plant of taraxaci herba) were between the lower and upper threshold values (700–5000 counts/60 s). We differentiated the 19 irradiated samples from the control samples by using their higher upper threshold values (5000 counts/60 s).The PPSL signals also showed higher upper threshold values in irradiated samples after 12 weeks of storage. The non-irradiated samples produced very low intensity in first TL glow curves (TL_1) at about 250-300 °C. A higher peak was observed in the irradiated samples (5-50kGy) at around 150-250 °C. TL ratios [ratio of the integrated areas of the first (TL_1) and second (TL_2) glow], measured after re-irradiation for the TL_1-tested samples at 1 kGy, were found to be less than 0.1 for the non-irradiated samples and higher than 0.1 for the irradiated ones. The all irradiated samples were distinguished from non-irradiated controls by the use of their TL ratio values after 12 weeks of storage under dark conditions at 23 ± 2 °C.

[#] This chapter was previously published in *Advances in Medicine and Biology. Volume 88,* edited by Leon V. Berhardt, New York: Nova Publishers Inc., 2015.
* Corresponding Author Email: jmsong@snu.ac.kr; Tel.:+82 2 880 7841; Fax: +82 2 871 2238.

In: Medicine Research Summaries. Volume 17
Editors: Zhongwen Liáng and Bibao Zhang

ISBN: 978-1-53612-751-5

Chapter 105

METABOLIC ACIDOSIS: CAUSES, DIAGNOSIS AND MANAGEMENT[#]

Luca Di Lullo*
Department of Nephrology and Dialysis, L. Parodi,
Delfino Hospital, Colleferro, Roma, Italy

RESEARCH SUMMARY

Metabolic acidosis is defined as a condition characterized by low arterial blood pH together with reduced serum bicarbonate (HCO_3) concentration; as a result, P_{CO2} decreases as respiratory compensation. If we can confirm a metabolic acidosis diagnosis, we have to provide an anion gap analysis representing the difference between plasma concentrations of the major cation (Na) and the major anions (Cl and HCO_3). Metabolic acidosis with normal anion gap can recognize renal or extra – renal causes. First ones become evident when renal bicarbonate production does not balance bicarbonate and other alkaline molecules loss consumed in normal endogenous acid production. This event is defined as renal tubular acidosis (RTA).

Extra – renal causes of normal anion gap acidosis occur when acid loads, endogenous acid production or bicarbonate loss are too high and exceed normal net acid excretion by the kidneys: the typical example is provided by chronic diarrhea.

Anion gap acidosis are mainly represented by lactic acidosis, diabetic ketoacidosis and drugs – induced acidosis as it occurs in salycilate poisoning.

This chapter was previously published in *Advances in Medicine and Biology. Volume 88,* edited by Leon V. Berhardt, New York: Nova Publishers Inc., 2015.

* Corresponding Author Email: dilulloluca69@gmail.com.

In: Medicine Research Summaries. Volume 17
Editors: Zhongwen Liáng and Bibao Zhang

ISBN: 978-1-53612-751-5

Chapter 106

Quality of Life in Brazilian Patients with Overweight and Obesity[#]

Alberto K. Arbex[1,3,*], Denise R. T. W. Rocha[1] and Valeria B. Braulio[2], PhD

[1]Endocrinology Department, Medical Institute for Teaching and Research, IPEMED, Belo Horizonte, Brazil
Internal Medicine/Nutrology by the Federal University of Rio de Janeiro, Rio de Janeiro, RJ, Brazil
[2]Federal University of Rio de Janeiro.
Internal Medicine by the Federal University of Rio de Janeiro, Rio de Janeiro, RJ, Brazil
[3]Harvard School of PublicHealth- HPSH, Boston, MA, US

Research Summary

Introduction: Excess weight is highly prevalent in developing countries. It is associated with substantial physical, as well as mental health problems. The aim of this study was to investigate how the excess of body weight influences health-related quality of life, among a subset of overweight and obese patients seeking treatment.

Methods: The Medical Outcomes Study Questionnaire Short-form Health Survey (SF-36) was applied to 113 overweight/obese patients under treatment, at the Federal University Hospital of Rio de Janeiro, and to a control group.

Results: The increase in body mass index (BMI) was inversely correlated with the SF-36 scores ($p = 0.0001$). The strength of this correlation was higher in physical aspects ($R = 0.470$, $p = 0.0001$). Patients with severe obesity showed significantly lower scores, when

---

[#] This chapter was previously published in *Advances in Medicine and Biology. Volume 88,* edited by Leon V. Berhardt, New York: Nova Publishers Inc., 2015.

[*] Corresponding Author: Alberto Krayyem Arbex, Head of the Endocrinology Dept.; Masters in Internal Medicine/Nutrology; Praça Vereador Rocha Leão, 10, Copacabana, Rio de Janeiro – RJ, Zip-Code: 22271-020. Brazil.

compared to controls ($p = 0.05$). Class 2 obese patients scored significantly lower than controls in six of eight subscales ($p<0.05$). Overweight patients were affected only in physical functioning ($p<0.05$). Increasing BMI was associated with deterioration of quality of life ($p = 0.0001$).

Conclusion: These results suggest that overweight and obesity are significantly associated with the worsening of quality of life. This correlation seems to be stronger among physical aspects, but it is also verified among some mental aspects of quality of life.

In: Medicine Research Summaries. Volume 17
Editors: Zhongwen Liáng and Bibao Zhang
ISBN: 978-1-53612-751-5

Chapter 107

HYDROXYCINNAMIC ACIDS (HCAS): STRUCTURE, BIOLOGICAL PROPERTIES AND HEALTH EFFECTS[#]

Juliana Vinholes[1], Branca M. Silva[2] and Luís R. Silva*[*,2,3,4]

[1]Embrapa Clima Temperado, Pelotas, Brazil
[2]CICS-UBI - Health Sciences Research Centre Faculty of Health Sciences, University of Beira, Covilhã, Portugal
[3]LEPAE, Departamento de Engenharia Química, Faculdade de Engenharia, Universidade do Porto, Porto, Portugal
[4]Instituto Politécnico de Castelo Branco, Escola Superior de Saúde Dr. Lopes Dias, Castelo Branco, Portugal

RESEARCH SUMMARY

Dietary polyphenols are beneficial to human health by exerting various biological effects. Hydroxycinnamic acids and derivatives are widely distributed in plant-derived food products. The main compounds of this class are caffeic, *p*-coumaric and ferulic acids, being present in nearly all plants, occurring mainly in bound, conjugated and esterified forms. These compounds play diverse roles in plant physiology and activities, which are correlated with protein synthesis, allelopathy and photosynthesis. The biological effects of hydroxycinnamic acids in humans are related to their antioxidants function, being reported to reduce or even prevent cardiovascular disorders, cancer, neurological disorders such as Alzheimer's and Parkinson's diseases. In addition antidiabetic, antigenotoxic and antimicrobial activities are

---

[#] This chapter was previously published in *Advances in Medicine and Biology. Volume 88,* edited by Leon V. Berhardt, New York: Nova Publishers Inc., 2015.

* Corresponding Author: Luís R. Silva. CICS-UBI - Health Sciences Research Centre Faculty of Health Sciences, University of Beira, Interior Av. Infante D. Henrique, 6201-506, Covilhã, Portugal. LEPAE, Departamento de Engenharia Química, Faculdade de Engenharia, Universidade do Porto, Rua Dr. Roberto Frias, s/n, 4200-465 Porto, Portugal. Instituto Politécnico de Castelo Branco, Escola Superior de Saúde Dr. Lopes Dias, Avenida do Empresário, Campus da Talagueira, 6000-767, Castelo Branco, Portugal. Tel.: + 351 272 340 560; fax number: +351 272 340 568. E-mail address: luisfarmacognosia@gmail.pt.

also reported for these compounds. The several biological functions of hydroxycinnamic acids suggest potential pharmacological activities. Thus, this chapter will be focused in the chemical structures, occurrence and biological importance of hydroxycinnamic acids providing new leads for the developments of pharmaceutical, food and agriculture products and applications to improve human nutrition and health.

In: Medicine Research Summaries. Volume 17
Editors: Zhongwen Liáng and Bibao Zhang
ISBN: 978-1-53612-751-5

Chapter 108

COUNTERFEIT DRUGS SET ALARM BELLS RINGING: COMPARATIVE ANALYSIS OF DRUG POLICIES[#]

Abdeen Mustafa Omer
Occupational Health Administration, Ministry of Health,
Khartoum, Sudan

RESEARCH SUMMARY

The strategy of price liberalisation and privatisation had been implemented in Sudan over the last decade, and has had a positive result on government deficit. The investment law approved recently has good statements and rules on the above strategy in particular to pharmacy regulations. Under the pressure of the new privatisation policy, the government introduced radical changes in the pharmacy regulations. To improve the effectiveness of the public pharmacy, resources should be switched towards areas of need, reducing inequalities and promoting better health conditions. Medicines are financed either through cost sharing or full private. The role of the private services is significant. A review of reform of financing medicines in Sudan is given in this communication. Also, it highlights the current drug supply system in the public sector, which is currently responsibility of the Central Medical Supplies Public Corporation (CMS). In Sudan, the researchers did not identify any rigorous evaluations or quantitative studies about the impact of drug regulations on the quality of medicines and how to protect public health against counterfeit or low quality medicines, although it is practically possible. However, the regulations must be continually evaluated to ensure the public health is protected against by marketing high quality medicines rather than commercial interests, and the drug companies are held accountable for their conduct.

[#] This chapter was previously published in *Advances in Medicine and Biology. Volume 88,* edited by Leon V. Berhardt, New York: Nova Publishers Inc., 2015.

In: Medicine Research Summaries. Volume 17
Editors: Zhongwen Liáng and Bibao Zhang
ISBN: 978-1-53612-751-5

Chapter 109

ROLE OF THE CLINICAL CHEMISTRY LABORATORY IN THE DIAGNOSIS AND MANAGEMENT OF METABOLIC ACIDOSIS[#]

Verena Gounden
MBChB, FCP(Chemical Pathology), MMed (Chemical Pathology)
Department of Chemical Pathology, University of KwaZulu Natal and National Institutes of Health, Inkosi Albert Luthuli Central Hospital, Cape Town, Johannesburg, Durban, South Africa

RESEARCH SUMMARY

Metabolic acidosis is a clinical disturbance characterized by a decreased blood pH. The condition is commonly recognized using laboratory investigations that include blood gas analysis and bicarbonate determination. Apart from detecting and confirming the presence of metabolic acidosis, laboratory investigations are important to assist in identifying the possible cause of the metabolic acidosis, determining the severity of the acidosis biochemically and monitoring response to treatment. In this chapter we review the utility and interpretation of common testing performed for the investigation metabolic acidosis such as arterial blood gas, serum electrolytes, anion and osmolar gaps as well as more specific and specialised testing that may assist in identifying the cause of the metabolic acidosis.

We also critically assess the methodologies that are utilized for analysis of these analytes. Additionally we describe the investigation of metabolic acidosis presenting in early childhood with particular emphasis on the laboratory investigation of inborn errors of metabolism.

[#] This chapter was previously published in *Advances in Medicine and Biology. Volume 88,* edited by Leon V. Berhardt, New York: Nova Publishers Inc., 2015.

In: Medicine Research Summaries. Volume 17
Editors: Zhongwen Liáng and Bibao Zhang

ISBN: 978-1-53612-751-5

Chapter 110

Tale Reading to Premature Babies in Neonatal Intensive Care Unit is a Further Step up in Caring for Them: Results Two Years Later[#]

Augusto Biasini[1,*], Fiorella Monti[2], Francesca Fiuzzi[1], Marcello Stella[1], Mariachiara China[1] and Erica Neri[2]

[1] Pediatric and Neonatal Intensive Care Unit
M.Bufalini Hospital Cesena, Italy
[2] Department of Psychology, University of Bologna, Italy

Research Summary

Introduction: The goal of this chapter was to examine the possible advantages of precocious tale reading to premature infants.

Methods: A picture book in one's native family language was given to newborn parents after their admission in the NICU and it was suggested that the parents read to their baby every time they thought it would be useful. On the discharge home, the same book followed the family. A questionnaire regarding the reading activity was administered and completed by parents 6-12 months after their infant's discharge. At 18 months of age, the level of infant hearing and language development was assessed by Griffiths Mental Development Scale.

Results: Overall, both in the NICU and after discharge, parents stated they liked reading to their infant and that it helped them feel closer to their babies. 64.5% of parents in the NICU and 39.2% after their baby was discharged read every day to the infant. In the first assessment, the Likert scale in the first two items ("reading helps both, we parents and our neonate" and "it makes us closer"), showed a higher score in families with very low birth weight infants (VLBW) than in those with low birth weight infants (LBW), (Fisher F (1,124)

[#] This chapter was previously published in *Health Communication: Advocacy Strategies, Effectiveness and Emerging Challenges*, edited by Rosemary M. Caron, New York: Nova Publishers Inc., 2015.

[*] Corresponding Author Email: abiasini@ausl-cesena.emr.it.

= 10,31; p=.002; F (1,123) = 16,23; p<.0005 respectively). In the same items, the Italian parents had a score significantly higher than foreign ones (F (1,24) = 6,40 p < .0005; F (1,23) = 13,76 p < .0005 respectively). Although in all the families, the frequency of reading tends to decrease in the second assessment (F 1,114 = 17,49 p < .0005), a significant positive correlation between the infant birthweight x time duration emerges (F (1,114) = 3,76 p 0,05): LBW parents say the act of reading helps them to be closer to their child only after discharge. Moreover, at 18-months of age, the intervention was associated with a higher Griffith index score in the language subscale (p = 0.011).

Conclusion: Parent book-reading intervention in the NICU enhances parent-infant interaction and promotes reading. These results suggest that starting reading in the NICU may have consistent benefits.

In: Medicine Research Summaries. Volume 17
Editors: Zhongwen Liáng and Bibao Zhang
ISBN: 978-1-53612-751-5

Chapter 111

PERSPECTIVES OF OLDER ADULTS ON HEALTH COMMUNICATION RELATED TO CANCER PREVENTION AND CARE [#]

Boaz Kahana[1,*], Eva Kahana[2], Jeong Eun Lee[2], Jeffrey Kahana[3] and Jiao Yu[2]

[1]Department of Psychology, Cleveland State University, Cleveland, OH, US
[2]Department of Sociology, Case Western Reserve University, Cleveland, OH, US
[3]Department of History, Mount Saint Mary College, Newburgh, NY, US

RESEARCH SUMMARY

The focus of this chapter is on perspectives of older adults regarding doctor-patient communication in ambulatory care visits, primarily related to cancer prevention and care. We synthesize data from several research projects conducted by the authors to illuminate older patient and primary care doctor interactions in the context of routine medical visits and visits related to cancer care. We reflect on the prevalence and effectiveness of patient proactivity for enhancing care that is responsive to patient preferences. We offer insights into the rationale of older patients in giving limited priority to goals of cancer prevention, relative to other objectives during medical visits. We provide original data about the negative impact of chronic illnesses and patient age on perceptions of physician responsiveness and on satisfaction with communication and care. Aggregate data from panel studies of community dwelling elders support propositions of the health care partnership model of communications that we propose.

[#] This chapter was previously published in *Health Communication: Advocacy Strategies, Effectiveness and Emerging Challenges*, edited by Rosemary M. Caron, New York: Nova Publishers Inc., 2015.
[*] Corresponding Author Email: Boaz.Kahana@csuohio.edu.

In: Medicine Research Summaries. Volume 17
Editors: Zhongwen Liáng and Bibao Zhang
ISBN: 978-1-53612-751-5

Chapter 112

PUBLIC HEALTH ADVOCACY STRATEGIES, EFFECTIVENESS, AND EMERGING ISSUES [#]

Ray Marks*

Department of Health and Behavior Studies, Program in Health Education,
Columbia University, Teachers College, and School of Health and Behavioral Sciences,
Department of Health, Physical Education and Gerontological Studies and Services,
City University of New York, York College, New York, US

RESEARCH SUMMARY

This chapter discusses advocacy strategies employed by public health professionals in the United States. It discusses the importance of advocacy as a strategy for enhancing public and private good, what is meant by advocacy, various advocacy strategies and strategies to foster the ability to advocate. While the effectiveness of advocacy is difficult to measure, emerging challenges that preclude a linear pathway from advocacy strategy to outcome are discussed.

This chapter was previously published in *Health Communication: Advocacy Strategies, Effectiveness and Emerging Challenges*, edited by Rosemary M. Caron, New York: Nova Publishers Inc., 2015.

* Corresponding Author: Department of Health and Behavior Studies, Box 114, 525W 120 St., New York, NY 10027; rm226@columbia.edu.

In: Medicine Research Summaries. Volume 17
Editors: Zhongwen Liáng and Bibao Zhang

ISBN: 978-1-53612-751-5

Chapter 113

WHAT ARE HEALTH CARE PROVIDERS TELLING PREGNANT WOMEN ABOUT FISH CONSUMPTION, *LISTERIA* AND FOOD SAFETY?[#]

Caroline L. Noblet[1,*], Amy M. Lando[2] and Mario F. Teisl[1]
[1]School of Economics, University of Maine, Maine, US
[2]Center for Food Safety and Applied Nutrition,
U.S. Food and Drug Administration, MD, US

RESEARCH SUMMARY

Pregnant women have unique nutritional and food safety needs and are advised to follow guidelines to promote the health of their babies. Since health care providers (HCPs) are an important source of nutrition and food safety information for pregnant women, we were interested in learning about their knowledge and perception of important food safety and nutrition topics. We used data from a national survey of OBGYNs, nurse practitioners, nurse midwifes, physician assistants, and WIC educators to examine the perceptions held by HCPs regarding their role to provide advice during pregnancy about fish consumption, *Listeria*, and general food safety. We found that healthcare providers are not systematically providing all recommended advice about each of these topics to their pregnant patients. Rather, within each category healthcare providers are more likely to supply some advice over others. These findings suggest that, especially in multi-provider practices, clarifying the role of providing food safety and nutrition information to patients is important.

[#] This chapter was previously published in *Health Communication: Advocacy Strategies, Effectiveness and Emerging Challenges*, edited by Rosemary M. Caron, New York: Nova Publishers Inc., 2015.

[*] Corresponding Author: 5782 Winslow Hall Orono, Maine 04469, US; Email: caroline.noblet@maine.edu.

In: Medicine Research Summaries. Volume 17
Editors: Zhongwen Liáng and Bibao Zhang

ISBN: 978-1-53612-751-5

Chapter 114

CBPR AND A MULTITRACK MODEL OF DEVELOPMENT: A CRITICAL ETHNOGRAPHY OF A COMMUNITY-BASED HEALTH COMMUNICATION PROJECT

Jeanette M. Dillon* and Kate Magsamen-Conrad
Bowling Green State University, Bowling Green, Ohio, US

RESEARCH SUMMARY

Scholars in development communication have called for a more participatory approach in development programs. However, the traditional, generally top-down approach associated with the modernization paradigm still dominates in practice [1]. The mere existence of participatory models has not been enough to move the participatory approach to prominence. Sparks has noticed the discrepancy between theory and practice observing that although the dominant paradigm has been disparaged and the participatory paradigm praised since the 1970s, researchers have been slow to adopt participatory methods [1]. This discrepancy may be because in practice, participation is difficult to manipulate, control, analyze and evaluate. We argue in this chapter that the participatory paradigm, specifically, community-based participatory research (CBPR), can contribute significantly to improving population health as it works in tandem with the dominant paradigm, despite seemingly antithetical epistemologies. To assess this contention, we propose interdisciplinary guidelines synthesizing various participatory approaches, and conduct a longitudinal critical ethnography of a CBPR project in a Midwestern university health communication class, as well as during subsequent student involvement across one year. Ultimately, in this chapter we seek to share

---

This chapter was previously published in *Health Communication: Advocacy Strategies, Effectiveness and Emerging Challenges*, edited by Rosemary M. Caron, New York: Nova Publishers Inc., 2015.

* Corresponding Author: Jeanette M. Dillon is a graduate student in the School of Media and Communication, Bowling Green State University, 302 West Hall, Bowling Green, OH, 43403, phone: (419) 372-8349, fax: (419) 372-0202, jmdillo@bgsu.edu.

lessons learned about CBPR by making connections between health and development communication within a pedagogical and community setting.

Reference

[1] Sparks, C. Globalization, development and the mass media. *Los Angeles: SAGE*, 2007.

In: Medicine Research Summaries. Volume 17
Editors: Zhongwen Liáng and Bibao Zhang
ISBN: 978-1-53612-751-5

Chapter 115

Health in All Policies (HiAP): Contributing to Healthy Communities#

Michelle McCarthy and Rosemary M. Caron*
University of New Hampshire, Durham, NH, US

Research Summary

Health in All Policies (HiAP) is an approach that utilizes the expertise of varied public and private sectors to consider the health implications for constituents who may reside in a geographic area for which a policy is being developed and implemented. The focus of HiAP is to maintain or improve the health status and equity of a population. HiAP is a new concept being adopted by many communities in different ways. Although there are different versions of the definition of HiAP, they all have the same goal of involving multiple sectors of the community when implementing policies to achieve the best quality of health for people. The purpose of this chapter is to review HiAP and discuss its key operating principles, procedural guidelines, goals and national and international examples where HiAP has been successfully implemented, as well as expanding HiAP to environmental issues and offer recommendations for action.

This chapter was previously published in *Health Communication: Advocacy Strategies, Effectiveness and Emerging Challenges*, edited by Rosemary M. Caron, New York: Nova Publishers Inc., 2015.

* Corresponding Author: Rosemary M. Caron, PhD, MPH, Professor, University of New Hampshire, Department of Health Management and Policy, 4 Library Way, #319 Hewitt Hall, Durham, NH, USA; Rosemary.Caron@unh.edu.

In: Medicine Research Summaries. Volume 17
Editors: Zhongwen Liáng and Bibao Zhang

ISBN: 978-1-53612-751-5

Chapter 116

USING THE MANY-TO-MANY CAPABILITIES OF SOCIAL MEDIA FOR PUBLIC HEALTH COMMUNICATION[#]

Mark J. Bonica*
University of New Hampshire, Durham, NH, US

RESEARCH SUMMARY

This chapter explores the use of many-to-many communications made possible by decreasing communications costs and the evolution of social media. The Triple Aim is discussed in the context of patient empowerment, and the opportunity for patient empowerment through many-to-many networks on social media platforms is explored. Many-to-many communications strategies for organizations are looked at from two axes: hybrid/virtual organizations vs. virtual-only organizations; and private social media platforms vs. public social media platforms. The four possible strategies are demonstrated using real organizational examples. The chapter concludes that many-to-many communication is a powerful complementary tool for the promotion of public health and public health leaders should explore using these strategies.

[#] This chapter was previously published in *Health Communication: Advocacy Strategies, Effectiveness and Emerging Challenges*, edited by Rosemary M. Caron, New York: Nova Publishers Inc., 2015.
[*] Corresponding Author: Mark J. Bonica, Ph.D., Department of Health Management and Policy, Hewitt Hall, 3 Library Way, Durham, NH 03834 Email: mark.bonica@unh.edu

In: Medicine Research Summaries. Volume 17
Editors: Zhongwen Liáng and Bibao Zhang

ISBN: 978-1-53612-751-5

Chapter 117

POPULATION HEALTH MANAGEMENT: CONSIDERATIONS FOR IMPLEMENTATION[#]

Hailey Bodwell and Rosemary M. Caron*
University of New Hampshire, Durham, NH, US

RESEARCH SUMMARY

Population health management (PHM) should not only consider the measurement and evaluation of health outcomes for a group of individuals but also conduct this action based on the monitoring of health status indicators and determinants. This base definition lends to the overall proposed definition of PHM, which is a health care delivery model focused on improving the overall health of a group of individuals through the integration of healthcare systems, community resources, professional and patient collaboration, and data management and exchange. While PHM requires a great deal of transformational change and resources, at the organization and community levels, proper identification and analysis of community needs prevents patient overuse and underuse of health system and community resources. This allows for the proper care to be provided for the right individuals at ideally a lower cost. The combination of improved community health and cost savings suggests that PHM is the future of sustainable healthcare and this chapter poses considerations for implementation in this new age of healthcare reform.

[#] This chapter was previously published in *Health Communication: Advocacy Strategies, Effectiveness and Emerging Challenges*, edited by Rosemary M. Caron, New York: Nova Publishers Inc., 2015.

* Corresponding Author: Rosemary M. Caron, PhD, MPH, Professor, University of New Hampshire, Department of Health Management and Policy, 4 Library Way, #319 Hewitt Hall, Durham, NH, USA; Rosemary.Caron@unh.edu.

In: Medicine Research Summaries. Volume 17
Editors: Zhongwen Liáng and Bibao Zhang

ISBN: 978-1-53612-751-5

Chapter 118

THE EVOLUTION OF HEALTH CARE COMMUNICATION IN THE 21ST CENTURY#

***Joseph E. Massey*[1], *Lisa Sparks*[2] *and Terrence D. Duncan*[*1]**
[1]Walden University, Minneapolis, MN, US
[2]Chapman University, Orange, CA, US

RESEARCH SUMMARY

Health care is changing. Changes in health communication mediums are pointing towards decreasing costs of health care at an individual systems level and improved access to health care information. In particular, various electronic health platforms and social media are promising to provide patients with more knowledge and access to health information, consequentially decreasing overall costs of health care. As the health care industry continues to evolve, continued challenges exist within the industry. Costs continue to escalate. Demographics of physicians trend towards an older age group and our aging population continues to grow. Different generations require different demands for proper care. The quality of care is strained with additional demands and a dwindling of resources. The challenges of the industry and physicians include determining how to improve health care quality and effective communication despite legislative changes, an aging workforce, and an increase of patients facing palliative care. Barriers to improve health care communication coupled with external challenges make operating and managing health care more complex, and more diverse than it has been decades past.

This chapter was previously published in *Health Communication: Advocacy Strategies, Effectiveness and Emerging Challenges*, edited by Rosemary M. Caron, New York: Nova Publishers Inc., 2015.

* Corresponding Author Email: terrence.duncan@waldenu.edu.

In: Medicine Research Summaries. Volume 17
Editors: Zhongwen Liáng and Bibao Zhang
ISBN: 978-1-53612-751-5

Chapter 119

Reducing the Gap: Provider Communication in the Context of Community Health and Low Health Literacy Patients[#]

Julie E. Miller-Cribbs[1*], Toni Hoberecht[2], Gloria Miller[1] and Jedediah Bragg[1]

[1]Anne and Henry Zarrow School of Social Work, University of Oklahoma, Tulsa
[2]Schusterman Library, University of Oklahoma, Tulsa

Research Summary

This chapter describes a community-based participatory research methodology (Photovoice) that was used to examine issues related to community health, conducted by a partnership between an interdisciplinary research team, a school of community medicine, and a local nonprofit organization, over a one year period. This chapter reports on a sub-set of findings from a larger community based study designed to examine issues related to health literacy and provider-patient communication. Findings reveal significant communication gaps between health professionals and community members related to health information. Several examples are provided and implications are discussed.

[#] This chapter was previously published in *Health Communication: Advocacy Strategies, Effectiveness and Emerging Challenges*, edited by Rosemary M. Caron, New York: Nova Publishers Inc., 2015.

[*] Corresponding Author Email: jmcribbs@ou.edu.

In: Medicine Research Summaries. Volume 17
Editors: Zhongwen Liáng and Bibao Zhang ISBN: 978-1-53612-751-5

Chapter 120

MEASURING HEALTH LITERACY IN SPANISH-SPEAKING ADULTS: A COMPARATIVE STUDY OF TWO INSTRUMENTS#

***Holly E. Jacobson*[1] *and Francisco Soto Mas*[*2]**
[1]Department of Linguistics, University of New Mexico, Albuquerque, New Mexico
[2]Department of Family and Community Medicine,
University of New Mexico School of Medicine, Albuquerque, New Mexico

RESEARCH SUMMARY

Although health literacy is a critical factor in medicine and public health, there are still many research gaps in the health literacy literature, including a lack of reliable instruments and consistent estimates of health literacy. This is particularly true of instruments used with Spanish speakers. The purpose of this cross-sectional study was to assess how the Spanish versions of two popular instruments compared in terms of assessing health literacy levels among Spanish-speaking adults. A total of 211 participants completed both the S-TOFHLA and the NVS, and estimates of health literacy level were determined. While S-TOFHLA scores placed more than 90% of participants at the "adequate functional health literacy" level, only 30% reached the "adequate literacy" level according to the NVS. Furthermore, the intercorrelation between S-TOFHLA and NVS total scores yielded a low coefficient ($r = 0.35$). Results indicate that the Spanish version of the S-TOFHLA and the NVS may not be used arbitrarily for assessing health literacy among Spanish-speaking adults. They measure different dimensions of health literacy, and are not comparable. Further research is recommended.

This chapter was previously published in *Health Communication: Advocacy Strategies, Effectiveness and Emerging Challenges*, edited by Rosemary M. Caron, New York: Nova Publishers Inc., 2015.
* Corresponding Author Email: FSotoMas@salud.unm.edu.

In: Medicine Research Summaries. Volume 17
Editors: Zhongwen Liáng and Bibao Zhang
ISBN: 978-1-53612-751-5

Chapter 121

INFLAMMATORY DISORDERS AND CARDIOVASCULAR PROGNOSIS[#]

Emmanuel Androulakis[1], Dimitris Tousoulis[2,*], and Theodoros Christophides[3]

[1]Cardiology Department, John Radcliffe Hospital, Oxford University Hospitals NHS Trust, Oxford, UK

[2]1st Cardiology Unit, Hippokration Hospital, Athens University Medical School, Greece

[3]Cardiology Department, Royal Free Hospital, Royal Free NHS Foundation Trust, London, UK

RESEARCH SUMMARY

Inflammation is increasingly being considered a fundamental mechanism to the pathogenesis of atherosclerosis and an important risk factor for vascular disease. Epidemiological and clinical data have shown consistent associations between markers of inflammation and risk of future cardiovascular (CV) events; however, the relationship between chronic inflammatory disorders and CV risk has only recently been recognized. A growing body of literature has suggested similar pathogenesis of autoimmune diseases, such as rheumatoid arthritis and systemic lupus erythematosus, to that of atherosclerosis. More importantly, it has been suggested that these patients may experience an increased risk for CV morbidity and mortality which cannot be fully explained by the presence of traditional risk factors. In accordance, recent data indicate that suppression of inflammation may reduce the risk of CV morbidity and mortality. Furthermore, the immunomodulatory and anti-inflammatory actions of statins may prove useful in the context of chronic inflammatory

---

[#] This chapter was previously published in *Advances in Medicine and Biology. Volume 89,* edited by Leon V. Berhardt, New York: Nova Publishers Inc., 2015

[*] Corresponding Author: Dimitris Tousoulis MD, PhD, FACC; 1st Cardiology Unit, Hippokration Hospital; Athens University Medical School; Athens, Greece; Tel: +30-210-7782446, Fax: +30-210-7784590; Email: drtousoulis@hotmail.com.

autoimmune disease, though the results are controversial. Therefore, further research consisting of large prospective cohort studies is needed to evaluate CV prognostic significance of inflammatory disorders and possible therapeutic opportunities.

In: Medicine Research Summaries. Volume 17
Editors: Zhongwen Liáng and Bibao Zhang

ISBN: 978-1-53612-751-5

Chapter 122

NON-ALCOHOLIC FATTY LIVER DISEASE (NAFLD): AN UP-TO-DATE IN THERAPEUTIC OPTIONS[#]

Fernando José Leopoldino Fernandes Candido[1], Alexandre Bueno Merlini[1,2], Caroline Tatim Saad Vargas[1] and Mário Rodrigues Montemor Netto[3]
[1]Division of Gastroenterology, Department of Medicine.
Universidade Estadual de Ponta Grossa. Ponta Grossa, Brazil
[2]Department of Critical Medicine, Hospital Israelita Albert Einstein. São Paulo, Brazil
[3]Division of Pathology, Department of Medicine.
Universidade Estadual de Ponta Grossa. Ponta Grossa, Brazil

RESEARCH SUMMARY

The non-alcoholic fatty liver disease (NAFLD) is defined by triglycerides accumulation in the liver, due to non-alcoholic causes. The NAFLD prevalence is considerably high, being up to 70% in obese patients, which is worrisome since it can lead to cirrhosis and liver failure. This study aims to review the literature recommended treatments for this condition, in adults as well as in children. One of the main points of the NAFLD pathogenesis is the insulin resistance, therefore the weight loss can be appointed as the main goal of the patient's management. Lifestyle changes, such as a healthy diet and regular physical activity, have been reported to improve the liver histology, when properly done, even though the optimal changes are yet unclear. On what concerns the drug treatment, the results are variable. The use of metformin, for instance, has not been reported to improve steatosis levels, whereas the thiazolidinediones can be used to treat NAFLD patients, when the lifestyle changes have failed. However, it must be noted that the use of these drugs have been related to increased risk of bladder cancer, bone loss, congestive heart failure in some studies, which may

[#] This chapter was previously published in *Advances in Medicine and Biology. Volume 89,* edited by Leon V. Berhardt, New York: Nova Publishers Inc., 2015

compromise its recommendation in a long term. Vitamin E, when correctly dosed, can be considered first-line pharmacotherapy in non-diabetic adults with NAFLD. Statins can be recommended if the patient presents some level of dyslipidemia. The use of some substances, such as angiotensin receptors blockers and omega-3 fatty acids is still controversial, and larger studies are needed, in order to achieve any conclusion. Bariatric surgery is reported to improve NAFLD levels, even though the lack of further evidence about the benefits and risks involved in the surgery prevents any conclusion about its recommendation. Finally, during childhood, the only NALFD treatment considered effective is lifestyle changes, since the drug therapy appears to not show better results than placebo.

In: Medicine Research Summaries. Volume 17
Editors: Zhongwen Liáng and Bibao Zhang

ISBN: 978-1-53612-751-5

Chapter 123

REGULATION OF TESTICULAR GLUCOSE METABOLISM IN (PRE)DIABETES AND ITS IMPLICATIONS TO MALE REPRODUCTIVE HEALTH

Maria J. Meneses[1,2], Raquel L. Bernardino[2], Mário Sousa[2,3], Branca M. Silva[1], Rosália Sá[2], Pedro F. Oliveira[1,2] and Marco G. Alves[1]

[1]Health Sciences Research Centre, University of Beira Interior, CICS-UBI, Covilhã, Portugal

[2]Department of Microscopy, Laboratory of Cell Biology, Unit for Multidisciplinary Research in Biomedicine, Abel Salazar Institute of Biomedical Sciences, University of Porto – UMIB/ICBAS/UP

[3]Centre for Reproductive Genetics Professor Alberto Barros, Porto, Portugal

RESEARCH SUMMARY

Diabetes mellitus (DM) represents one of the most prevalent chronic diseases nowadays. It comprehends a group of metabolic disorders characterized by chronic hyperglycaemia resulting from defects in insulin secretion, insulin action, or both. Type 1 DM is a chronic autoimmune disease that results from the pathogenic action of T lymphocytes on pancreatic beta cells leading to impaired insulin production. On the other hand, the cause for type 2 DM (T2DM) is a combination between insulin resistance and insufficient insulin secretion. The complexity of DM led to the establishment of a transitional condition, known as pre-diabetes. This intermediate state is a reversible condition in which the progression to T2DM can be prevented or, at least delayed by drug-based and lifestyle interventions.

This chapter was previously published in *Advances in Medicine and Biology. Volume 89,* edited by Leon V. Berhardt, New York: Nova Publishers Inc., 2015

It is well known that the metabolic cooperation established between testicular cells, particularly concerning glucose metabolism, is crucial for the occurrence of a normal spermatogenesis and consequently, for male fertility potential. Therefore, it is crucial to unveil these mechanisms in diabetic individuals and how they are affected by the disease and alter the fertility of the males. In the recent years, several studies have provided new information concerning pre-diabetes and DM-induced alterations in male reproductive health. Moreover, it was highlighted that testicular cells have several mechanisms that react to hormonal fluctuations and to counteract hyper- and hypoglycemic events. In this chapter, we will discuss the effects of pre-diabetes and DM in the regulation of testicular glucose metabolism and its implication in male reproductive health.

In: Medicine Research Summaries. Volume 17
Editors: Zhongwen Liáng and Bibao Zhang

ISBN: 978-1-53612-751-5

Chapter 124

NEAR-INFRARED SPECTROSCOPY AS A METHOD OF MEASURING RESPIRATORY MUSCLE OXYGENATION CHANGES[#]

Tyler M. Saumur[1,*]***, W. Darlene Reid***[1]
and Nada Basoudan[2]
[1]Department of Physical Therapy, University of Toronto, Canada
[2]Department of Physical Therapy, University of British Columbia, Vancouver, Canada

RESEARCH SUMMARY

Near-infrared spectroscopy (NIRS) is a non-invasive tool that has been used to measure changes in tissue oxygenation and blood volume or flow. Its application to the respiratory muscles over the past 20-plus years has provided insight related to compromised muscle oxygenation during exercise and disease. During tidal ventilation, healthy individuals have no impairment in respiratory muscle oxygenation; however, by manipulating oxygen availability and work rate, different trends appear. For example, during graded exercise there can be competition for blood flow between the respiratory muscles and locomotor muscles depending on the degree of stress placed on the respiratory system. This can be altered by increasing breathing resistance. The sternocleidomastoid, the main accessory muscle recruited, appears to undergo deoxygenation during incremental inspiratory loading; this deoxygenation can be further accentuated in the presence of a reduced fraction of inspired oxygen. People with chronic obstructive pulmonary disease and chronic heart failure experience similar deoxygenation changes during exercise as those induced by hypoxia in healthy individuals. Potential mechanisms could be due to inadequate gas exchange, and consequent inability to adequately regulate blood flow and provide sufficient oxygen to working muscles. Understanding these pathophysiological alterations in these populations will facilitate optimal rehabilitation and training protocols. In the near future, NIRS will

[#] This chapter was previously published in *Advances in Medicine and Biology. Volume 89,* edited by Leon V. Berhardt, New York: Nova Publishers Inc., 2015
[*] Corresponding Author Email: tyler.saumur@utoronto.ca.

likely be a technology applied to clinical settings when the demand between oxygen supply and demand to muscle is compromised such as in intensive care patients and in those with cardiac or respiratory disorders.

In: Medicine Research Summaries. Volume 17
Editors: Zhongwen Liáng and Bibao Zhang
ISBN: 978-1-53612-751-5

Chapter 125

TRAUMATIC RETINAL INJURIES[#]

Steven S. Saraf*[*], *Robert A. Prinzi, Daniel D. Kim, Ankit Desai, Nitin Kumar and Uday R. Desai
Henry Ford Hospital, Department of Ophthalmology,
Detroit, Michigan, US

RESEARCH SUMMARY

We review common retinal injuries, their incidence, prognosis, and management. Macular hole formation and choroidal rupture are discussed, which result from anteroposterior compression of the globe from a blunt force. Advances in surgical techniques have shown good outcomes in addressing traumatic macular holes that do not close spontaneously. Commotio retinae and macular hemorrhages are other common injuries. The mainstay of management for commotio retinae is observation. New advances in surgical techniques have allowed recovery of vision in patients with certain types of macular hemorrhages. Retinal detachments and dialyses require prompt surgical intervention. Additional topics include retinal pigment epithelium tears, retinal contusion, retinal concussion, retinitis sclopetaria and whiplash retinopathy.

[#] This chapter was previously published in *Advances in Medicine and Biology. Volume 89,* edited by Leon V. Berhardt, New York: Nova Publishers Inc., 2015

[*] Corresponding Author Email: SSARAF1@hfhs.org; Phone: (607) 342-8705.

In: Medicine Research Summaries. Volume 17
Editors: Zhongwen Liáng and Bibao Zhang

ISBN: 978-1-53612-751-5

Chapter 126

RESOLVING ENURESIS: FACTORS AFFECTING OUTCOMES[#]

Abigail E. Kennedy and William J. Warzak
Munroe-Meyer Institute, University of Nebraska Medical Center, Omaha, Nebraska, US

RESEARCH SUMMARY

Elimination disorders are a common childhood occurrence, and bedwetting, known as enuresis, affects millions of families. Enuresis is the elimination of urine into bed or clothing at least twice a week for at least three consecutive months in children who are chronologically or developmentally five years of age or older (American Psychiatric Association, 2013). Enuresis contributes to familial sleep disruption (Friman & Warzak, 1990), is a drain on family expenses (e.g., Mercer, 2011; Pugner & Holmes, 1996) and may interfere with effective psychosocial development (Longstaffe, Moffatt, & Whalen, 2000; Von Gontard, Baeyens, Van Hoecke, Warzak & Bachman, 2011; Warzak, 1993). In accord with the most recent terminology of the International Children's Continence Society (Hjalmas et al., 2004), enuresis denotes only nocturnal enuresis, or bedwetting. Diurnal enuresis, or combined nocturnal and diurnal wetting, is denoted as urinary incontinence.

Estimates of enuresis prevalence vary, primarily as a function of selection bias inherent in the age of the sample and the operational definition of enuresis (Hellström, Hanson, Hansson, Hjälmås, & Jodal, 1990; Järvelin, Vikeväinen-Tervonen, Moilanen, & Huttunen, 1988). Nevertheless, the findings of a number of cross-sectional, longitudinal, and population based studies of children are largely consistent. Enuresis estimates of seven year-old children may be the most relevant because these children have entered school and the social consequences of enuresis are greater and more limiting than in younger children (Hjalmas et al., 2004).

For example, Järvelin et al. (1988) sampled 3206 seven-year-old children to ascertain the prevalence of enuresis with associated somatic and genetic risk factors. They reported the overall prevalence of enuresis to be 9.5% with higher rates reported for children with

[#] This chapter was previously published in *Advances in Medicine and Biology. Volume 89,* edited by Leon V. Berhardt, New York: Nova Publishers Inc., 2015

developmental delays consistent with clinical experience (Cicero, 2012). Hellström, Hanson, Hansson, Hjälmås, and Jodal (1990) reported on the micturition habits of over 3500 seven-year-old Swedish youngsters. Isolated bedwetting was found to be 7.0% for boys and 2.8% for girls. Nocturnal incontinence of at least "once every three months" was reported to be 7.1% of girls and 11.9% of boys. In a similar study, Ferguson, Hons, Horwood, and Shannon (1986) surveyed a cohort of eight year-old New Zealand children and reported that 7.4% of the sample experienced enuresis. Finally, Butler, Golding, Northstone, and ALSPAC Study Team (2005) obtained surveys from over 8,000 families of 7.5 year old children, suggesting that the overall prevalence of bedwetting was high (15%) but the prevalence of those children who met DSM IV criteria for enuresis was much lower (2.6%). Untreated, enuresis has a spontaneous cure rate of 14-16% per year, with a very small percentage remaining enuretic as adults (Forsythe & Redmond, 1974).

The preeminent evidence-based intervention for enuresis is the urine alarm (e.g., Gimpel, Warzak, Kuhn & Walburn, 1998; Glazener, Evans, & Peto, 2005; Mellon & McGrath, 2000), first brought to prominence by Mowrer and Mowrer in 1938. Approximately two-thirds of enuretic children have become dry with alarm use and over half of these children have remained dry upon follow-up (Glazener et al., 2005).

Pharmacological treatments, primarily desmopressin (DDAVP), also are commonly prescribed despite their low curative effect and potential side effects (Vogel, Young, & Primack, 1996; Von Gontard & Néveus, 2006). This chapter describes treatments for enuresis with an emphasis on the urine alarm. Pharmacological treatments are briefly considered. To help elucidate factors affecting treatment results, we briefly discuss bladder physiology, various alarms available to practitioners, behavioral factors that influence success or failure of the alarm, as well as conceptualizations regarding the behavioral mechanism of the alarm. We conclude with suggestions for future research.

References

American Psychiatric Association. (2013). *Diagnostic and statistical manual of mental disorders (5th ed.)*. Washington, DC: Author.

Butler, R. J., Golding, J., Northstone, K., & ALSPAC Study Team. (2005). Nocturnal enuresis at 7.5 years old: Prevalence and analysis of clinical signs. *British Journal of Urology International*, *96*, 404–410.

Cicero, F. (2012). *Toilet training success: A guide for teaching individuals with developmental disabilities.* New York, NY: DRL Books.

Ferguson, D. M., Hons, B. A., Horwood, L. J., & Shannon, F. T. (1986). Factors related to the age of attainment of nocturnal bladder control: An 8-year longitudinal study. *Pediatrics, 78,* 884-890.

Forsythe, W. I., & Redmond, A. (1974). Enuresis and spontaneous cure rate. *Archives of Disease in Childhood, 49*, 259-263.

Friman, P. C. & Warzak, W. J. (1990). Nocturnal enuresis: a prevalent, persistent, yet curable parasomnia. *Pediatrician*, 17, 38–45.

Gimpel, G.A., Warzak, W.J., Kuhn, B.R., & Walburn, J.N. (1998) Clinical perspectives in primary nocturnal enuresis. *Clinical Pediatrics*, 37, 23-29.

Glazener, C. M. A., Evans, J. H. C., & Peto, R.E. (2005). Alarm interventions for nocturnal enuresis in children. *Cochrane Database of Systematic Reviews,* Issue 2.

Hellström, A. L., Hanson, E., Hansson, S., Hjälmås, K., & Jodal, U. (1990). Micturition habits and incontinence in 7-year-old Swedish school entrants. *European Journal of Pediatrics, 149,* 434-437.

Hjalmas, K., Arnold, T., Bower, W., Caione, P., Chiozza, L.M., von Gontard, A., Yeung, C. K. (2004). Nocturnal enuresis: An international evidence based management strategy. *Journal of Urology, 171,* 2545-2561.

Järvelin, M. R., Vikeväinen-Tervonen, L., Moilanen, I., & Huttunen, N. P. (1988). Enuresis in Seven-Year-Old Children. *Acta Paediatrica, 77,* 148-153.

Longstaffe, S., Moffatt, M. E. K., & Whalen, J. (2000). Behavioral and self-concept changes after six months of enuresis treatment: A randomized, controlled trial [Supplemental material]. *Pediatrics, 105,* 935-940.

Mellon, M. W., & McGrath, M. L. (2000). Empirically supported treatment in pediatric psychology: Nocturnal enuresis. *Journal of Pediatric Psychology, 25,* 193-214.

Mercer, R. (2011). *Seven steps to nighttime dryness.* Ashton, MD: Brookeville Media.

Mowrer, O.H., & Mowrer, W. M. (1938). Enuresis -- A method for its study and treatment. *American Journal of Orthopsychiatry, 8,* 436–459.

Pugner, K., & Holmes, J. (1996). Nocturnal enuresis: economic impacts and self-esteem preliminary research results [Supplemental material]. *Scandinavian Journal of Urology and Nephrology.183,* 65-69.

Vogel, W., Young, M., & Primack, W. (1996). A survey of physician use of treatment methods for functional enuresis. *Developmental and Behavioral Pediatrics, 17,* 90-93.

Von Gontard, A., Baeyens, D., Van Hoecke, E., Warzak, W., & Bachman, C. (2011). Psychological and psychiatric issues in bladder disturbances. *Journal of Urology, 185,* 1432-1437.

Von Gontard, A., & Néveus, T. (2006). *Management of disorders of bladder and bowel control in childhood.* London: Mac Keith Press.

Warzak, W. J. (1993). Psychosocial implications of nocturnal enuresis [Special issue]. *Clinical Pediatrics, 32,* 38-40.

In: Medicine Research Summaries. Volume 17
Editors: Zhongwen Liáng and Bibao Zhang

ISBN: 978-1-53612-751-5

Chapter 127

RADIOFREQUENCY ABLATION (RFA): POTENTIAL COMPLICATIONS (SKIN BURN)#

Keita Ogake[1], Hiroya Iida[2], Tsukasa Aihara[3], Shin-ichi Ikuta[3], Takayoshi Nakajima[3], Hidehiko Waki[4] and Naoki Yamanaka[3]

[1]Meiwa General Hospital, Nishinomiya, Hyogo, Japan
[2]Department of Surgery, Kansai Medical University, Osaka, Japan
[3]Department of Surgery, Meiwa General Hospital, Nishinomiya, Hyogo, Japan
[4]Department of Clinical Laboratory, Meiwa General Hospital, Nishinomiya, Hyogo, Japan

RESEARCH SUMMARY

Radiofrequency ablation (RFA) can cause a complication of thermal skin injuries. This chapter reports our experienced 2 cases of skin burns caused by grounding pad detachment and damage onthermal insulating coating surrounding RF needle. It was identified that impedance (IMP) hadan abrupt increase in the point of skin burn caused by detachment of grounding pad and an abrupt decrease by damage of the insulating coating. Hence, we monitor the tissue IMPwave during RFA as a countermeasure to prevent the complication.

This chapter was previously published in *Advances in Medicine and Biology. Volume 89,* edited by Leon V. Berhardt, New York: Nova Publishers Inc., 2015

In: Medicine Research Summaries. Volume 17
Editors: Zhongwen Liáng and Bibao Zhang
ISBN: 978-1-53612-751-5

Chapter 128

GRASSHOPPER IN WOUND HEALING ACCORDING TO ETHNOPHARMACOLOGICAL PREMISES: STUDY OF THE EFFECT OF GRASSHOPPER'S ABDOMINAL SECRETION ON WOUND HEALING[#]

Magdalena Buszewska-Forajta, Danuta Siluk and Roman Kaliszan
Medical University of Gdańsk,
Department of Biopharmaceutics and Pharmacodynamics, Gdańsk, Poland

RESEARCH SUMMARY

Modern drug discovery process involves the search of biologically active compounds derived from different sources. According to the knowledge on drugs of natural origin, active compounds were discovered in plants, insects and natural products (poisons, oils, proteins) and have been used in folk medicine since ages. The current trend in research is to identify biologically active compounds in insects. In the last decade, an impressive number of active compounds were isolated from insects, especially peptides with miotropic and antifungal properties. Moreover, the therapeutic properties of compounds derived from insects were highlighted in etnopharmacological premises. Some of these properties are observed in grasshoppers' abdominal secretion and were proposed in the treatment of wart and melanoma. Other reports concerned the use of grasshopper in the process of wound healing. Recent studies, based on etnopharmaceutical knowledge, have been dedicated to the use of grasshopper's abdominal secretion in wound healing. The folk tales from Westcentral Poland have reported that hard-to-heal wounds were treated with an ointment-like material squeezed out from abdomen of grasshoppers. For this reason, searching for a rationale beyond the etnopharmacological practice in terms of biological effect of insect's secretion, seems justified.

[#] This chapter was previously published in *Advances in Medicine and Biology. Volume 89,* edited by Leon V. Berhardt, New York: Nova Publishers Inc., 2015

While searching for the biologically active compounds, three major species of grasshoppers occurring in Poland were tested. The qualitative analysis of grasshoppers' ointment composition was carried out with the use of gas chromatography coupled with mass spectrometry (GC-MS) and enabled to obtain the main profile of secretion. Moreover, the beneficial influence of grasshopper abdominal secretion on wound healing was tested in pharmacological models. The obtained results demonstrate that grasshopper abdominal secretion helps to heal the wounds.

In: Medicine Research Summaries. Volume 17
Editors: Zhongwen Liáng and Bibao Zhang

ISBN: 978-1-53612-751-5

Chapter 129

FISH COLLAGEN: A SUBSTITUTE FOR MAMMALIAN COLLAGEN IN FOOD PRODUCTS[#]

Sushil Anand and Andreas L. Lopata[1,2]
[1]School of Applied Sciences, RMIT University, Melbourne, Australia
[2]College of Public Health, Medical and Veterinary, Centre for Biodiscovery and Development of Molecular Therapeutics, James Cook University, Townsville, Queensland, Australia

RESEARCH SUMMARY

Collagen is widely used in food, biomedical and pharmaceutical applications worldwide. Recently, collagen from marine sources has drawn attention to find an alternative to mammalian collagen (porcine and bovine) since the outbreak of BSE and FMD has dampened consumer and manufacturer confidence in collagen derived from mammalian sources. The fish processing industry generates vast amounts of fish waste (skin, bone and scale), which is a very good source of fish collagen. Moreover, many fish collagens have demonstrated to have similar biochemical and physical properties as to mammalian collagen, indicating the possible application in the food and pharmaceutical industry. However, fish collagen properties are influenced by the living habitats of fish species, therefore, collagens from warm water fish and cold water fish exhibit differences in their properties, implying to be utilized for different applications in food products.

[#] This chapter was previously published in *Advances in Medicine and Biology. Volume 89,* edited by Leon V. Berhardt, New York: Nova Publishers Inc., 2015

In: Medicine Research Summaries. Volume 17
Editors: Zhongwen Liáng and Bibao Zhang
ISBN: 978-1-53612-751-5

Chapter 130

LICHEN PLANUS: GENERAL CHARACTERISTICS[#]

Fernanda Mombrini Pigatti*[1]**, DDS, MsC,
Luís Antônio de Assis Taveira*[2]*, DDS, MsC, PhD
and João Adolfo Costa Hanemann*[3]*, DDS, MsC, PhD
[1]Department of Oral Pathology, School of Dentistry,
University of São Paulo, São Paulo, São Paulo, Brazil
[2]Department of Oral Pathology, Bauru School of Dentistry,
University of São Paulo, Bauru, São Paulo, Brazil
[3]Department of Clinic and Surgery, School of Dentistry,
Federal University of Alfenas, Alfenas, Minas Gerais, Brazil

RESEARCH SUMMARY

Lichen planus is a chronic inflammatory mucocutaneous disease of unknown cause, rarely observed in young individuals primarily affecting women between the fifth and sixth decades of life. Although its pathogenesis is unclear, several studies suggest this is a persistent immune disorder where the basal keratinocytes are probably attacked by T lymphocytes. In the skin free from hair, the lichen planus lesion is characterized by small flat-topped papules that may coalesce into plaques that may be localized or extensive. The papules often show a network of white lines known as Wickham's striae. Pruritus is usually pronounced and has a predilection for the inside of the wrists, legs, torso, or genitals. The lichen planus oral has distinct features and is easy to identify, appearing in two main forms: reticular and erosive. Other forms of the disease are not rare and four other shapes were described: papular, plake-like, bullous and atrophic. The reticular form is usually asymptomatic and involves the posterior buccal mucosa bilaterally. The erosive, although in a lesser proportion, is the most significant for the patient since they are often symptomatic lesions ranging from mild discomfort to severe pain episodes. The treatment of patients with

---

[#] This chapter was previously published in *Lichen Planus: Epidemiology, Symptoms and Treatment*, edited by Yvonne L. Summers, New York: Nova Publishers Inc., 2015.

* Corresponding Author E-mail: fer.pigatti@gmail.com.

lichen planus must be individualized. Most of recent reviews suggest that the best treatment remains high-potency topical corticosteroids, whereas systemic corticosteroids may be occasionally indicated.

In: Medicine Research Summaries. Volume 17
Editors: Zhongwen Liáng and Bibao Zhang

ISBN: 978-1-53612-751-5

Chapter 131

ORAL LICHEN PLANUS#

Vanja Vucicevic Boras[1,•], Kruna Valter[2], Meliha Solak Mekić[3] and Dragana Gabric[4]

[1]Department of Oral Medicine, School of Dental Medicine and Clinical Hospital Center Zagreb, Zagreb, Croatia
[2]Private Dental Practice, Zagreb, Croatia
[3]Clinic for Tumours, Clinical Hospital Centre Sisters of Mercy, Zagreb, Croatia
[4]Department of Oral Surgery, School of Dental Medicine, University of Zagreb, Croatia

RESEARCH SUMMARY

Oral lichen planus (OLP) is a chronic inflammatory oral mucosal disease mediated through T- lymphocytes albeit still of unknown etiology [1, 2, 3]. OLP is characterized by periods of acute disease and remission period [4]. Oral lichen planus is more frequent than skin lichen planus, it lasts longer and is more reluctant to treatment [5, 6]. Rarely, the dissapearance of OLP is seen. Numerous studies point out malignant potential of OLP [6, 7]. Prevalence of OLP is 0.5-2.2% within general population. Most frequently OLP affects persons aged 30-60 years, and more often women [4, 8]. OLP female to male ratio is 2:1 [2, 9, 10, 11]. Oral lichen planus rarely affects children [12, 13]. Approximately 16% patients with OLP have concomitant skin lesions, while genital lesions are seen in 25% of females with OLP and in 2-4% of males with OLP. Other extraoral lichen planus lesions such as esophageal, nail ones are rarely seen together with OLP [14, 15].

This chapter was previously published in *Lichen Planus: Epidemiology, Symptoms and Treatment*, edited by Yvonne L. Summers, New York: Nova Publishers Inc., 2015.

• Corresponding Author Email: boras@sfzg.hr.

References

[1] Chainani-Wu N., Silverman S., Lozada-Nur F., Mayer P., Watson J. J. Oral lichen planus: patient profile, disease progression and treatment responses. *J. Am. Dent. Assoc.*, 2001; 132: 901-9.

[2] Eisen D., Carrozzo M., Bagan-Sebastian J. V., Thongprasom K. Number V. Oral lichen planus: clinical features and management. *Oral Dis.,* 2005; 11: 338-49.

[3] Sugerman P. B., Savage N. W., Walsh L. J., Zhao Z. Z., Zhou X. J., Khan A., et al. The pathogenesis of oral lichen planus. *Crit. Rev. Oral Biol. Med.,* 2002; 13: 350-65.

[4] van der Waal I. Oral lichen planus and oral lichenoid lesions; a critical appraisal with emphasis on the diagnostic aspects. *Med. Oral Patol. Oral Cir. Bucal.*, 2009; 14: 310-4.

[5] Mollaoglu N. Oral lichen planus: a review. *Brit. J. Oral Maxillofacial Surg.*, 2000; 38: 370-7.

[6] Zhang L., Michelsen C., Cheng X., Zeng T., Priddy R., Rosin M. P. Molecular analysis of oral lichen planus. *Am. J. Pathol.,* 1997; 151: 323-7.

[7] Lanfranchi H. E., Aguas S. C., Sano S. M. Malignant transformation of atypical oral lichen planus: a review of 32 cases. *Med. Oral.*, 2003; 8: 2-9.

[8] Escudier M., Ahmed N., Shirlaw P., Setterfield J., Tappuni A., Black M. M., et al. A scoring system for mucosal disease severity with special reference to oral lichen planus. *Brit. J. Derm.*, 2007; 157: 765-70.

[9] McGrath C., Hegarty A. M., Hodgson T. A., Porter S. R. Patient-centered outcome measures for oral mucosal disease are sensitive to treatment. *Int. J. Oral Maxillofac. Surg.*, 2003; 32: 334-6.

[10] Hegarty A. M., McGrath C., Hodgson T. A., Porter S. R. Patient centered outcome measures in oral medicine: are they valid and reliable? *Int. J. Oral Maxillofac. Surg.*, 2002; 31: 670-4.

[11] Scully C., Beyli M., Ferreiro M. C., Ficarra G., Gill Y., Griffiths M., et al. Update on oral lichen planus: etiopathogenesis and management. *Crit. Rev. Oral Biol. Med.*, 1998; 9: 86-122.

[12] Laeijendecker R., Van Joost T., Tank B., Oranje A. P., Neumann H. A. Oral lichen planus in childhood. *Pediatr. Dermatol.*, 2005; 22: 299 - 304.

[13] Patel S., Yeoman C. M., Murphy R. Oral lichen planus in childhood: a report of three cases. *Int. J. Paediatr. Dent.*, 2005; 15: 118-22.

[14] Eisen D. The evaluation of cutaneous, genital, scalp, nail, esophageal and ocular involvement in patients with oral lichen planus. *Oral Surg. Oral Med. Oral Pathol. Oral Radiol. Endod.*, 1999; 88: 431-6.

[15] Rogers R. S. 3rd, Eisen D. Erosive oral lichen planus with genital lesions: the vulvovaginal-gingival syndrome and the peno-gingival syndrome. *Dermatol. Clin.*, 2003; 21: 91-8.

In: Medicine Research Summaries. Volume 17
Editors: Zhongwen Liáng and Bibao Zhang

ISBN: 978-1-53612-751-5

Chapter 132

ORAL LICHEN PLANUS: ETIOPATHOGENIC, CLINICAL, HISTOPATHOLOGICAL AND TREATMENT CONSIDERATIONS[#]

Mônica Ghislaine Oliveira Alves* and Janete Dias Almeida
Department of Biosciences and Oral Diagnosis,
Institute of Science and Technology, UNESP - Univ Estadual Paulista,
São José dos Campos, São Paulo, Brazil

RESEARCH SUMMARY

Oral lichen planus (OLP) is a chronic autoimmune disease characterized by type IV hypersensitivity, which manifests as a cell response to antigen changes that occur in the lining oral mucosa. Among patients affected by this systemic disease, 25% only have lesions in the mouth and 50% simultaneously exhibit lesions in the oral mucosa and on the skin. Oral lichen planus is more common in adult middle-aged women in their 5th and 6th decades of life. The lesions are usually bilateral, symmetrical and multifocal, and the buccal mucosa is the most commonly affected site. Six clinical forms of OLP have been described, which usually coexist: reticular, papular, plaque-like, atrophic, erosive, and bullous. In 2005, the World Health Organization classified OLP as a potentially malignant disorder. However, there is still much controversy about this classification. Several epidemiological, retrospective and prospective studies conducted over the last 20 years in different parts of the world suggest the probability of a lesion initially diagnosed as OLP to progress to squamous cell carcinoma to be 0.65 to 1.9%. Nevertheless, some authors highlight the difficulty in diagnosing OLP. Others report the lack of a universal and specific standard method for the diagnosis of this disease, which can often be confused with lesions of epithelial cell atypias exhibiting a

[#] This chapter was previously published in *Lichen Planus: Epidemiology, Symptoms and Treatment*, edited by Yvonne L. Summers, New York: Nova Publishers Inc., 2015.

* Corresponding Author: Mônica Ghislaine Oliveira Alves, 777 Engenheiro Francisco José Longo Avenue, São Dimas. São José dos Campos, SP, Brazil. Zip code: 12245-000. Fax number: +55 1239479010. Phone number: + 55 1232072962 / + 55 1281278200. E-mail: mgoliveiraalves@gmail.com.

lichenoid appearance. Hence, clinical and histopathological criteria need to be taken into consideration for the diagnosis of OLP. There is no specific treatment. Oral lichen planus should be treated when the patient manifests symptoms, since no standardized management exists that is completely satisfactory and definitive. Since most patients do not complain of symptoms, periodical follow-up for reassessment of the lesions should be performed. Moreover, the erosive and atrophic forms are almost always symptomatic and professional follow-up at shorter intervals is necessary in these cases. Corticosteroids are the most widely used drugs for the management of symptomatic lesions.

In: Medicine Research Summaries. Volume 17
Editors: Zhongwen Liáng and Bibao Zhang
ISBN: 978-1-53612-751-5

Chapter 133

Association of Oral Lichen Planus with Systemic Diseases and Amalgam Restorations: A 7 Year Retrospective Case-Control Analysis in a Northern Serbia Population [#]

Marija Bokor-Bratic[1,*] and Milos Cankovic
[1]Clinic for Dentistry, Faculty of Medicine, University of Novi Sad, Novi Sad, Serbia
[2]Faculty of Medicine, University of Novi Sad, Novi Sad, Serbia

Research Summary

Oral lichen planus (OLP) is a still poorly understood and relatively common chronic inflammatory disease of oral mucosa. A connection between OLP and certain diseases have been reported in the past, such as diabetes, hypertension, hepatitis C infection (HCV), thyroid disease, and malignant diseases. The most previous studies reporting an association between amalgam restorations and OLP /oral lichenoid lesions (OLL) suffer from absence of the control group. There is still insufficient evidence to support routine removal of all amalgam fillings in patients with OLP/OLL. This study has two objectives, first was to investigate associated systemic diseases in OLP patients, and second to estimate association between amalgam restoration and the prevalence of OLP. A total of 99 patients (74 females and 25 males, mean age 59.4 ± 13.9) with clinical and histopathological proven OLP, along with 99 matched controls without oral mucosa lesions were included in the study. This was a retrospective case-control study conducted in patients who had visited the Dental Clinic, Faculty of Medicine, University of Novi Sad, between January 2007 and December 2014.

[#] This chapter was previously published in *Lichen Planus: Epidemiology, Symptoms and Treatment*, edited by Yvonne L. Summers, New York: Nova Publishers Inc., 2015.

[*] Corresponding Author: Marija Bokor-Bratic, Clinic for Dentistry, Faculty of Medicine, Hajduk Veljkova 12, Novi Sad, Serbia, Tel : (+381) 21 661 2222, Fax: (+381) 21 526 120, E-mail: mbokor@uns.ac.rs.

Clinical characteristics of OLP lesions, other oral mucosal diseases, presence of cutaneous LP, history of allergies, medical history with special regard to their systemic diseases and medication intake, number, class (Black's classification) of amalgam restoration and its contact with lesion were recorded. The electric potential difference was measured using digital milivoltmeter, while the measurement of salivary pH was determined using pH paper indicator strips. Significant association regarding systemic diseases was found in prevalence of thyroid, autoimmune and cardiovascular diseases. We did not find any significance regarding the presence of OLP and other coexisting diseases. The mean number of amalgam restoration per patient and electric potential difference in OLP group was 4.7 ± 3.0 and 88.7 ± 76.8, and in control group was 3.6 ± 2.9 and 97.5 ± 84.7 respectively. Analysis showed that there were no significant differences in the number, class, electrical potential and salivary pH between the tested groups. This study indicates connection between thyroid gland disorders (especially hypothyroidism) and OLP. There is a need for further investigations as a screening for asymptomatic OLP in woman over the 40 years old with thyroid gland disorders, particularly hypothyroidism. There is no association between amalgam restoration and OLP, as well. Thus, result of this study does not support routine removal of all amalgam restorations in patients with OLP.

In: Medicine Research Summaries. Volume 17
Editors: Zhongwen Liáng and Bibao Zhang
ISBN: 978-1-53612-751-5

Chapter 134

QUALITATIVE EVALUATION OF AN OBESITY PREVENTION PROGRAM FOR ELEMENTARY SCHOOL-AGE CHILDREN[#]

Laura A. Nabors*, PhD, Teminijesu John Ige, MBCHB, MPH, Patrice D. DeLeon, MEd, Paige Young and Mary E. Devlin
Health Promotion and Education Program,
School of Human Services, University of Cincinnati, Cincinnati, OH, US

RESEARCH SUMMARY

Risk for being overweight is a very real health concern for our nation's children. Improving knowledge about the impact of obesity prevention programs in novel school settings, such as after-school programs, is important as time constraints may preclude health programming during the school day. After-school programs are important targets for delivery of prevention programs as there is the potential to reach children who might not have access to health programming and activities in their communities as both their parents may be working. The current paper presents information about program delivery and evaluation of the Children's Healthy Eating and Exercise Program, which was delivered in an after-school program, where children could elect to participate in the program, with parent permission as a pre-requisite. Participants for the current study were elementary school-age youth. Healthy eating lessons involved explanation of the Traffic Light Diet and providing information about MyPlate, nutrition (eating vegetables and whole grains), portion size, as well as label reading. Children reviewed information presented in lessons through art activities. After the healthy eating lesson, children participated in exercise time, involving games such as tag, relay races, basketball, Frisbee toss, developing and using their own obstacle course, etc. Children

---

[#] This chapter was previously published in *Advances in Medicine and Biology. Volume 90,* edited by Leon V. Berhardt, New York: Nova Publishers Inc., 2015.

* Corresponding Author: Laura Nabors, Ph.D., Mail Location 0068, CRC Building, Health Promotion and Education Program, School of Human Services, College of Education, Criminal Justice, and Human Services, University of Cincinnati, Cincinnati Ohio, 45221.

completed videotaped interviews to discuss what they learned in the program and whether it changed their behaviors. Qualitative methods were used to analyze interview data for themes. Children indicated that they were learning to eat more green foods and were exercising more at home. Future research should endeavor to examine change in the intervention group relative to a control group and to determine ways to transfer knowledge and behavior change in the home setting.

In: Medicine Research Summaries. Volume 17
Editors: Zhongwen Liáng and Bibao Zhang

ISBN: 978-1-53612-751-5

Chapter 135

FOREIGN BODY INGESTION IN CHILDREN: EPIDEMIOLOGY, CLINICAL MANIFESTATIONS AND MANAGEMENT#

Chiara Mameli[1], Dario Dilillo[1], Erica Galli[1], Giulia Ramponi [2], Fabio Meneghin[2], Francesca Penagini[1] and Gian Vincenzo Zuccotti[1]
[1]Department of Pediatrics, University of Milan,
V. Buzzi Hospital, Milan, Italy
[2]Department of Pediatrics, University of Milan,
Luigi Sacco Hospital, Milan, Italy

RESEARCH SUMMARY

More than 100,000 foreign body (FB) ingestions are reported to American Poison Control Centers each year and about 80% of these occur in children younger than 5 years. Presenting symptoms depend on the FB type, location, size relative to the patient's age and duration of impaction. Spontaneous object passage through the gastrointestinal system occurs in 80%-90% of cases that seek medical attention, around 10%-20% requires endoscopic removal, and less than 1% requires surgery for complications. Over 75% of all cases, FB impaction occurs at the upper third oesophagus and may be asymptomatic or present with unspecific symptoms. A detailed history, an accurate clinical examination along with appropriate imaging studies are the cornerstone of diagnosis. Biplane radiographs of neck, chest and abdomen should be performed. Moreover x-ray with a water-soluble contrast, computed tomography, ultrasonography, magnetic resonance imaging and metal detector may be useful to identify radiolucent FBs. The management depends on patient's age and clinical conditions, foreign object type, size and shape, anatomic location and which removal techniques are available. Usually the treatment of first choice is flexible endoscopy. Other

---

This chapter was previously published in *Advances in Medicine and Biology. Volume 90,* edited by Leon V. Berhardt, New York: Nova Publishers Inc., 2015.

techniques such as Foley catheter and Bougienage are used in particular for coins and blunt objects impacted in the upper oesophagus. Surgery is recommended for complications and should be considered in case of multiple magnets or lead ingestion, sharp or large FBs that don't pass through the gastrointestinal tract. Ingestion of high lead content objects, magnets and button batteries may be harmful and require specific management.

In: Medicine Research Summaries. Volume 17
Editors: Zhongwen Liáng and Bibao Zhang

ISBN: 978-1-53612-751-5

Chapter 136

IDENTIFICATION OF SOMATOSENSORY DORSAL ROOT GANGLIA NEURONS THROUGH FLUORESCENT TRACER RETROGRADE LABELING[#]

Yao-Qing Yu[1,2,*]
[1]Institute for Biomedical Sciences of Pain, Tangdu Hospital,
The Fourth Military Medical University, China
[2]Key Laboratory of Brain Stress and Behavior, PLA, China

RESEARCH SUMMARY

Dorsal root ganglion (DRG) neurons are known as nociceptor and widely used to explore the mechanism of pain. However, dorsal root ganglias contain different subtypes of neurons conducting a variety of sensory information from diverse tissues including skin, muscle, bone as well as visceral organs. To investigate the properties of one DRG neuron, it's necessary to firstly clarify the neuron and its innervating tissue. Here, I show the evidence that fluorescent tracer DiI (1, 1'-dioctadecyl-3, 3, 3', 3'-tetramethyl-indocarbo-cyanine perchlorate) can retrogradely label cutaneous somatosensory DRG neurons innervating the injected tissue. Diluted DiI (17 mg/ml, 20 μl) was subcutaneously injected at three to five sites in glabrous skin of rat hindpaw. Two weeks later, DiI fluorescent showed in both acutely dissociated lumber DRG neurons and perfusion fixed DRG tissues. Further immunohistochemical stains showed that DiI-labeled DRG neurons were transient receptor potential vanilloid (TRPV1) receptor positive small-sized and NF200 positive medium- and large-sized neurons. However, DiI rarely labeled DRG neurons of parvalbumin, a highly specific molecular marker for proprioceptors. The results support that the fluorescent tracer DiI can retrogradely label somatosensory DRG neurons, but not primary proprioceptors in DRG through muscle spindle afferent. The method is valuable to clarify the cutaneous sensory DRG neurons innervating injection site from the mixture of diverse primary afferent neurons.

This chapter was previously published in *Advances in Medicine and Biology. Volume 90,* edited by Leon V. Berhardt, New York: Nova Publishers Inc., 2015.

* Corresponding Author: Yao-Qing Yu, MD, PhD, Institute for Biomedical Sciences of Pain, The Fourth Military Medical University, 569 Xinsi Road, Baqiao, Xi'an, 710038, PR China, E-mail: yyq7803@163.com.

In: Medicine Research Summaries. Volume 17
Editors: Zhongwen Liáng and Bibao Zhang
ISBN: 978-1-53612-751-5

Chapter 137

PGE2 Induced Nociceptor Sensitization and Potentiation Contribute to Chronic Pain Conditions[#]

Weiya Ma*
Douglas Mental Health University Institute and Department of Psychiatry, McGill University, Montreal, Quebec, Canada

Research Summary

Chronic pain conditions including inflammatory and neuropathic pain severely deteriorate the quality of life of millions of individuals around the world and impose a heavy financial burden on the health care systems of our society. It is generally believed that chronic pain is developed from acute pain due to augmented peripheral and central sensitization. Peripheral sensitization refers to the hyper-excitability of nociceptive dorsal root ganglion (DRG) neurons (nociceptors) and their innervating axonal endings while central sensitization usually refers to that of nociceptive neurons in spinal dorsal horn and brain regions along pain transmission pathway.

Peripheral sensitization is a prerequisite for central sensitization. It is usually triggered by pain mediators abundantly produced in injured or inflamed tissues. Once nociceptive neurons are sensitized, their thresholds to innocuous and noxious stimuli are lowered to be hyper-excitable.

Prostaglandin E2 (PGE2) is one of the well-known pain mediators enriched in injured or inflamed tissue. By acting on its four EP receptors (EP1-4) expressed in dorsal root ganglion (DRG) neurons, PGE2 exerts both acute and chronic sensitizing effects on nociceptors. These sensitizing effects facilitate both short- and long-term plasticity in DRG neurons, thus

---

This chapter was previously published in *Advances in Medicine and Biology. Volume 90,* edited by Leon V. Berhardt, New York: Nova Publishers Inc., 2015.

* Corresponding Author: Weiya Ma, PhD, MD. Douglas Mental Health University Institute and Department of Psychiatry, McGill University, 6875 LaSalle Boulevard, Verdun, Montreal, Quebec, Canada, H4H 1R3. Tel: 514-761-6131- ext. 2935, fax. 514-762-3034, e-mail: Weiya.ma@douglas.mcgill.ca, weiya.ma2@mcgill.ca, weiyama2010@gmail.com.

contributing to peripheral sensitization in various acute and chronic pathological pain states. This book chapter summarized the progress in this field over the past two decades. Some acute nociceptor sensitizing effects of PGE2 has been well known. For example, PGE2 directly excites Na^+ and Ca^{++} channels and reduces K+ channel current, stimulates the release of pain-related neuropeptides such as substance P (SP) and calcitonin gene-related peptide (CGRP) from DRG neurons and potentiates the sensitizing effects of other pain mediators such as ATP, bradykinin and capsaicin. We and others have made recent progresses in the acute sensitizing effects of PGE2 on nociceptors by showing that PGE2 stimulates the cell surface trafficking of EP receptors and pain-related channels such as transient receptor potential vanilloid-1 (TRPV1) and Nav1.8. These acute sensitizing effects of PGE2 on nociceptors occur at the functional or the post-translational level.

We and others have reported that persistent high levels of PGE2 cause chronic sensitizing effects on nociceptors by stimulating the synthesis of numerous pain mediators such as SP, CGRP, interleukin-6 (IL-6), brain-derived neurotrophic factor (BDNF), TRPV1, P2X3, Nav1.8 and EP4 in DRG neurons. These chronic sensitizing effects of PGE2 on nociceptors occur at the transcriptional and translational levels, which lead to the long lasting peripheral sensitizations, thus contributing to the maintenance of hyperalgesia and allodynia. The broad acute and chronic sensitizing effects of PGE2 on nociceptors have laid the basis of wide application of the inhibitors of non-selective cyclooxygenase (COX), also called as non-steroid anti-inflammatory drugs (NSAIDs), and the selective COX2 inhibitors in the clinic to treat both acute and chronic pain conditions. However, duo to the serious adverse effects of NSAIDs and COX2 inhibitors in clinical applications, the antagonists of EP receptors, particularly EP4, have emerged as potential therapeutic targets downstream of COX2/ PGE2 signaling pathway to treat chronic pain conditions in the preclinical studies.

In: Medicine Research Summaries. Volume 17
Editors: Zhongwen Liáng and Bibao Zhang

ISBN: 978-1-53612-751-5

Chapter 138

ULTRASOUND GUIDED NERVE BLOCK FOR TRIGEMINAL NEURALGIA[#]

Kenichi Takechi*[*], *Kotaro Kikuchi and Takumi Nagaro
Department of Anesthesia and Perioperative Medicine
Ehime University Graduate School of Medicine, Toon, Japan

RESEARCH SUMMARY

Trigeminal neuralgia is a neuropathic disorder characterized by episodes of intense pain in the face, originating from the trigeminal nerve. Drug therapy with carbamazepine is the first choice of treatment. However, in cases where carbamazepine or similar drugs have no effect, or cannot be tolerated, neurosurgical interventions are not readily available, or the patient is too old and too feeble to tolerate an invasive treatment such as microvascular decompression or radiofrequency thermo-lesion, a peripheral trigeminal nerve block can be a useful treatment option for the acute paroxysmal period of trigeminal neuralgia.

With recent advances in sonography and the easy access of pain physicians to it, many peripheral-nerve blocks have become quite amenable to performance with ultrasound guidance. The technique of ultrasound-guided trigeminal nerve block has been reported in a small case series of trigeminal neuralgia, postherpetic neuralgia, atypical facial pain and oral and maxillofacial surgery with a high success rate with minor, transient side effects.

In this chapter, we discuss current reports concerning the ultrasound guided trigeminal nerve block for trigeminal neuralgia.

[#] This chapter was previously published in *Advances in Medicine and Biology. Volume 90,* edited by Leon V. Berhardt, New York: Nova Publishers Inc., 2015.

[*] Corresponding Author Email: ntakechi@me.com.

In: Medicine Research Summaries. Volume 17
Editors: Zhongwen Liáng and Bibao Zhang

ISBN: 978-1-53612-751-5

Chapter 139

Postoperative Monitoring after Free Tissue Transfer: Current Technologies[#]

Christopher S. Crowe, Simone W. Glaus and Gordon K. Lee
Division of Plastic and Reconstructive Surgery,
Stanford School of Medicine, Stanford, CA, US

Research Summary

Tissue transfer techniques (aka "flaps") are used in reconstructive surgery to rebuild parts of the body that may be missing as a result of trauma, cancer, or infection. A common example of this is the transfer of abdominal skin and fat to reconstruct a breast after a mastectomy to remove it due to cancer. In lower extremity traumatic wounds, muscle and skin tissue can be transferred from the back or thigh to cover exposed bony fractures and avoid amputation. A potentially devastating complication of these complex procedures is the lack of tissue perfusion, which may be caused by clot ("thrombosis") or twisting/kinking of the blood vessels associated with the tissue flap. When devoid of tissue perfusion and oxygenation, the tissue flaps undergo cell death and necrosis. Therefore, the monitoring of tissue flap perfusion and oxygenation is critical due to the time-sensitive nature of ischemic complications. This chapter discusses the various methods that are currently used, as well as lesser-known modalities that have been trialed. We discuss the characteristics of an ideal monitoring tool, and explore the advantages and disadvantages of current monitoring techniques. Such monitoring tools include clinical, photoelectric, metabolic, and dye- and image-based modalities. Clinical examination remains the gold standard for assessing flap viability and comprises evaluation of skin color and turgor, temperature, capillary refill, and bleeding. However, clinical exam can be labor intensive as it requires an in-person examination and requres experience of the healthcare provider. Examination can be supplemented by photoelectric flow measurement that involves the use of ultrasound or laser Doppler probes to assess blood velocity through target tissue. Metabolic methods have been

[#] This chapter was previously published in *Advances in Medicine and Biology. Volume 90,* edited by Leon V. Berhardt, New York: Nova Publishers Inc., 2015.

used primarily experimentally in laboratory settings, and include those that aim to measure tissue oxygenation, either directly (e.g., partial pressure or oxygen or oxygen saturation) or indirectly (e.g., pH monitoring). Dyes and radioactive tracers are imaged within a flap to serve as indicators of the degree of circulation within the tissue. Other imaging modalities have been trialed to assess for vascular compromise but have not yet found routine use in the operating room or hospital ward. Research in this area is primarily focused on developing automated methods to assess tissue oxygenation that does not require a healthcare provider to be present. Digital assessment may allow for real-time measurement of tissue oxygenation that can sense compromises in tissue perfusion and promptly alert the healthcare provider of potential compromise in perfusion through remote Wi-Fi communication.

In: Medicine Research Summaries. Volume 17
Editors: Zhongwen Liáng and Bibao Zhang

ISBN: 978-1-53612-751-5

Chapter 140

MOBILIZATION, COLLECTION AND TRANSFUSION OF GRANULOCYTES[#]

Rainer Moog*[*] *and Naska Moog
German Red Cross Blood Donor Service North-East,
Institute Cottbus and the University of Rostock, Institute of Biology, Germany

RESEARCH SUMMARY

Bacterial and fungal infections are a main cause of morbidity and mortality in neutropenic patients, especially in patients undergoing stem cell transplantation. The transfusion of granulocytes to restore host defences in severely neutropenic patients has been studied for decades. In the past inadequate dosage of granulocytes and inconsistent efficacy has limited the usage of these transfusions. The introduction of mobilizing agents such as granulocyte-colony stimulating factor (G-CSF) has renewed interest in these treatment modalities. There are some studies that have shown a benefit in neutropenic patients transfused with high doses of granulocyte concentrates. A battery of tests of granulocyte function can be performed in the laboratory to assess the quality of granulocyte concentrates, which may be useful to optimise granulocyte collection and storage. Studies that have examined granulocyte function focused on the assessment of viability, chemotaxis, phagocytosis and oxidative burst and showed that G-CSF mobilized granulocytes can be stored prior to transfusion thereby optimizing the logistics of patients' supportive hemotherapy. However, the efficacy of granulocyte transfusion is still a matter of debate and randomised controlled trials are necessary to prove the efficacy of granulocyte transfusion in the era of improved antibacterial and antifungal agents.

[#] This chapter was previously published in *Advances in Medicine and Biology. Volume 90,* edited by Leon V. Berhardt, New York: Nova Publishers Inc., 2015.

[*] Corresponding Author: Prof. Dr. Rainer Moog, German Red Cross Blood Donor Service North-East, Institute Cottbus, Thiemstr. 105, D-03050 Cottbus, Germany, Phone: +49355/4995101, Fax: +49355/4995103, Email: r.moog@blutspende.de.

In: Medicine Research Summaries. Volume 17
Editors: Zhongwen Liáng and Bibao Zhang
ISBN: 978-1-53612-751-5

Chapter 141

DEFECTS OF GRANULOCYTES AND GRANULOPOIESIS[#]

Faiza Basheer[1], Clifford Liongue[1,2], Sarah Shigdar[1,2] and Alister C. Ward[1,2,*]
[1]School of Medicine and
[2]Centre for Molecular and Medical Research, Deakin University,
Geelong, Victoria, Australia

RESEARCH SUMMARY

Granulocytes represent essential components of the immune system. Consisting of neutrophils, eosinophils and basophils, these cell populations play key roles in combatting infection by bacteria, parasites, certain fungi and viruses, as well as participating in various inflammatory processes. The functions of these cells are largely mediated by specific enzymes and other proteins found in their distinctive cytoplasmic granules or on their cell surface. The lifespan of granulocytes is limited and so they must be continuously generated throughout life via the process of granulopoiesis. This is a complex process under the control of both intrinsic and extrinsic factors. Mutations in specific components of either type of control can lead to defects in granulopoiesis, including deficiencies and excesses. In addition, mutations in key functional components of mature granulocytes can disrupt their function. This review describes granulocytes and granulopoiesis at the molecular level, and how specific gene mutations disrupt the function and/or production of granulocytes leading to severe clinical consequences.

[#] This chapter was previously published in *Advances in Medicine and Biology. Volume 90,* edited by Leon V. Berhardt, New York: Nova Publishers Inc., 2015.

[*] Corresponding Author: Prof. Alister C. Ward, School of Medicine, Deakin University, Pigdons Road, Waurn Ponds, Victoria 3217, Australia, Phone: +61-3 5227 2041, Fax: +61-3 5227 2945, Email: award@deakin.edu.au.

In: Medicine Research Summaries. Volume 17
Editors: Zhongwen Liáng and Bibao Zhang
ISBN: 978-1-53612-751-5

Chapter 142

NEAR INFRARED SPECTROSCOPY: THE NEXT STANDARD OF CARE IN NEONATAL CLINICAL MONITORING[#]

Stephanie M. Cruz, Adesola C. Akinkuotu and Oluyinka O. Olutoye
Division of Pediatric Surgery, Texas Children's Hospital,
The Michael E. DeBakey Department of Surgery,
Baylor College of Medicine, Houston, TX, US

RESEARCH SUMMARY

The management of newborns is challenging and monitoring systems that can detect changes in their health status will have an important impact on patient care. Current standard bedside monitoring systems in the Neonatal Intensive Care Unit (NICU) are not optimized to anticipate or detect early signs of clinical deterioration. To detect clinical changes, it is often necessary to analyze and integrate multiple physiological variables.

The utilization of near infrared spectroscopy (NIRS) to measure cerebral and somatic tissue oxygenation is gaining recognition as a potential tool for clinical monitoring in neonatology. NIRS has been found to be an effective form of monitoring in infants with congenital heart disease by measuring cerebral hypoperfusion. This technology evaluates the tissue oxygen saturation (rSO2) of various organs (i.e., brain, muscle and kidney) and detects states of low organ perfusion.

Animal and neonatal studies have shown a correlation between regional tissue oxygen saturation and low flow state. NIRS studies on piglets have demonstrated that a low abdominal rSO2 within 24 hours of life and a greater variability from baseline are early predictors of the onset of necrotizing enterocolitis (NEC). This low abdominal rSO2 value within the first hours of life and greater variability trend were also observed in premature infants diagnosed with NEC. In a study of neonates on extracorporeal membrane oxygenation, an algorithm was designed to detect early changes in cerebral rSO2 that were

[#] This chapter was previously published in *Advances in Medicine and Biology. Volume 90,* edited by Leon V. Berhardt, New York: Nova Publishers Inc., 2015.

indicative of low perfusion states and form the basis of an alert system of impending respiratory distress within 1 hour prior to the event.

In conclusion, NIRS shows promise as a continuous monitoring system and early detector of hypoperfusive states and respiratory distress in the pediatric population.

In: Medicine Research Summaries. Volume 17
Editors: Zhongwen Liáng and Bibao Zhang
ISBN: 978-1-53612-751-5

Chapter 143

APPLICATION OF NEAR INFRARED SPECTROSCOPY IN THE FOOD AND PHARMACEUTICAL INDUSTRIES[#]

Aderval S. Luna[*] and Jéssica S. A. Pinho
Rio de Janeiro State University, Department of Analytical Chemistry,
Maracanã, Rio de Janeiro, Brazil

RESEARCH SUMMARY

Demand for high levels of quality and safety in food and pharmaceutical production requires high standards in quality assurance and process control; satisfying this demand in turn requires appropriate analytical tools for products analysis both during and after production. Desirable features of such tools include speed easy-of-use, minimal or no sample preparation and the avoidance of sample destruction. These features are characteristic of a range of spectroscopy techniques including the near infrared. Therefore, near infrared spectroscopy is a fast and non-destructive analytical technique, and when associated with chemometrics, it becomes a powerful tool for food and pharmaceutical analysis. Indeed, near infrared spectroscopy is suitable for analysis of solids, liquids, pharmaceutical forms and food products.

Moreover, near infrared spectroscopy can be implemented during product development, in the production of process monitoring or quality control laboratories. This chapter focuses on the application of near infrared spectroscopy coupled with chemometric techniques in food and pharmaceutical products. The following topics are covered qualitative and quantitative analyze methods and on-line applications. Theoretical and practical aspects are described with food and pharmaceutical examples of near infrared spectroscopy applications associated with classification and modeling chemometric techniques.

[#] This chapter was previously published in *Advances in Medicine and Biology. Volume 90,* edited by Leon V. Berhardt, New York: Nova Publishers Inc., 2015.

[*] Corresponding Author Email: asluna@uerj.br.

In: Medicine Research Summaries. Volume 17
Editors: Zhongwen Liáng and Bibao Zhang
ISBN: 978-1-53612-751-5

Chapter 144

SARCO (ENDO) PLASMIC RETICULUM CALCIUM-ATPASES (SERCAS) AND MICRORNAS[#]

Emanuela Boštjančič[1,*] and Damjan Glavač[1]
[1]Department of Molecular Genetics, Institute of Pathology, Faculty of Medicine, University of Ljubljana, Slovenia

RESEARCH SUMMARY

Sarco(endo)plasmic reticulum calcium ATPases (SERCAs) promote muscle contraction and relaxation and are some of the major players in calcium signaling. The Ca2 +-sequestering activities of SERCAs facilitate the relaxation of cardiac and skeletal muscle. Calcium, which is released from intracellular stores into the cytoplasm, is important for signaling and leads to specific cellular responses; SERCAs pump calcium back into the endoplasmic reticulum to refill its internal storage. SERCAs are also responsible for achieving an appropriate calcium concentration within the endoplasmic reticulum to maintain the calcium-rich environment required for protein processing.

There are three major types of SERCAs (SERCA1, SERCA2 and SERCA3) encoded by three genes (ATP2A1, ATP2A2 and ATP2A3, respectively) with more than 10 distinct isoforms expressed in various tissues. SERCA regulation is clinically relevant, as deregulated SERCA function and mutations in ATP2A1-3 have been implicated in the pathology of several disease states, including Brody disease, Darier disease, heart failure and predispositions to squamous cell carcinoma and type II diabetes mellitus.

The activity of SERCAs is regulated at the level of protein content; however, the main regulators of SERCAs are believed to be the endogenous proteins phospholamban (PLB) and sarcolipin (SLN). Post-transcriptional regulation by microRNAs (miRNAs) is believed to be a novel mechanism of controlling Ca2+ transport activity. Although there is no evidence yet

---

[#] This chapter was previously published in *Advances in Medicine and Biology. Volume 90,* edited by Leon V. Berhardt, New York: Nova Publishers Inc., 2015.

* Corresponding Author Email: emanuela.bostjancic@mf.uni-lj.si.

that SLN is regulated by miRNA, there are several studies investigating the expression of miRNAs after silencing PLB in cardiomyocytes.

Similarly to SLN, no correlation has yet been observed between the expression of SERCA1 or SERCA3 and miRNA and the regulation of these two SERCAs' genes by miRNA.

However, the majority of studies performed examined SERCA2 and miRNAs, predominantly in the context of heart disease (miR-25, miR-328, miR-22, miR-1 and several other predicted and deregulated miRNAs), myoblast proliferation and differentiation (miR-151-3p) and chromosome 22q11 deletion syndrome (miR-185, miR-25). The purpose of this review is to summarize the current knowledge of the influence of miRNAs on SERCA regulation.

In: Medicine Research Summaries. Volume 17
Editors: Zhongwen Liáng and Bibao Zhang
ISBN: 978-1-53612-751-5

Chapter 145

Assessment of Vascular Supply to the Skin: A Review of Methodologies[#]

Gloria R. Sue, MD* and Gordon K. Lee, MD, FACS
Division of Plastic and Reconstructive Surgery, Department of Surgery,
Stanford University School of Medicine, California, US

Research Summary

The skin is the largest organ in the body, and represents a major barrier to microorganisms to prevent infection, allows for thermoregulation of the body's temperature, prevents loss of water, and more. The skin maintains its viability through a network of blood vessels, the subdermal plexus, which has both arteries and veins that circulate blood, oxygen, and nutrients. Surgical incisions that alter and manipulate the skin can disrupt the blood supply. Fortunately, the large plexus of vessels allow surgery to be performed without the development of necrosis, or tissue death. Nevertheless, the vascular supply to the skin is an important consideration following surgery involving the skin. Insufficient vascular supply leads to necrosis of the skin, which could require subsequent wound care, debridement, or re-operation. The assessment of vascular supply to the skin is particularly relevant following mastectomy, in which mastectomy skin flap necrosis is a costly complication, and following a free flap reconstruction containing a cutaneous component.

Mastectomy is a surgical procedure performed for breast cancer. It involves the dissection and elevation of skin flaps off of the underlying breast tissue. In this way, the surgeon can remove the entire breast tissue with the associated malignancy. However, a major complication is mastectomy skin flap necrosis, which can be a significant problem following breast reconstruction. The development of skin flap necrosis can delay postmastectomy oncologic treatment, require the need for prolonged wound care, increase healthcare costs, and create unsightly scarring. Salvage rates are inversely related to the interval between

[#] This chapter was previously published in *Advances in Medicine and Biology. Volume 91,* edited by Leon V. Berhardt, New York: Nova Publishers Inc., 2015.
* Corresponding Author Email: gsue@stanford.edu.

ischemia onset and clinical recognition, therefore early detection and ideally, avoidance and prevention are key.

Several modalities have been developed to assess the vascular supply to mastectomy skin flaps and free flaps. These methods include clinical assessment (skin color, turgor, capillary refill), non-invasive monitoring, and invasive monitoring methodologies. Non-invasive monitoring includes the use of handheld vascular Doppler, laser Doppler flowmetry, near-infrared spectroscopy, and visible light spectroscopy. Invasive monitoring includes the implantable Doppler system and microdialysis. Fluorescein dye and fluorescent angiography with indocyanine green dye are used to directly visualize blood flow to the skin.

There is no clear ideal method for skin flap assessment. In this chapter, we discuss the relative pros and cons of the above listed flap assessment methods.

In: Medicine Research Summaries. Volume 17
Editors: Zhongwen Liáng and Bibao Zhang
ISBN: 978-1-53612-751-5

Chapter 146

THE IMPLEMENTATION OF THE EU ISOTRETINOIN PREGNANCY PREVENTION PROGRAMME IN THE NETHERLANDS -HEALTHCARE PROFESSIONAL SURVEYS: A DESCRIPTIVE STUDY[#]

Ineke Crijns[1,2], Aukje Mantel-Theeuwisse[3], Rudi Bloemberg[1], Eldridge Pinas[2], Sabine Straus[2,4] and Lolkje de Jong-van den Berg[1]
[1]University of Groningen, Department of Pharmaco Epidemiology and Pharmaco Economics, Research Institute for Health Research (SHARE), Groningen, the Netherlands
[2]Medicines Evaluation Board, Utrecht, the Netherlands
[3]Pharmacoepidemiology and Clinical Pharmacology, Utrecht Institute for Pharmaceutical Sciences (UIPS), Faculty of Science, Utrecht University, Utrecht, the Netherlands
[4]Department of Medical Informatics, Erasmus Medical Center, Rotterdam, the Netherlands

RESEARCH SUMMARY

Background: The current EU isotretinoin Pregnancy Prevention Programme (PPP) has been implemented in 2003-2004, however still pregnancies occur. Health care professionals are involved in the performance of this PPP and have an important role.

Objective: The aim of performing two surveys with pharmacists and one survey with dermatologists was to explore the compliance with the PPP by community pharmacists and dermatologists, in the Netherlands. The two surveys among pharmacists have been conducted in 2007 and 2011, allowing assessment of improvement over time.

[#] This chapter was previously published in *Advances in Medicine and Biology. Volume 91,* edited by Leon V. Berhardt, New York: Nova Publishers Inc., 2015.

Methods: The three surveys were circulated via e-mail with an online link. Two surveys were send to pharmacists. In 2007, a survey was send to approximately 1000 pharmacies who are member of the Utrecht Pharmacy Panel for Education and Research (UPPER) network. In 2011, the second survey was send to the Dutch Association of Pharmacists (KNMP), especially the specific research group of the Association (n = 556 pharmacists). In 2010, a survey was sent to 564 practicing dermatologists and dermatologists in training registered to the Dutch Association of Dermatology and Venereology (NVDV).

Results: Response rates of both pharmacists questionnaires were 20% and 28% of the dermatologist questionnaire.

Pharmacists: Dispensing checks on the limitation of 30 days for isotretinoin remained stable (82%) over the years. The seven day validity of the prescription check decreased from 61% to 53%. Only 15% of the pharmacists asked the patient for a negative pregnancy test before each dispensing, and the use of prescribed contraception was checked before each dispensing by 44-49% of the pharmacists, which remained stable over time. The majority of the pharmacists (72-74%) considered that the main responsibility for the isotretinoin PPP with the prescriber.

Dermatologists: Contraception will be prescribed by 105 dermatologists (64%), in addition 35 dermatologists (22%) prescribe contraceptives after checking whether the patient is already on contraception or refer these patients to a gynaecologist or general practioner for contraception. 93% of the dermatologists were of the opinion that he/she adhered to the PPP. Analysis of the response on adherence to the different elements of the PPP showed however that 41 (25%) actually were compliant with the PPP.

Conclusion: The observed non-adherence to the isotretinoin PPP by health care professionals calls for careful evaluation of proposed risk minimisation plans and participation of all stakeholders in the developmental phase of these plans.

In: Medicine Research Summaries. Volume 17
Editors: Zhongwen Liáng and Bibao Zhang
ISBN: 978-1-53612-751-5

Chapter 147

PRESCRIPTIVE CONTRACEPTIVE USE AMONG WOMEN OF CHILDBEARING POTENTIAL USING ISOTRETINOIN IN THE NETHERLANDS COMPARED WITH FEMALE ISOTRETINOIN NON-USERS: A DRUG UTILISATION STUDY#

Hubertina J. M. J. Crijns[1,2], Nienke van Rein[1], Christine C. Gispen-de Wied[2], Sabine M. Straus[2,3] and Lolkje T. W. de Jong-van den Berg[1]
[1]University of Groningen, Department of PharmacoEpidemiology and PharmacoEconomics, Groningen, the Netherlands
[2]Medicines Evaluation Board, Utrecht, the Netherlands
[3]Department of Medical Informatics, Erasmus Medical Center, Rotterdam, the Netherlands

RESEARCH SUMMARY

Background: Pregnancy Prevention Programme (PPP) for teratogenic drugs impose contraceptive methods on the use by women of childbearing potential (WCBP). Isotretinoin has a PPP.

Objective: Evaluation of contraceptive use among WCBP using isotretinoin to assess the compliance with contraceptive methods concerning the isotretinoin PPP.

Methods: A drug utilisation study was performed using data from a drug prescription database (containing Dutch community pharmacy data) covering a population of 500,000 patients. Contraceptive use in WCBP using isotretinoin (aged 15-49 years) and in a reference group of female isotretinoin non-users (aged 15-49 years) was compared using data covering 1999 until 2006 in two year periods.

This chapter was previously published in *Advances in Medicine and Biology. Volume 91,* edited by Leon V. Berhardt, New York: Nova Publishers Inc., 2015.

Results: A proportion of 52-54% of WCBP using isotretinoin (n = 651) received contraceptives in strict accordance to the PPP - used before, during and after discontinuation of isotretinoin, compared to 39-46% in the reference group.

If a minimum of one prescription of a contraceptive during isotretinoin use was considered, contraceptives use among WCBP using isotretinoin was 61-64%. Similar patterns were seen when data were broken down in age groups. WCBP using isotretinoin prescribed by GPs versus specialists had a higher proportion of contraceptive use.

Conclusion: The intended 100% compliance with contraceptive use was not found. Reasons clarifying this low compliance are of importance before further measures are taken.

In: Medicine Research Summaries. Volume 17
Editors: Zhongwen Liáng and Bibao Zhang

ISBN: 978-1-53612-751-5

Chapter 148

NEW APPROACHES TO THE TREATMENT AND DIAGNOSIS OF ONYCHOMYCOSIS[#]

Ana Paula da Silva*, Vanderlei S. Bagnato and Natalia M. Inada
São Carlos Institute of Physics, University of São Paulo,
São Carlos, SP, Brazil

RESEARCH SUMMARY

Onychomycosis is the most common nail disease, constituting approximately half of all nail infection cases. Conventional treatment consists in the administration of systemic antifungals and antibiotics. There are a variety of clinical forms of onychomycosis and etiologic agents which may be dermatophytes, yeasts and non-dermatophytic fungi. The treatment is usually long, ranging from weeks to months.

In this chapter we discuss incidence, methods used for diagnosis and management of onychomycosis. We propose the use Photodynamic Therapy for elimination of microorganism causing of the onychomycosis, using curcumins as photosensitizer (PS). We are presenting a case of a patient treated using the curcumin. The light source is a LEDs (light emitting diodes) device emitting at 450 nm and with an output intensity of 35 mW/cm^2. The clinical result demonstrated.

This chapter was previously published in *Advances in Medicine and Biology. Volume 91,* edited by Leon V. Berhardt, New York: Nova Publishers Inc., 2015.

* Corresponding Author: Fax: +55 16 3373 9811; E-mail: paulalsir@yahoo.com.br.

In: Medicine Research Summaries. Volume 17
Editors: Zhongwen Liáng and Bibao Zhang
ISBN: 978-1-53612-751-5

Chapter 149

Onychomycosis: Prevalence, Diagnosis and Management[#]

Héctor Ricardo Galvan García*, MD
University of Guadalajara, Jalisco, Mexico

Research Summary

Onychomicosis refers to the fungal infection of nail and is the most common nail disease encountered in dermatology practice (1). In the USA, the prevalence is 14%, in differents countries 2 – 32.7%, most frequently affecting 20 – 40 year olds. 70% in foot nails, 27% hand nails and 3% in both locations (2).

T.rubrum is the causal agent in 50-85% of cases; the fast and easy diagnosis is KOH (60-80% VS 30-60% for cultures) first (3, 4, 5); second: dermatoscopy (Onychoscopy) present "jagged edge" and "longitudinal striae" at 95-100% cases (6, 7), both tests are performed in the same first consultation. Management in the past could be either medical, topical, systemic, or a combination, with many side effects and medium to poor results.

At present, laser treatment for onychomycosis is considered common practice because it is simple, quick, and no complications (8, 9); one session, 95-100% in all cases.

References

[1] Archana Singal, Deepshikha Khanna. Dermatophytic Onychomycosis. *Nail & its Disorders*. Jaypee 2013; Chapter 11: 119 – 148.
[2] Arenas Guzman Roberto. *Onicopatias.* Mc Graw Hill. 2012; Capitulo 9: 99 – 124.
[3] Mireles TEF, Rocha MFG, Brilhant RSN et al. Sucessive mycological nail testing for onychomycosis: a strategy for efficient diagnosis. *Braz J Infect Dis*. 2008; 12: 333 – 7.

[#] This chapter was previously published in *Advances in Medicine and Biology. Volume 91,* edited by Leon V. Berhardt, New York: Nova Publishers Inc., 2015.
* Corresponding Author: Dermoquirurgica .phone number: 52+3336163215/3315.

[4] Shemer A. Trau H, Davidovici B. et al. Nail sampling in onychomycosis: comparative study of curettage from three sites of the infected nail. *J Dtsch Dermatol Ges*. 2007; 5: 1108- 11.
[5] Weinberg JM, Koestenblatt EK, Tutrone WD et al. Comparison of diagnostic methods in the evaluation of onychomycosis. *J Am Acad Dermatol*. 2003; 49:193 – 7.
[6] Piraccini B.M., Balestri R., Starace M., Rech G. Nail digital dermoscopy (onychoscopy) in the diagnosis of onychomycosis. *Journal of the European Academy of Dermatology and Venerology*. 2013; 27,509 – 513.
[7] Kamraan Z., Chong David. Dermatoscopy of onychomicosis. *International Journal of Dermatology*. 2014; 53: e80 – e157.
[8] Tosti Antonella. *Dermoscopy of the hair and nails*. CRC Press. 2016; cap. 26: 179 – 181.
[9] Feldstein Stephanie, BA, Troti Christine, MAS, Frallon Friedlander Sheila. Antifungal Therapy for onychomycosis in children. Clinics in Dermatology. *Pediatric Dermatology*: Part II. 2015; vol. 33, num.3, May/June: 333 – 339.

In: Medicine Research Summaries. Volume 17
Editors: Zhongwen Liáng and Bibao Zhang

ISBN: 978-1-53612-751-5

Chapter 150

ONYCHOMYCOSIS TREATMENT: NEW EMERGING THERAPIES AND CHALLENGES[#]

Lívia Neves Borgheti-Cardoso[1], Tamara Angelo[2], Guilherme Martins Gelfuso[2], Stephânia Fleury Taveira[3] and Tais Gratieri[2,*]

[1]Faculdade de Ciências Farmacêuticas de Ribeirão Preto,
Universidade de São Paulo Avenida do Café, Ribeirão Preto, SP, Brazil
[2]Faculdade de Ciências da Saúde, Universidade de Brasília
Campus Universitário Darcy Ribeiro, Brasília, DF, Brasil
[3]Faculdade de Farmácia, Universidade Federal de Goiás, Setor Leste Universitário,
Goiânia, GO - Brazil

RESEARCH SUMMARY

Onychomycosis is a fungal infection of the fingernails or toenails caused by dermatophytes, non-dermatophytes, molds, and yeasts. It is one of the most common nail disorders affecting 10-30% of world population with a reinfection rate of 10-50%. Onychomycosis is not just a cosmetic concern. It can disturb daily activities, negatively influencing quality of life, and sporadically resulting in significant pain and discomfort. In diabetic patients, this infection increases the risk of limb amputation and local and systemic secondary bacterial infection. To date, there are several oral and topical therapies available, however, treatment is complicated due to the very anatomy and physiology of the nail: a formidable barrier to drug permeation rich in proteins. In addition, its low blood supply reduces bioavailability of orally administered antifungal drugs, leading to serious side effects in longer duration treatments. In this scenario, current research are mainly focused on two strategies: (i) synthesis of newer antifungal compounds to increase efficacy and decrease side effects and (ii) application of new therapies based on chemical and physical enhancement

[#] This chapter was previously published in *Advances in Medicine and Biology. Volume 91,* edited by Leon V. Berhardt, New York: Nova Publishers Inc., 2015.
[*] Corresponding Author Email: taisgratieri@gmail.com.

methods to surpass topical administration challenges. In this chapter the challenges for topical nail administration are discussed, presenting the human nail structure and different types of onychomycosis. The new therapies under research are discussed regarding the advantages and challenges of each for the effective treatment of onychomycosis.

In: Medicine Research Summaries. Volume 17
Editors: Zhongwen Liáng and Bibao Zhang

ISBN: 978-1-53612-751-5

Chapter 151

PLATELET-ASSOCIATED REGULATORY SYSTEM (PARS)[#]

József Bódis[1,*], Szilárd Papp[1,†], István Vermes[2,‡], Endre Sulyok[3,§], Péter Tamás[1,§], Bálint Farkas[1,¶], Katalin Zámbó[4,•], Ioannis Hatzipetros[1] and Gábor L. Kovács[5,#]

[1]Department of Obstetrics and Gynecology, University of Pécs, Hungary
[2]Instiitute of Diagnostics, Faculty of Health Sciences, University of Pécs, Hungary
[3]Faculty of Health Sciences, University of Pécs, Hungary
[4]Department of Nuclear Medicine, University of Pécs, Hungary
[5]Department of Laboratory Medicine, University of Pécs, Hungary

RESEARCH SUMMARY

Background: Blood platelets play an essential role in hemostasis, thrombosis and coagulation of blood. Beyond these classic functions their involvement in inflammatory, neoplastic and immune processes was also investigated. It is well known, that platelets have an armament of soluble molecules, factors, mediators, chemokines, cytokines and neurotransmitters in their granules, and have multiple adhesion molecules and receptors on their surface.

[#] This chapter was previously published in *Advances in Medicine and Biology. Volume 91,* edited by Leon V. Berhardt, New York: Nova Publishers Inc., 2015.

[*]bodis.jozsef@pte.hu.
[†]Correspondence Author: Tel: +36/ 20/569-4475, Fax: +36/72/536 372; E mail: karakot@freemail.hu.
[‡] Corresponding Author Email: i.vermes@home.nl.
[§] Corresponding Author Email: esulyok@t-online.hu.
[§] Corresponding Author Email: tamas.peter@pte.hu.
[¶] Corresponding Author Email: farkas.balint@pte.hu.
[•] Corresponding Author Email:zambo.katalin@pte.hu.
[#] Corresponding Author Email:kovacs.l.gabor@pte.hu.

Methods: Selected relevant literature and own views and experiences as clinical observations have been used.

Results: Considering that platelets are indispensable in numerous homeostatic endocrine functions, it is reasonable to suppose that a *platelet-associated regulatory system(PARS)* may exist; internal or external triggers and/or stimuli may complement and connect regulatory pathways aimed towards target tissues and/or cells. The signal (PAF, or other tissue/cell specific factors) comes from the stimulated (by the e.g., hypophyseal hormones, bacteria, external factors, etc.) organs or cells, and activates platelets. Platelet activation means their aggregation, sludge formation, furthermore the release of the for-mentioned biologically very powerful factors, which can locally amplify and deepen the tissue specific cell reactions. If this process is impaired or inhibited for any reason, the specifically stimulated organ shows hypofunction. When PARS is upregulated, organ hyperfunction may occur that culminate in severe diseases.

Conclusion: Based on clinical and experimental evidences we propose that platelets modulate the function of hypothalamo-hypophyseal-ovarian system. Specifically, hypothalamic GnRH releases FSH from the anterior pituitary, which induces and stimulates follicular and oocyte maturation and steroid hormone secretion in the ovary. At the same time follicular cells enhance PAF production. Through these pathways activated platelets are accumulated in the follicular vessels surrounding the follicle and due to its released soluble molecules (factors, mediators, chemokines, cytokines, neurotransmitters) locally increase oocyte maturation and hormone secretion. Therefore we suggest that platelets are not only a small participant but may be the conductor or active mediator of this complex regulatory system which has several unrevealed mechanisms. In other words platelets are corpuscular messengers, or are more than a member of the family providing hemostasis.

In: Medicine Research Summaries. Volume 17
Editors: Zhongwen Liáng and Bibao Zhang

ISBN: 978-1-53612-751-5

Chapter 152

Thromboxane A_2 and Endothelial Dysfunction: Experimental Analysis on Isolated Blood Vessels[#]

Miroslav Radenković
Department of Pharmacology, Clinical Pharmacology and Toxicology,
Faculty of Medicine, University of Belgrade, Belgrade; Serbia

Research Summary

It is known that production of certain isoprostanes is notably increased in different cardiovascular pathological conditions or endocrine-metabolic disorders related to endothelial dysfunction, which is primarily characterized by decreased activity of endothelial nitric oxide synthase, reduced formation of nitric oxide and distinctive oxidative stress.

What is more, pathological activation of endothelial cells was consistently associated with enhanced release of endothelial contractile factors, such as thromboxane A_2, an autacoid with autocrine or paracrine actions, which further contributes to vascular smooth muscle cells proliferation and hypertrophy, as well as dysregulation of vascular tone and haemostasis.

Knowing that thromboxane A_2 has vasoconstrictor properties, growing pieces of evidence suggest that direct inhibition of thromboxane A_2/prostaglandin (TP)-receptors may positively affect endothelial dysfunction and vascular tone regulation, as well. Correspondingly, it appears that decrease of thromboxane A_2 could be associated with inhibition of oxidative stress.

Thus, an improvement of endothelial dysfunction related to pharmacological inhibition of thromboxane A_2 actions could correspond to an additional therapeutic approach in treatment of certain cardiovascular and metabolic disorders. Accordingly, our experimental experience on isolated blood vessels underlying the role of thromboxane A_2 in transduction mechanisms of different vasoactive substances and possible connection with endothelial (dys)function was briefly presented.

[#] This chapter was previously published in *Advances in Medicine and Biology. Volume 91,* edited by Leon V. Berhardt, New York: Nova Publishers Inc., 2015.

In: Medicine Research Summaries. Volume 17
Editors: Zhongwen Liáng and Bibao Zhang

ISBN: 978-1-53612-751-5

Chapter 153

MEASLES PROBLEMS CURRENTLY[#]

Vanda Bostik[1], Radek Sleha[1], Rudolf Kukla[2], Miloslav Salavec[3] and Petr Prasil[4]

[1]Department of Epidemiology, Faculty of Military Health Sciences, University of Defence, Hradec Králové, Czech Republic
[2]Department of Clinical Microbiology, University Hospital, Hradec Kralove, Czech Republic
[3]Department of Dermatology, Charles University Medical School and University Hospital, Hradec Králové, Czech Republic
[4]Department of Infectious Diseases
[3]Charles University Medical School and University Hospital, Hradec Králové, Czech Republic

RESEARCH SUMMARY

Mass gathering events represent a risk for the spread of communicable diseases such as measles. For example during 2011 more than 12,000 cases of measles have been identified by ECDC through epidemic intelligence activities. The majority of case reports are un-vaccinated individuals. Cases amongst healthcare workers have also been reported. The importance of pre-travel health advice in case of mass gathering events is well-known. persons travelling can be exposed to infectious diseases such as measles and carry the acquired infections back to their home countries where they infect other people. On the other hand, visitors can bring infections from their home country, and as such, expose fellow visitors and nationals. In this context, ECDC continues to stress the importance for European citizens to be vaccinated against measles if they have not already been vaccinated or have not previously had measles. The vaccine should be administered according to their national authority recommendations.

[#] This chapter was previously published in *Advances in Medicine and Biology. Volume 91,* edited by Leon V. Berhardt, New York: Nova Publishers Inc., 2015.

In: Medicine Research Summaries. Volume 17
Editors: Zhongwen Liáng and Bibao Zhang

ISBN: 978-1-53612-751-5

Chapter 154

A Striking Increase in Seroprevalence of Measles-Specific Immunoglobulin G among Native Japanese Healthcare Students: The Impact of a Five-Year Measles-Rubella Vaccination Catch-Up Campaign in Japan[#]

Takao Kimura[1,2,*], Ai Takeichi[2], Toshiya Inoue[2], Chiaki Suto[2], Katsuhiko Tsunekawa[1,2], Makoto Nara[1,3], Yutaka Tokue[3] and Masami Murakami[1,2,3]

[1]Department of Clinical Laboratory Medicine,
Gunma University Graduate School of Medicine, Maebashi, Gunma, Japan
[2]Clinical Laboratory Center, Gunma University Hospital, Gunma, Japan
[3]Infection Control and Prevention Center, Gunma University Hospital, Gunma, Japan

Research Summary

In Japan, a measles epidemic occurred during the summer of 2007. In 2008, the Japanese government implemented a 5-year measles–rubella vaccination catch-up campaign for individuals aged 13 and 18 years old, with the goal to eliminate measles by 2012. The aim of the present study was to determine the impact of the 5-year vaccination campaign by monitoring the seroprevalence of measles-specific and rubella-specific immunoglobulin (IgG) among Japanese healthcare students from 2007-2014. A total of 2328 Japanese medical, nursing, and paramedical students from the Gunma University were serologically screened once a year at the time of admission. Our study demonstrated that the vaccination campaign

---

This chapter was previously published in *Advances in Medicine and Biology. Volume 91,* edited by Leon V. Berhardt, New York: Nova Publishers Inc., 2015.

* Corresponding Author: Takao Kimura. E-mail: tkimura@gunma-u.ac.jp; Department of Clinical Laboratory Medicine, Gunma University Graduate School of Medicine, 3-39-15 Showa-machi, Maebashi, Gunma 371-8511, Japan.

caused a dramatic increase in the seroprevalence of measles-specific IgG, from 52.7% in 2007 to 96.6% in 2013. The seroprevalence remained > 90% during 2009–2013, and then decreased to 86.2% in 2014. On the other hand, the seroprevalence of rubella antibodies remained >90%, except in 2008 (85.6%), and ended at 95.2% in 2014. In conclusion, the campaign raised the seroprevalence of measles-specific IgG by > 50% during the 2007–2014 study period. In contrast, the measles–rubella vaccination campaign did not improve the protection against rubella because the seroprevalence was already > 95% in 2007. Nonetheless, a substantial number of healthcare students remain susceptible to vaccine-preventable infectious diseases. Because their profession will involve frequent interactions with patients, including immigrants and travelers, we propose a nationwide targeted immunization program for Japanese healthcare students using serological screening prior to clinical training.

In: Medicine Research Summaries. Volume 17
Editors: Zhongwen Liáng and Bibao Zhang
ISBN: 978-1-53612-751-5

Chapter 155

PHOSPHOLIPASE D: A MAJOR PLAYER IN PATHOPHYSIOLOGICAL DISEASES[#]

***Chaithanya Chelakkot*[1], *Jaewang Ghim*[2], *Jin-Hyeok Jang*[2], *Pann-Ghil Suh*[3] *and Sung Ho Ryu*[4,*]**

[1]Division of Integrative Biosciences and Biotechnology, Pohang University of Science and Technology, Pohang, Republic of Korea
[2]Department of Life Science, Pohang University of Science and Technology, Pohang, Republic of Korea
[3]School of Life Science, Ulsan National Institute of Science and Technology, Ulsan, Republic of Korea
[4]School of Interdisciplinary Bioscience and Bioengineering, Pohang University of Science and Technology, Pohang, Republic of Korea
Department of Life Science, and Division of Molecular and Life Sciences, Pohang University of Science and Technology, Pohang, Republic of Korea

RESEARCH SUMMARY

Phospholipase D (PLD), a member of the phospholipase superfamily of lipid-signaling enzymes, catalyzes the hydrolysis of phosphatidyl choline to generate a key signaling metabolite, phosphatidic acid (PA). Multiple extracellular signals and growth factors can induce PLD activation, and through the production of PA or by binding with its binding partners, PLD can mediate a plethora of cellular functions such as proliferation, migration, endocytosis, and actin cytoskeleton remodeling. Although PLD regulated molecular and cellular functions have already been widely studied, the in vivo functions of PLD at the

---

[#] This chapter was previously published in *Advances in Medicine and Biology. Volume 91,* edited by Leon V. Berhardt, New York: Nova Publishers Inc., 2015.

[*] Corresponding Author: Sung Ho Ryu. School of Interdisciplinary Bioscience and Bioengineering, Pohang University of Science and Technology, Pohang 790-784, Republic of Korea. Department of Life Science, and Division of Molecular and Life Sciences, Pohang University of Science and Technology, Pohang 790-784, Republic of Korea. E-mail: sungho@postech.ac.kr.

organismal level have not yet been fully evaluated. Gene knockout studies using animal models have identified the critical role of PLD in several pathological conditions including Alzheimer's disease, ischemia, myocardial diseases, angiogenesis, and cancer. Considering these recent advancements concerning the pathological role of PLD, in this review, we attempt to address the plausible role of PLD in human diseases. Several recent studies have reported increased expression of PLD in cancer; and have emphasized the unambiguous involvement of PLD in pathophysiological conditions such as cancer progression and development of neurodegenerative diseases. Therefore, a thorough understanding of the full potential of PLD in pathological and disease conditions is imperative and may provide insight into the potential use of PLD as a robust therapeutic target for various diseases. The recent development of isotype-specific inhibitors may prove to be a more advantageous therapeutic approach in this regard.

In: Medicine Research Summaries. Volume 17
Editors: Zhongwen Liáng and Bibao Zhang
ISBN: 978-1-53612-751-5

Chapter 156

THE BRAZILIAN HUMAN MILK BANKS NETWORK AND THE PARTNERSHIP WITH THE BRAZILIAN MILITARY FIREFIGHTERS CORPS: FIGHTING FOR LIFE[#]

Lucienne Christine Estevez de Alencar [*]
and Dirce Bellezi Guilhem [†]
University of Brasilia, College of Health Sciences, Department of Nursing,
Campus Universitário Darcy Ribeiro, Asa Norte Brasília, DF, Brasil

RESEARCH SUMMARY

Introduction: The Brazilian Human Milk Banks Network represents great acquisition for the Brazilian Health System. It is a result from a historical process of citizenship's construction and seeks to promote the quality of processes and procedures based on the experience and accumulated knowledge by the Human Milk Bank of Fernandes Figueira Institute, Rio de Janeiro. Its mission is to "Promote health of women and children by integrating and building partnerships with federal agencies, units of the federation, municipalities, private sector and society, under the action of Human Milk Banks."

Objective: To analyze the partnership established between the Human Milk Banks and the Brazilian Military Firefighters Corps.

Method: Documental and literature analysis to verify the establishment of the historical and practical construction of this partnership.

Results: In Brazil, several Human Milk Banks developed projects or programs of cooperation with the Brazilian Military Firefighters Corps of states and cities. The fireman going on routinely in the homes of donors to collect frozen human milk. This contact

---

[#] This chapter was previously published in *Advances in Medicine and Biology. Volume 91,* edited by Leon V. Berhardt, New York: Nova Publishers Inc., 2015.

[*] Corresponding Author Email: luciennealencar@unb.br; luciennealencar@terra.com.br.

[†] Corresponding Author Email: guilhem@unb.br; dirceguilhem@gmail.com.

contributes to strengthening human links, offers the opportunity to remove doubts and give social support to the donor.

Conclusion: This type of cooperation offers flexibility to the process of collecting, processing and distribution of human milk, which helps to increase survival of preterm babies and who needs it.

In: Medicine Research Summaries. Volume 17
Editors: Zhongwen Liáng and Bibao Zhang
ISBN: 978-1-53612-751-5

Chapter 157

RISK FACTORS IN OVARIAN CANCER: A BRIEF OVERVIEW#

Ludek Zavesky[1,*], Eva Jandakova[2] and Radovan Turyna[3]
[1]Institute of Biology and Medical Genetics, First Faculty of Medicine, Charles University Prague and General University Hospital in Prague, Prague, The Czech Republic
[2]Institute of Pathology, University Hospital Brno, Brno, The Czech Republic
[3]Institute for the Care of Mother and Child, Prague, The Czech Republic

RESEARCH SUMMARY

The exact causes of the sporadic cases of the most malignant gynecological cancer, ovarian carcinoma, are still difficult to ascertain. However, they account for the vast majority of ovarian cancer cases (~ 85%). The remaining cases may be attributed to genetic alterations in genome, chromosomes, genes and regulatory factors. Within this group, germline mutations in BRCA1/2 and DNA mismatch repair genes are the best known genetic risk factors. The aim of the epidemiological studies is to find out the risk or protective factors, associated with the ovarian cancer. In this review, we focus on a brief survey of these factors, with emphasis put particularly on the genetic alterations, reproductive factors and life style factors along with dietary factors. Unfortunately, there is no factor found to be fully protective. On the other hand, there is also no factor known to result in 100% risk of development of ovarian cancer. Further investigations of factors associated with ovarian cancer are warranted, similarly as the search for novel diagnostic markers and improved treatment options.

This chapter was previously published in *Handbook on Ovarian Cancer: Risk Factors, Therapies and Prognosis*, edited by Bethany R. Collier, New York: Nova Publishers Inc., 2015.

* Corresponding Author Email: ludek.zavesky@gmail.com.

In: Medicine Research Summaries. Volume 17
Editors: Zhongwen Liáng and Bibao Zhang

ISBN: 978-1-53612-751-5

Chapter 158

Ovarian Cancer: New Therapies, Potential Risk Factors and Prognostic Values for Improving Survival Outcomes in Women#

Luiz Gustavo de Almeida Chuffa[1,*], Fábio Rodrigues Ferreira Seiva[2], João Paulo de Arruda Amorim[3] and Luiz Antonio Lupi Júnior[1]

[1]Department of Anatomy - IBB/UNESP, Institute of Biosciences of Botucatu, Univ. Estadual Paulista, SP, Brazil
[2]Department of Biology and Technology – UENP/CLM - Universidade Estadual do Norte do Paraná, PR, Brazil
[3]Department of Anatomy - UNIOESTE/FB – Universidade Estadual do Oeste do Paraná, PR, Brazil

Research Summary

Ovarian cancer (OC) is the third most diagnosed gynecologic cancer and the first leading cause of death from all of gynecological malignancies. OC presents with the highest mortality rate, largely due to its advanced stage at the time of diagnosis. About 90% of these cases are epithelial ovarian cancer (EOC), and 70% are diagnosed with widespread intra-abdominal or distant metastases. Unfortunately, the frequency of invasive and advanced EOC is mostly due to the lack of a suitable and sufficiently reliable screening tool at the moment of diagnosis. Despite new strategies and improvements in surgical techniques and chemotherapeutic options, a 5-year survival rate for invasive EOC is approximately 46%. The main symptoms reported from OC include abnormal vaginal bleeding, pelvic and abdominal pain, weight loss,

---

This chapter was previously published in *Handbook on Ovarian Cancer: Risk Factors, Therapies and Prognosis*, edited by Bethany R. Collier, New York: Nova Publishers Inc., 2015.

* Corresponding Author: Luiz Gustavo de Almeida Chuffa. E-mail: guchuffa@yahoo.com.br. Department of Anatomy, Institute of Biosciences of Botucatu, Univ. Estadual Paulista, SP. Address: Distrite of Rubião Júnior s/n, Botucatu - São Paulo/SP.

back pain, urinary urgency, and fatigue, which contribute to the difficulties of an early diagnosis, thereby resulting in low prognosis and survival rates. The treatment of early stage OC involves surgical resection followed by chemotherapy; clinical trials show an overall survival rate with adjuvant platinum-based chemotherapy, but this treatment in sub-groups of patients may vary according to different prognosis. Many risk factors associated with breast cancer are also related to the risk of other gynecologic cancers, such as OC. They include current age, age at menarche, parity, and first-degree family history with a wide inter-individual genetic variations in the susceptibility of OC. Recent studies regarding genome-wide association have reported several single nucleotide polymorphisms that confer low-penetrance susceptibility to EOC. In addition, mutations in BRCA gene, the gene that produces breast cancer-linked protein, are strongly associated with hereditary forms of OC. Hormone replacement therapy is further associated with increased risks of OC, mainly long duration use of both unopposed estrogens and estrogens plus progestins, regardless of treatment regimen. Independent prognostic factors are often considered including those described by International Federation of Gynecology and Obstetrics (FIGO), such as stage, tumor grade, volume of residual OC, and specific biomarkers for predicting survival in ovarian tumor patients. This chapter will discuss the new therapies, major risk factors in early and advanced ovarian cancer stage, and most prognostic factors as a tool for improving the survival rate outcomes in women.

In: Medicine Research Summaries. Volume 17
Editors: Zhongwen Liáng and Bibao Zhang

ISBN: 978-1-53612-751-5

Chapter 159

MICRORNAS IN DIAGNOSIS OF OVARIAN CANCER: POTENTIAL, CHALLENGES, PITFALLS[#]

Ludek Zavesky[1,*], Eva Jandakova[2], Lucie Langmeierova[3], Vit Weinberger[4] and Lubos Minar[4]

[1]Institute of Biology and Medical Genetics, First Faculty of Medicine, Charles University Prague and General University Hospital in Prague, Prague, The Czech Republic
[2]Institute of Pathology, University Hospital Brno, Brno, The Czech Republic
[3]Faculty Transfusion Centre, General University Hospital in Prague, Prague, The Czech Republic
[4]Department of Obstetrics and Gynecology, University Hospital Brno, Brno, The Czech Republic

RESEARCH SUMMARY

Ovarian cancer is the most deadly gynecological cancer. High mortality of the patients is usually associated with the progression of the disease. Most of the patients are diagnosed within the advanced stages due to lacking relevant diagnostic and screening markers. Achieving the diagnosis in the early stages of disease is a prerequisite of the more successful treatment of ovarian cancer. In this review, we focus on the recent progress in research focused on circulating, particularly cell-free microRNAs expression in diagnostically relevant samples such as blood, plasma/serum and urine. More research will be needed to establish circulating and extracellular microRNAs as the novel diagnostic markers for ovarian cancer.

[#] This chapter was previously published in *Handbook on Ovarian Cancer: Risk Factors, Therapies and Prognosis*, edited by Bethany R. Collier, New York: Nova Publishers Inc., 2015.

[*] Corresponding Author Email: ludek.zavesky@gmail.com.

In: Medicine Research Summaries. Volume 17
Editors: Zhongwen Liáng and Bibao Zhang
ISBN: 978-1-53612-751-5

Chapter 160

IMMUNOTHERAPY AND TARGET THERAPY: NEW APPROACHES IN OVARIAN CANCER[#]

Rosekeila Simões Nomelini[1]*, Millena Prata Jammal[1], Agrimaldo Martins Filho[1] and Eddie Fernando Candido Murta[1]
[1]Discipline of Gynecology and Obstetrics, Oncological Research Institute (IPON), Federal University of the Triângulo Mineiro, Uberaba, MG, Brazil

RESEARCH SUMMARY

Ovarian cancer remains the leading cause of death among gynecological malignancies. Surgery should be performed in adnexal masses suspected of ovarian cancer for diagnosis, staging and treatment. The debulking surgery is still the main surgical approach in advanced primary ovarian cancer. The adjuvant treatment is performed with taxanes and platinum-based chemotherapy. The addition of the bevacizumab, an anti-angiogenic agent, is recommended. Adjuvant treatment in ovarian cancer in advanced stage leads to an improvement in disease-free survival in approximately 10-30% of patients, depending on the stage and residual disease. Retrospective data show better outcomes in patients who underwent complete cytoreduction. Immunotherapy can be insufficient to eliminate all tumor when used alone. However, the use after surgery and chemotherapy can be useful to eliminate remaining tumor cells.

In recent years, there was an increase in the use of immunohistochemical markers in ovarian cancer. Most of the published data refers to the use of antibodies for diagnosis, some markers also has prognostic value.

[#] This chapter was previously published in *Handbook on Ovarian Cancer: Risk Factors, Therapies and Prognosis*, edited by Bethany R. Collier, New York: Nova Publishers Inc., 2015.

* Corresponding Author: Prof. Rosekeila Simões Nomelini, Oncological Research Institute (IPON)/Discipline of Gynecology and Obstetrics, UFTM, Av. Getúlio Guaritá, s/n, Bairro Abadia, 38025-440 Uberaba-MG, Brazil. E-mail: rosekeila@terra.com.br.

In general, when immunohistochemistry is utilized for diagnosis markers panels provide better information than the use of a single antibody. Ovarian cancer is a heterogeneous disease; each of the subtypes is associated with different genetic risk factors and molecular events during oncogenesis. Each subtype responds differently to chemotherapy.

The tendency of ovarian cancer treatment is moving toward different therapies for their specific subtypes. It is likely that a panel of tumor markers will be required to detect all subtypes of the disease. The ovarian cancer subtypes should be considered as distinct diseases in biomarker studies and clinical trials, in order to relate the biomarker, diagnosis and prognosis.

The main aim of this chapter is to provide an update of the current treatments in ovarian cancer. The section also demonstrates the potential targets of future therapies, such as immunotherapy and target therapies.

In: Medicine Research Summaries. Volume 17
Editors: Zhongwen Liáng and Bibao Zhang
ISBN: 978-1-53612-751-5

Chapter 161

DOPAMINE RECEPTOR: A TREATMENT TARGET FOR OVARIAN CANCER[#]

Min Yong, Jinyan Li, Lina Hu and Tinghe Yu*
Key Medical Laboratory of Obstetrics and Gynecology,
The Second Affiliated Hospital,
Chongqing Medical University, Chongqing, China

RESEARCH SUMMARY

The physiological actions of dopamine (DA) are mediated by five receptors (DR) that are divided into two major groups: D1 and D2. The D1-like subtypes (DR1 and DR5) can activate the adenylate cyclase thereby increasing the cAMP level, but the D2-like subtypes (DR2, DR3 and DR4) lead to the opposite effect (i.e., decreasing the cAMP level). The role of DA and DR in cancer therapy remains unclear. Human ovarian cancer cells express all DR except DR3. The DR2-mediated inhibition of the Src activation can reverse the permissive microenvironment for tumor growth attributable to chronic stress. DA favors the uptake of cisplatin via stabilizing tumor blood vessels, which results from DR1-mediated activation of the cAMP–kinase A signaling pathway. An antagonist of DR2 can inhibit tumor growth by targeting the VEGFR-2/PI3K/mTOR pathway. The blockage of D2-family proteins inhibits growth of cancer cells (including cancer stem cells). Therefore, DR2 can be a target for cancer treatments.

[#] This chapter was previously published in *Handbook on Ovarian Cancer: Risk Factors, Therapies and Prognosis*, edited by Bethany R. Collier, New York: Nova Publishers Inc., 2015.

[*] Corresponding Author Email: yutinghe@hotmail.com.

In: Medicine Research Summaries. Volume 17
Editors: Zhongwen Liáng and Bibao Zhang
ISBN: 978-1-53612-751-5

Chapter 162

MALIGNANT OVARIAN GERM CELL TUMORS: TREATMENT AND PROGNOSIS[#]

R. Díaz-Murillo, M. Lombarte-García, J. de Santiago and I. Zapardiel*
Gynecologic Oncology Unit, La Paz University Hospital-IdiPAZ,
Madrid, Spain

RESEARCH SUMMARY

Malignant ovarian germ cell tumors are a very uncommon disorder. The incidence is estimated in 0.5/100000 women. They represent only a 5 percent of ovarian cancers overall. Mostly, ovarian germ cell neoplasms affect women aged between 10-30 years and they constitute in this collective the most frequent ovarian tumor (around 70%).

These type of neoplasms have their origin on the primordial ovarian cells. There are different hystological subtypes: they can be divided into embryo-like neoplasms (immature teratoma and dysgerminoma) and placenta-like neoplasms (similar than extraembrionic fetal-derived cell population), or a mixture. The main malignant ovarian germ cell are: *immature teratoma, dysgerminoma, endodermal sinus (yolksac) tumors, embryonal cell carcinoma, choriocarcinoma, polyembrioma and mixed germ cell tumors.*

Basically, patients' present abdominal pain with abdominal enlargement, abnormal vaginal bleeding and/or precocious puberty. Tumor marker tester can be increased, as AFP, beta-HCG, inhibin, CA 125, LDH.

Malignant ovarian germ cell tumors are staged by the International Federation of Gynecology and Obstetrics (FIGO) into: stage I, confined to the ovarian; stage II extension into other pelvic organs; stage III, disease extended into the abdmen or retroperitoneal lymphnodes; stage IV, metastatic disease beyond the abdomen or affecting the liver. Frequently, the tumor is diagnosed at stage I.

[#] This chapter was previously published in *Handbook on Ovarian Cancer: Risk Factors, Therapies and Prognosis*, edited by Bethany R. Collier, New York: Nova Publishers Inc., 2015.

* Corresponding Author Email: ignaciozapardiel@hotmail.com.

Treatment involves primary surgery, depending on the preferences of the patient to conserve or not her fertility. Fertility-sparing surgery must be done laparoscopically with an intraoperative frozen section evaluation. At advanced stages, chemotherapy can be involved to complete the treatment. Malignant ovarian germ cell tumors have an excellent prognosis: 5-years survival after complete suitable treatment is more than 85%.

In this chapter, treatment and prognosis are going to be explained, according to the official international guidelines.

In: Medicine Research Summaries. Volume 17
Editors: Zhongwen Liáng and Bibao Zhang

ISBN: 978-1-53612-751-5

Chapter 163

CONTROVERSIES IN THE MANAGEMENT OF OVARIAN CANCER#

Grace Hwei Ching Tan[1] and Melissa Ching Ching Teo[2*]
[1]MBBS (London), MRCS (Edinburgh),
Division of Surgical Oncology, National Cancer Centre Singapore
[2]MBBS, FRCS (Edinburgh), MPH (Johns Hopkins),
Division of Surgical Oncology,
National Cancer Centre Singapore

RESEARCH SUMMARY

Ovarian cancer is one of the commonest malignancy in women worldwide and has an annual incidence of 239 000 [1, 2]. It is the most lethal of all the gynaecological malignancies, the fifth leading cause of cancer death, and claimed 151 917 lives in 2012 [1, 2]. Ovarian cancer often presents at an advanced stage, with the involvement of the peritoneal surface either at the initial diagnosis or at recurrence. Despite the advances made in the surgical techniques and chemotherapeutic options regarding agents, schedule, and route of administration, majority of the patients recur and eventually succumb to their disease. The change in the surgical approach, in a bid to attain optimal cytoreduction with no gross residual disease, has seen improvement in the survival, as has the use of intraperitoneal chemotherapy in combination with intravenous agents. Cytoreductive surgery (CRS) and hyperthermic intraperitoneal chemotherapy (HIPEC) provide the combined benefits of surgical eradication and effective chemotherapy, and can be performed with acceptable morbidity and mortality [7]. Further trials are being undertaken to examine its role in the

This chapter was previously published in *Handbook on Ovarian Cancer: Risk Factors, Therapies and Prognosis*, edited by Bethany R. Collier, New York: Nova Publishers Inc., 2015.

* Corresponding Author: Head and Senior Consultant Division of Surgical Oncology; Adj. Associate Prof Melissa Teo Ching Ching, Email: Melissa.teo.c.c@nccs.com.sg, Address: 9 Hospital Drive, Singapore 169612, Tel:(65) 6436 8000, Fax: (65) 6225 6283

primary, as well as recurrent settings of advanced ovarian cancer and to determine the ideal drug combinations and dosages [8-10]. We aim to discuss these increasing controversies.

References

[1] Ferlay J, Soerjomataram I, Ervik M, et al. GLOBOCAN 2012 v1.0, *Cancer incidence and mortality worldwide: IARC CancerBase* No. 11 [Internet]. Lyon, France: International Agency for Research on Cancer; 2013. Available from: http://globocan.iarc.fr

[2] Bernard W. Stewart and Christopher P. Wild. *World cancer report* 2014. IARC publication; 2014.

[3] Coleman RL, Monk BJ, Sood AK, et al. Latest research and treatment of advanced-stage epithelial ovarian cancer. *Nat. Rev. Clin. Oncol.* 2013; 10: 211–224. doi: 10.1038/nrclinonc.2013.5.

[4] Horner MJ, Ries LA, Kracho M, et al. *SEER cancer statistics review*, 1975-2006. Bethesda, MD: National Cancer Institute; 2009. http://seer.cancer.-gov/csr/1975_2006/. AQ5

[5] Deraco M, Baratti D, Laterza B, et al. Advanced cytoreduction as surgical standard of care and hyperthermic intraperitoneal chemotherapy as promising treatment in epithelial ovarian cancer. *Eur. J. Surg. Oncol.* 2011; 37:4–9.

[6] Herter P, Hahmann M, Lueck HJ, et al. Surgery for recurrent ovarian cancer: role of peritoneal carcinomatosis: exploratory analysis of the DESKTOP 1 trial about risk factors, surgical implications, and prognostic value of peritoneal carcinomatosis. *Ann. Surg. Oncol.* 2009; 16:1324–1330.

[7] Chan DL, Morris DL, Rao A, Chua TC. Intraperitoneal chemotherapy in ovarian cancer: a review of tolerance and efficacy. *Cancer Manag Res.* 2012; 4:413–422.

[8] Chia TC, Liauw W, Robertson G, et al. Towards randomized trials of cytoreductive surgery using peritonectomy and hyperthermic intraperitoneal chemotherapy for ovarian cancer peritoneal carcinomatosis. *Gynaecol. Oncol.* 2009; 114: 137–139.

[9] Classe JM, Muller M, Frenel JS, et al. Intraperitoneal chemotherapy in the treatment of advanced ovarian cancer. *Mem A′ cad Nat Chir* 2009; 8: 86–90.

[10] OVHIPEC trial. ClinicalTrials.gov identifier. NCT0042657. http://clinical-trials.gov/ct2/show/nct0042657.

In: Medicine Research Summaries. Volume 17
Editors: Zhongwen Liáng and Bibao Zhang

ISBN: 978-1-53612-751-5

Chapter 164

SPLENECTOMY AS PART OF CYTOREDUCTIVE SURGERY FOR ADVANCED STAGE AND RELAPSED OVARIAN CANCER[#]

***N. Bacalbasa*[1,*] *and Irina Balescu*[2]**
[1]"Carol Davila" University of Medicine and Pharmacy, Bucharest
[2]Ponderas Hospital, Bucharest, Romania

RESEARCH SUMMARY

Ovarian cancer is the second most common gynecologic malignancy among women worldwide after endometrial cancer and the most common cause of death in women with gynecologic malignancies. Because of the increasing life expectancy experienced worldwide it is estimated that the incidence of this aggressive disease will significantly increase in the next few decades. Among all cases diagnosed with ovarian cancer the histopathological subtype consisting of epithelial tumors represents the largest part and has been widely studied. However, there is still an important number of patients who are diagnosed in an advanced stage of the disease, when disseminated bulky tumors are already present. It has been demonstrated that the most frequent patterns of spread are represented by the peritoneal, hematogenous and lymphatic route, all of them being responsible in different proportions for the presence of upper abdominal burden which sometimes is present from the moment of initial diagnosis. In all these cases the therapeutic mainstay remains cytoreductive surgery, followed by taxanes and platinum based adjuvant chemotherapy. When it comes to long term outcomes, among various prognostic factors such as age, stage at diagnosis, histopathological subtype, differentiation grade and residual disease, only residual disease has been widely demonstrated to strongly impact survival; at the same time, the amount of residual tumor burden at the end of debulking surgery is the only parameter which is influenced by the

---

This chapter was previously published in *Handbook on Ovarian Cancer: Risk Factors, Therapies and Prognosis*, edited by Bethany R. Collier, New York: Nova Publishers Inc., 2015.

* Corresponding Author: Nicolae Bacalbasa, Address: Dimitrie Racovi'ă Street, no. 2, Bucharest, Romania. Phone number: +40723540426. Mail address: nicolae_bacalbasa@yahoo.ro.

treating physician's experience. The presence of upper abdominal disseminations has been considered for a long period of time to be the sign of a tumor with a more aggressive biology and was considered as a poor prognostic factor. The main invaded organs in the upper abdomen consist of liver and porta hepatis, diaphragm, and less common, the spleen. While in cases presenting hepatic involvement the presence of hematogenous disease has been accepted as a poor prognosis factor and was classified the disease as FIGO stage IV, there was no explicit specification whether parenchimatous splenic involvement should be classified as part of the same FIGO stage. Initially a poorer outcome was reported for patients submitted to splenectomy as part of debulking surgery for advanced stage epithelial ovarian cancer, this fact being related to a more aggressive biological behaviour of the tumor. Other studies have stipulated the fact that the presence of splenic metastases is an independent poor prognosis factor but they could not distinguish whether the poorer outcome is related to the presence of hematogenous involvement of the upper abdominal parenchimatous viscera or to the co-existence of bulky left quadrant upper abdominal tumoral burden.

However, the initial results were strongly influenced by the small number of cases included and by the different characteristics of the included patients. For example patients submitted to splenectomy as part of primary and secondary cytoreduction were included in the same study so the results were also influenced by the moment of performing the surgery.

More recently, a significant difference in terms of survival was reported for hematogenous versus peritoneal splenic metastases and concluded that their presence should be considered as an explicit criterion for FIGO stage IV disease. Although it is a safe and effective surgical procedure, performing a splenectomy as part of cytoreductive surgery for advanced stage or relapsed ovarian cancer might associate a higher rate of postoperative morbidity rather due to the fact that in these cases ovarian cancer becomes a systemic disease with multiple visceral involvements, imposing multiple visceral resections in order to achieve an R0 resection; in all these cases the postoperative outcomes are influenced by a cumulative postoperative risk related to each performed resection in part.

However, since splenectomy can be safely performed with acceptable rates of postoperative complications it should be routinely performed in cases presenting splenic tumoral involvement in order to increase the rate of complete cytoreduction. This chapter focuses on the patterns of spread, prognostic factors of patients with splenic involvement, safety and effectiveness of splenectomy as part of cytoreductive surgery for advanced stage and relapsed epithelial ovarian cancer.

In: Medicine Research Summaries. Volume 17
Editors: Zhongwen Liáng and Bibao Zhang

ISBN: 978-1-53612-751-5

Chapter 165

LIVER SURGERY IN OVARIAN CANCER LIVER METASTASES#

***N. Bacalbasa*[1,*] *and Irina Balescu*[2]**
[1]"Carol Davila" University of Medicine and Pharmacy, Bucharest, Romania
[2]Ponderas Hospital, Bucharest, Romania

RESEARCH SUMMARY

Ovarian cancer is one of the most aggressive gynecologic malignancies and represents a major cause of death for women worldwide. This aggressive behavior is especially related to the fact that most patients are diagnosed in an advanced stage of the disease when disseminated tumoral burden is already present. Although the intraperitoneal route seems to be the most common pattern of spread, ovarian cancer can also develop distant metastases by hematogenous route and throughout lymphatic channels, the most commonly affected sites by hematogenous spread including the lungs and liver. Historically, patients with liver involvement have been considered as having a systemic, uncontrollable disease and were considered as candidates for supportive care or palliative chemotherapy.

Although the presence of liver metastases at the moment of diagnosis is usually associated with an altered tumor biology and aggressive disease, there was no convincing evidence that cytoreduction in the presence of liver metastases is less efficacious. Starting from this hypothesis, hepatic resection for ovarian cancer liver metastases has been proposed.

However, at this moment it is estimated that the number of patients submitted to liver resection for hepatic metastases from gynecological cancer represent less than 1% of the total resected liver metastases, the role of surgery in patients with ovarian cancer liver metastases being still in question. The main reason for this paucity of hepatectomies in ovarian cancer liver metastases is related to the fact that usually these kinds of tumors develop liver

---

This chapter was previously published in *Handbook on Ovarian Cancer: Risk Factors, Therapies and Prognosis*, edited by Bethany R. Collier, New York: Nova Publishers Inc., 2015.

* Corresponding Author: Nicolae Bacalbasa, Address: Dimitrie Racoviă Street, no. 2, Bucharest, Romania. Phone number: +40723540426. Mail address: nicolae_bacalbasa@yahoo.ro.

metastases in the settings of obvious systemic or regional dissemination which is not suitable for a complete macroscopic resection. Patients presenting resectable, isolated and limited to liver metastases are rather an exception than a rule in the setting of ovarian cancer. However this small subgroup of patients with isolated hepatic lesions has been initially considered to suit best to liver resection.

According to this principle, initially the main indication for resection in ovarian cancer liver metastases was the presence of solitary liver lesions with no extrahepatic tumoral burden as the best results in terms of survival had been obtained in such cases. More recently, it has been demonstrated that the presence of extrahepatic tumoral burden does not represent a significant prognostic factor for a poorer outcome in all patients and allowed to identify the subsets of patients with extrahepatic tumor burden who could benefit most from liver resections.

A crucial step in studying the long term outcomes after liver resection for ovarian cancer hepatic metastases was demonstrating the different outcomes between the two distinct patterns of hepatic involvement: peritoneal and hematogenous spread. Metastases originating from peritoneal seeding with parenchimatous invasion of at least 2 cm were classified as peritoneal lesions while lesions entirely surrounded by liver parenchyma were considered to have hematogenous origins. Significant differences in terms of survival between patients with peritoneal versus hematogenous lesions submitted to complete resections were observed. Based on these findings, it has been largely accepted that the presence of peritoneal seeding involving the liver included the case in FIGO stage IIIC while the presence of hematogenous liver involvement should be classified as FIGO stage IV.

When it comes to the role of liver resection as part of secondary or even tertiary cytoreduction, literature data is even scarcer, the presence of liver metastases being considered for long time as an exclusion criterion when establishing whether a patient is a candidate for optimal cytoreduction at the moment of surgery for recurrent disease. In time, improved understating of hepatic anatomy in association with the improvement of surgical techniques and postoperative care transformed hepatic resection in a more frequent associated surgical procedure in serial resections for ovarian cancer relapse. Once liver resection has been successfully associated as part of cytoreduction for relapsed ovarian cancer, attention was focused on determining other potential prognostic factors which might influence survival such as initial FIGO stage, disease free survival or histopatologic subtype of the tumor.

This chapter focuses on the subject of liver resection as part of cytoreductive surgery for advanced stage or relapsed ovarian cancer. The influence of different patterns of spread, the safety and effectiveness of performing anatomical or extended liver resections are also presented.

In: Medicine Research Summaries. Volume 17
Editors: Zhongwen Liáng and Bibao Zhang
ISBN: 978-1-53612-751-5

Chapter 166

POTENTIAL OF PHYTOCHEMICALS AND THEIR DERIVATIVES IN THE TREATMENT OF OVARIAN CANCER[#]

Wen-Wu Li*[*], Okiemute Rosa Johnson-Ajinwo and Fidelia Ijeoma Uche
Institute for Science and Technology in Medicine, Keele University, Staffordshire, UK

RESEARCH SUMMARY

Ovarian cancer is the leading cause of death in the gynaecologic cancers within the UK and US. Presently the standard treatment for ovarian cancer entails the use of chemotherapy drugs paclitaxel and carboplatin after aggressive surgical reduction in order to prolong the patient's life for multiple years. However, prolonged use of platinum-based chemotherapy often leads to drug resistance, which causes the ovarian cancer patient to relapse and potential death. Therefore there is an urgent medical need for breakthrough drugs with an effective therapeutic impact on ovarian cancer. Phytochemicals (plant-derived natural products) have been used for thousands of years as treatment for various diseases, because of their huge chemical diversity and wide range of biological activities.

In this review, the role of phytochemicals as chemo-preventive compounds, potential sources of new drugs for ovarian cancer and the benefits of their adoption as mono-therapeutic agents or as chemosensitizers when used in-conjunction with the conventional anti-cancer drugs is highlighted. We will describe the phytochemicals: 1) clinically approved drugs such as paclitaxel and camptothecin including its semi-synthetic derivatives topotecan and irinotecan; 2) currently in clinical trials such as epipodophyllotoxin derivatives etoposide and teniposide, ventfolide, phenoxodiol, and combretastatins; 3) in preclinical trials such as quercetin, baicalein, baicalin, thymoquinone, betulinic acid and tetrandrine; and novel

[#] This chapter was previously published in *Handbook on Ovarian Cancer: Risk Factors, Therapies and Prognosis*, edited by Bethany R. Collier, New York: Nova Publishers Inc., 2015.
[*] Corresponding Author: Dr. Wen-Wu Li, e-mail: w.li@keele.ac.uk.

compounds which have high potency (IC_{50} less than 10 μM) and have been discovered recently (last 15 years). In particular, several new compounds including bufatrienolides, ipomoeassin D, 2'-(R)-O-acetylglaucarubinone, and molvizarin have IC_{50}s lower than 100 nM in ovarian cancer cells and might have different mechanisms of action from those of platinum derivatives/paclitaxel, therefore providing potential ways to attack multidrug resistance in ovarian cancer without jeopardising the patient's treatment.

In: Medicine Research Summaries. Volume 17
Editors: Zhongwen Liáng and Bibao Zhang
ISBN: 978-1-53612-751-5

Chapter 167

MOLECULAR ALTERATIONS CHEMORESISTANCE-RELATED IN OVARIAN CANCER PATIENTS AND RELATED TARGET THERAPIES[#]

Lucrezia Amoroso, Francesca De Iuliis and Susanna Scarpa
Experimental Medicine Department, Sapienza University of Rome, Italy

RESEARCH SUMMARY

Introduction. Ovarian cancer has the highest rate of mortality among gynecological malignancies and it is the fifth leading cause of cancer-related death in women of developed countries. It is often diagnosed at late stage, therefore, despite optimal cytoreduction by debulking surgery and adjuvant chemotherapy, recurrence is frequent.

New therapeutic strategies are needed to treat relapses and advanced stage chemoresistant ovarian cancer. Ovarian cancer is characterized by different molecular phenotypes, and it can be classified in five tumor types with different clinical, pathologic and prognostic properties, and with different chemosensitivity.

Objective. This review will focus on molecular alterations involved in ovarian cancer carcinogenesis, which may become new targets for therapy in the future. Biological therapies can impact on the prognosis, especially in advanced chemoresistant ovarian cancer patients.

Discussion. The most important pathways involved in ovarian cancer chemoresistance are PI3K/ AKT/ mTOR, KRAS/ MAPK/ ERK, BRCA1/BRCA2, Notch and Forkhead Box M1 pathways.

The amplification of PI3K is more frequent in high-grade ovarian tumors rather than in low grade ones, together with AKT phosphorylation, contributing to disease progression.

KRAS mutations are frequent in low-grade ovarian tumors, and their expression varies in different histopathological types. Loss of PTEN is frequently present in high-grade serous carcinomas and correlates with a poor prognosis.

[#] This chapter was previously published in *Handbook on Ovarian Cancer: Risk Factors, Therapies and Prognosis*, edited by Bethany R. Collier, New York: Nova Publishers Inc., 2015.

Several protein kinases and other signaling molecules, such as KRAS, BRAF, PI3KCA and CTNNB1, have been evaluated and their mutations have been correlated with prognosis. Epigenetic modifications are promising targets for ovarian cancer treatment. Several studies on molecular alterations have been conducted on ovarian cancer tissue, but further studies are needed to tailor every therapy to the specific histotype of ovarian cancer.

Actually, the approved biological therapies currently used in ovarian cancer patients are only three: Bevacizumab (a monoclonal antibodies directed against VEGF, usually utilized in platinum-pretreated patients), Pazopanib (tyrosine) and Olaparib (PARP-inhibitor, utilized in BRCA1/2 mutated patients).

Further studies are needed to better evaluate different chemoresistance related pathways, and to find new targets on which to focus clinical research.

Conclusions. Among the analyzed studies, only molecular alterations of PI3KI seem to have the strongest correlation with prognosis. These mutations could be future targets of therapy for chemoresistant patients, but more studies are required.

In: Medicine Research Summaries. Volume 17
Editors: Zhongwen Liáng and Bibao Zhang
ISBN: 978-1-53612-751-5

Chapter 168

PRIMARY CYTOREDUCTION IN EPITHELIAL OVARIAN CANCER[#]

E. Delgado, M. Martín-Cameán and I. Zapardiel [*]
Gynecologic Oncology Unit, La Paz University Hospital, Madrid, Spain

RESEARCH SUMMARY

Worldwide, ovarian cancer is the seventh cancer in frequency and the eighth cause of death from cancer in women. Epithelial ovarian cancer is also the leading cause of death among gynaecologic malignancies. Nowadays, the standard management of epithelial ovarian cancer is the correct surgical staging and optimal tumor cytoreduction followed by platinum plus taxane-based chemotherapy. Standard surgical treatment for early stages consists on peritoneal washings, total hysterectomy and bilateral anexectomy, inspection all organs and peritoneum surface, taking samples of suspicious areas, omentectomy and pelvic and para-aortic lymphadenectomy. Laparoscopic approach allows to do this surgical staging with less morbidity and mortality than a more aggressive laparotomy approach. After this complete surgical staging, the International Federation of Gynaecology and Obstetrics (FIGO) staging system for ovarian cancer ought to be applied to determine the management and prognosis of the patient. In advanced stages complete tumor cytoreduction has demonstrated survival advantage compared to incomplete debulking. The morbidity associated with the debulking surgery does not increase mortality. However, some patients with advanced epithelial ovarian cancer undergo debulking surgery but complete cytoreduction is not achieved, with an increase of the morbidity and no improvement in overall survival. There are some criteria to predict the cytoreduction outcomes, based on serum biomarkers levels, preoperative imaging techniques and laparoscopic based scores. Optimization of patient selection for primary cytoreduction would determine which patients could benefit from a complete cytoreduction or which ones might benefit from neoadjuvant chemotherapy and interval surgery.

[#] This chapter was previously published in *Handbook on Ovarian Cancer: Risk Factors, Therapies and Prognosis*, edited by Bethany R. Collier, New York: Nova Publishers Inc., 2015.

[*] Corresponding Author: Ignacio Zapardiel, Gynecologic Oncology Unit, La Paz University Hospital, Madrid, Spain, ignaciozapardiel@hotmail.com.

In: Medicine Research Summaries. Volume 17
Editors: Zhongwen Liáng and Bibao Zhang

ISBN: 978-1-53612-751-5

Chapter 169

SENSITIZING CHEMOTHERAPY WITH ULTRASOUND[#]

Li Luo[1], Jinyan Li[1], Meijiao Wang[1], Lin Yu[2] and Tinghe Yu[1,*]

[1]Key Medical Laboratory of Obstetrics and Gynecology,
The Second Affiliated Hospital, Chongqing Medical University, Chongqing, China
[2]Department of Otolaryngology, The First Affiliated Hospital,
Chongqing Medical University, Chongqing, China

RESEARCH SUMMARY

Chemotherapy is limited by toxicity to noncancerous tissues and the development of chemoresistance. Here we discuss the use of low intensity ultrasound to modulate chemotherapy against ovarian cancer. Ultrasound can enhance the action of certain drugs, including circumvention of chemoresistance. Ultrasonic cavitation plays the leading role in sonochemotherapy, which permeabilizes the cell membrane favoring the influx of drugs. Recent trials suggest that ultrasound can modulate chemotherapy via multiple pathways, and synergize the sensitization due to a chemical modulator such as verapamil and cyclosporin A. Ultrasound can be efficiently delivered to the preselected volume within the body thus realizing a targeted therapy. This technique can be specifically developed as a non-drug technique to improve the therapeutic outcome of chemotherapy against ovarian cancer.

This chapter was previously published in *Handbook on Ovarian Cancer: Risk Factors, Therapies and Prognosis*, edited by Bethany R. Collier, New York: Nova Publishers Inc., 2015.

* Corresponding Author Emal: yutinghe@hotmail.com.

In: Medicine Research Summaries. Volume 17
Editors: Zhongwen Liáng and Bibao Zhang
ISBN: 978-1-53612-751-5

Chapter 170

Elderly Ovarian Cancer Patients: Treatment Options#

Francesca De Iuliis, Lucrezia Amoroso and Susanna Scarpa
Experimental Medicine Department, Sapienza University of Rome, Italy

Research Summary

Introduction. Ovarian cancer, the main cause of death among gynaecological malignancies, affects half of women in postmenopausal age. With the increase in older population, this tumor will be more frequent in elderly women, but not all the elderly patients can undertake standard treatments, due to comorbidities and less functional organ reserves.

New therapeutic approaches are needed to obtain an amendable overall survival and quality of life in this kind of patients.

Objective. Our aim is to propose the best management of elderly ovarian cancer patients, taking account of biological age over chronologic age, with the aim to assure suitable treatments with a better overall survival.

Discussion. Carboplatin-paclitaxel doublet is the standard treatment in patients with ovarian cancer; elderly patients are less treated with this therapy, due both to comorbidities and to the major toxicity. When the standard schedule every 21 days is administered in elderly patients, dose delay or previous stop for toxicity is frequent.

Furthermore, elderly are not candidate for intraperitoneal chemotherapy and HIPEC (hyperthermic intraperitoneal chemotherapy), due to highest toxicity. Chemotherapy is often the only possible choice for these patients, because a surgical debulking can be too much aggressive and associated with several morbidities.

Elderly have the same chemosensitivity than younger: geriatric assessment is fundamental to screen elderly population fitting for chemotherapy, and new strategies with less toxicity have to be investigated. Older patients with ovarian cancer have been

---

This chapter was previously published in *Handbook on Ovarian Cancer: Risk Factors, Therapies and Prognosis*, edited by Bethany R. Collier, New York: Nova Publishers Inc., 2015.

underrepresented in clinical trials, so the few clinical studies with this kind of population must be evaluated.

It's not clear whether doublets or single agents are better in the treatment of elderly ovarian cancer patients. Single agent options for elderly patients include liposomal doxorubicin, topotecan, gemcitabine and vinorelbine. Doublet combinations every 21 days have been largely investigated, but only small clinical trials have been conducted on weekly schedule. Weekly carboplatin and paclitaxel have demonstrated an optimal compliance among elderly patients.

For what concern targeted therapies, there are no elderly-specific data on PARP inhibitors, but they appear to be well tolerated, on the opposite to antiangiogenic agents, which require more caution in the older population.

Metronomic chemotherapy and weekly schedules are the best solutions for elderly patients, for their efficacy and tolerability, contributing to quality of life.

Conclusions. Metronomic therapy, comprising weekly schedules, can be an optimal option for elderly ovarian cancer patients. Prospective studies are needed to develop further strategies for these women.

In: Medicine Research Summaries. Volume 17
Editors: Zhongwen Liáng and Bibao Zhang
ISBN: 978-1-53612-751-5

Chapter 171

INSOMNIA IN CHILDREN: SYMPTOMS, DIAGNOSIS AND THERAPY[#]

Benjamin Putois[1,*], Wendy Leslie[2,†], MSc and Patricia Franco[3,‡], MCU-PH

[1]Cognitive Sciences, Psychology, Formation Universitaire A Distance, Study Centre of Sierre, CH, Sierre, Switzerland
[2]Clinical Health Psychology, University of Ulster, Coleraine, Londonderry, UK
[3]Head of the Pediatric Sleep Unit, Epilepsy, Sleep, Neuropediatric Functional Explorations Service, Hôpital Femme Mère Enfant, Bron, France

RESEARCH SUMMARY

Insomnia is very common in children under 5 years old. It can impact a child's behavior, emotional regulation and learning and furthermore have consequences for their family members' quality of life and their parents' sleep. Diagnosing insomnia in a child requires a developmental understanding of the symptoms and a multidimensional exploration of potential etiologies: diet, environment, rhythm, psychology, parental background, organic diseases or conditioning. Aspects of differential diagnosis, along with potential treatments for insomnia in children, especially behavioral therapies, are all presented in this chapter.

This chapter was previously published in *Advances in Medicine and Biology. Volume 92,* edited by Leon V. Berhardt, New York: Nova Publishers Inc., 2016.

* Corresponding Author: Benjamin Putois, Doctor of Cognitive Sciences, Psychologist, Lecturer in Psychology; Email: bputois@gmail.com.
† Corresponding Author Email: wendyanneleslie@yahoo.fr.
‡ Corresponding Author: Patricia Franco, Head of the Pediatric Sleep Unit, Email: Patricia.Franco@chu-lyon.frs.

In: Medicine Research Summaries. Volume 17
Editors: Zhongwen Liáng and Bibao Zhang
ISBN: 978-1-53612-751-5

Chapter 172

INSOMNIA IN ADULTS: SYMPTOMS, DIAGNOSIS AND THERAPY[#]

Mélinée Chapoutot[1]*, MSc, Thierry Faivre[2], MD, Wendy Leslie[3], MSc and Benjamin Putois[4]

[1]Cognitive Psychology, Institut de Psychologie du Sommeil, France
[2]Sleep Unit, Clinique Lyon-Lumière, Meyzieu, France
[3]Clinical Health Psychology, University of Ulster, Coleraine, UK
[4]Cognitive Sciences, Formation Universitaire á Distance Suisse, Study Centre of Sierre, Sierre, Switzerland

RESEARCH SUMMARY

Chronic insomnia is the most common sleep disorder among adults, and remains considerably under-treated. As such, insomnia represents a major public-health problem associated with higher rates of medical and psychiatric comorbidity, decrease in work performance, poor general quality of life and a financial cost of billions of dollars every year. Insomnia is defined as the "chronic inability to obtain the amount of sleep needed for optimal functioning and well-being." It is a complex disorder often associated with numerous organic diseases and mental health problems, or can result from a sleep-wake regulatory system dysfunction, or even without any known origin. Insomnia therefore requires accurate diagnosis and appropriate treatment.

Sleep drugs constitute the first, and in most cases only, treatment for insomnia. This is despite the fact that most countries do nevertheless recognize behavioral therapies, mainly Cognitive Behavioral Therapy (CBT), to be the preferred and most efficient treatment to implement. Possible explanations for this could be that insomniacs' healthcare pathways do not lead them to CBT. Another reason could be the fact that such treatment can be challenging and is therefore often not well tolerated by insomniacs. The aim of the present

---

[#] This chapter was previously published in *Advances in Medicine and Biology. Volume 92,* edited by Leon V. Berhardt, New York: Nova Publishers Inc., 2016.

* Corresponding Author: Mélinée Chapoutot, Sleep Psychologist; Email: Mel.chapoutot@gmail.com.

chapter is to critically review insomnia treatments and propose a new therapy avenue which may be well-tolerated by patients and which directly targets the consequences of insomnia on patients' lives.

After first presenting the different types of insomnia and their repercussions on quality of life, the present chapter will initially review the evidence on insomnia treatments with a particular focus on CBT for insomnia (CBT-I). Then, we will present some of the limitations and obstacles inherent to following a CBT-I treatment. Finally, we will introduce Acceptation and Commitment Therapy, arguing that it may represent an effective solution for the broad range of clinical issues associated with insomnia and has demonstrated very promising results according to several studies on treatment for insomnia.

In: Medicine Research Summaries. Volume 17
Editors: Zhongwen Liáng and Bibao Zhang

ISBN: 978-1-53612-751-5

Chapter 173

COMMUNITY-BASED EARLY INTERVENTIONS FOR ACUTE TMJMD PATIENT SETTINGS[#]

Angela Liegey Dougall[1], PhD, Celeste Sanders[1], PhD, Rob Haggard[1], MS, LPC-S; BSN, RN, Peter Buschang[2], PhD, Steve Karbowski[2], DDS, Richard Riggs[3], DDS and Robert J. Gatchel[*,1], PhD, ABPP

[1]The University of Texas at Arlington, Arlington, Texas, US
[2]Baylor College of Dentistry, The Texas A&M System, Texas, US
[3]Private Dental Practice, Richardson, Texas, US

RESEARCH SUMMARY

Biobehavioral interventions have previously been shown to relieve joint and muscle dysfunction that occurs in Temporomandibular Joint and Muscle Disorders (TMJMD) in academic clinical settings. A large, randomized controlled trial was undertaken to examine the effectiveness of these interventions when they were implemented in community-based clinics.

Participants with symptoms of acute TMJMD were assessed for risk of developing a chronic condition, and high-risk patients were randomized to either a Biobehavioral group (n = 168) or a Self-Care group (n = 131), and compared with a Low-Risk/Non-Intervention group (n = 136). It was hypothesized that the early biopsychosocial intervention would be more therapeutically effective in these community settings, relative to the attention control intervention, at post-intervention and at the one-year and two-year follow-ups. While most patients reported improvements across multiple domains (e.g., self-reported pain, pain during a chewing performance task, depressive symptoms, nonspecific physical symptoms, limitations in jaw opening, and physical health-related quality of life), patients in the High-

[#] This chapter was previously published in *Advances in Medicine and Biology. Volume 92,* edited by Leon V. Berhardt, New York: Nova Publishers Inc., 2016.

[*] Corresponding Author: Dr. Robert J. Gatchel; gatchel@uta.edu.

Risk/Biobehavioral intervention reported quicker improvement rates and were more likely to improve to levels equivalent to the Low-Risk group (even though the Low Risk group was improving as well). In contrast, the High-Risk/Self-Care group was slower to display improvements with levels that were more likely to stay higher than the Low Risk group or improve but rebound by two years. Both Biobehavioral and simpler, Self-Care interventions can be effective at improving dysfunction associated with TMJMD. However, Biobehavioral intervention appears to produce faster results that are more enduring. These findings may be used to inform the implementation of future interventions.

In: Medicine Research Summaries. Volume 17
Editors: Zhongwen Liáng and Bibao Zhang

ISBN: 978-1-53612-751-5

Chapter 174

The Pharmacological and Therapeutical Potential of Scorpion Venoms and Their Toxins#

J. Bhavya[1], Sunil S. More[2*] and B.L. Dhananjaya[3*]
[1]Department of Biochemistry, Centre for Post Graduate Studies, Bengaluru, Karnataka, India
[2]Department of Basic and Applied Sciences, Dayananda Sagar University, Kumaraswamy Layout, Bengaluru, Karnataka, India
[3]Centre for Emerging Technologies (CET), Jain University, Bangalore, Karnataka, India

Research Summary

Scorpions are widely distributed throughout the world. The biological molecules present in the venoms are predominately proteins and peptide toxins, including ion-channel toxins. These ion-channel toxins modulate the ion channels either by blocking the pore of the channel or by altering the voltage gating. Molecules which block the pores have been useful in deciphering the structure of the ion channels. The scorpion toxin which inhibited the K^+ channel by blocking the pore; led to the identification of pore forming region (P region) of K^+ channel proteins. Some of the toxins includes, Iberiotoxin isolated from *B. tumulus* venom, which is a specific blocker of the high-conductance calcium-activated potassium channel. Tamulus toxin is another toxin isolated from *B. tumulus* venom and acts on potassium channels. Chlorotoxins isolated from the venom of *Leiurus quinquestraitus* could bind to voltage gated Cl^- channels and bring about various changes in cell physiology. Chlorotoxins are known to be toxic to the insects but not to the mammalian system. This toxin binds to the

---

This chapter was previously published in *Advances in Medicine and Biology. Volume 92,* edited by Leon V. Berhardt, New York: Nova Publishers Inc., 2016.

* Corresponding Authors: Dr. Sunil S. More and Dr. B. L. Dhananjaya. Dayananda Sagar University and Jain University, Karnataka, India. Phone no: +91 8197324276, official phone no: +91 80 2757 7200, telefax +91 80 2757 7199, e-mail address; sunilacr@ yahoo.co.in, chandu_greeshma@rediffmail.com.

matrix metaloproteinase -2(MMP-2) of the glioma cells which are expressed in many types of cancer and prevent their activity. Many scorpion toxins have already being used for probing the voltage gated sodium channels and studying their activation and inactivation processes.

The unique ability of scorpion toxins to discriminate between vertebrate and invertebrate channels has led more applications of them as specific pharmacological tools, particularly as insecticidal toxins. The toxins show therapeutic properties namely antimicrobial activity, anticancer activity, used to treat autoimmune diseases and cardiovascular effects. Chlorotoxins is used as a non invasive tool for the detection of skin, cervical, esophageal, colon and lung cancers. BmK I toxin is believed to modulate cardiac contraction Many such toxins are isolated, characterized which possess properties that are applicable and useful in the field of medicine. The chapter briefly describes the various scorpion toxins therapeutic potential in biomedical application.

In: Medicine Research Summaries. Volume 17
Editors: Zhongwen Liáng and Bibao Zhang

ISBN: 978-1-53612-751-5

Chapter 175

NON-ANTICOAGULANT OLIGOSACCHARIDES OF ENOXAPARIN RELIEVE CHEMICAL-INDUCED ACUTE COLITIS[#]

Qi Ying Lean[1,2], Nuri Gueven[1], Rajaraman D. Eri[3], Gregory M. Peterson[1,4,5] and Rahul P. Patel[1,*]
[1]Pharmacy, School of Medicine, Faculty of Health,
University of Tasmania, Hobart, Tasmania, Australia
[2]Faculty of Pharmacy, University of Technology MARA,
Puncak Alam, Selangor, Malaysia
[3]School of Health Sciences, Faculty of Health,
University of Tasmania, Launceston, Tasmania Australia
[4]Breathe Well Centre of Research Excellence for Chronic Respiratory Disease and Lung Ageing, School of Medicine, Faculty of Health, University of Tasmania, Hobart, Tasmania, Australia
[5]Health Services Innovation Tasmania, School of Medicine,
Faculty of Health, University of Tasmania, Hobart, Tasmania, Australia

RESEARCH SUMMARY

Enoxaparin, a low molecular weight heparin, is commonly used for the treatment and prophylaxis of thromboembolic disorders. Apart from its anticoagulant properties, enoxaparin is known to possess anti-inflammatory activities and therefore could potentially be useful for the management of chronic inflammatory conditions. However, the clinical use of enoxaparin in inflammation is deterred by the risk of bleeding, attributed to the presence of anticoagulant

---

[#] This chapter was previously published in *Advances in Medicine and Biology. Volume 92,* edited by Leon V. Berhardt, New York: Nova Publishers Inc., 2016.

[*] Corresponding Author: Dr Rahul Patel; Pharmacy, School of Medicine, Faculty of Health, University of Tasmania; Private Bag 26, Hobart, 7001 TAS, Australia. Rahul.Patel@utas.edu.au; +61 3 6226 1079 (phone); +61 3 6226 2870 (fax).

oligosaccharides. It is proposed that non-anticoagulant oligosaccharides of enoxaparin are predominantly responsible for its anti-inflammatory activity. We isolated oligosaccharides of enoxaparin using ion-exchange chromatography and the anti-inflammatory potential of oligosaccharides was evaluated in a mouse model of acute colitis. Male C57BL/6 mice were administered dextran sulphate sodium through drinking water and were subsequently treated orally with oligosaccharides of enoxaparin. Compared to untreated animals, oral enoxaparin oligosaccharide-treated mice showed reduced severity of colitis. Importantly, since the oligosaccharides of enoxaparin with no or minimal anticoagulant activity were found to be responsible for this protective effect, these molecules could be developed as novel therapeutic agents for the management of ulcerative colitis.

In: Medicine Research Summaries. Volume 17
Editors: Zhongwen Liáng and Bibao Zhang

ISBN: 978-1-53612-751-5

Chapter 176

CHEMOKINE RECEPTOR CXCR7: A NEW DRUG TARGET FOR ATHEROSCLEROSIS[#]

Jianzhong Shen[*] and Wanshu Ma
Department of Drug Discovery and Development,
Harrison School of Pharmacy, Auburn University,
Auburn, Alabama, US

RESEARCH SUMMARY

Objective: The discovery of CXCR7 as a new receptor for SDF-1 places many previously described SDF-1 functions attributed to CXCR4 in question, though whether CXCR7 acts as a signaling or "decoy" receptor has been in debate. It is known that CXCR7 is not expressed in normal blood leukocytes; however, the potential role of leukocyte CXCR7 in disease states has not been addressed. The aim of this study was to determine the expression and function of macrophage CXCR7 linked to atherosclerosis.

Results and Discussion: Here we show that CXCR7 was detected in macrophage-positive area of aortic atheroma of *ApoE*-null mice, but not in healthy aorta. During monocyte-to-macrophage differentiation, CXCR7 was up-regulated at mRNA and protein levels, with more expression in M1 than in M2 phenotype. In addition, CXCR7 induction was associated with a SDF-1 signaling switch from pro-survival ERK and AKT pathways in monocytes to pro-inflammatory JNK and p38 pathways in macrophages. The latter effect was mimicked by CXCR7-selective agonist TC14012, and abolished by siRNA knockdown of CXCR7. Moreover, CXCR7 activation increased macrophage phagocytic activity, which was suppressed by CXCR7 siRNA silencing or by inhibiting either the JNK or p38 pathways, but was not affected by blocking CXCR4. Activation of CXCR7 by I-TAC showed a similar signaling and phagocytic activity in macrophages with no detectable CXCR3. Additional study found that CXCR7 activation promotes macrophage adhesion and migration, which are

[#] This chapter was previously published in *Advances in Medicine and Biology. Volume 92,* edited by Leon V. Berhardt, New York: Nova Publishers Inc., 2016.

[*] Corresponding Author Email: jzs0019@auburn.edu.

involved in vascular inflammation and atherosclerosis. Finally, we found that the induced CXCR7 expression during monocyte-to-macrophage differentiation was significantly suppressed by atorvastatin treatment.

Conclusion: CXCR7 is induced during monocyte-to-macrophage differentiation, which is required for SDF-1 and I-TAC signaling to JNK and p38 pathways, leading to enhanced macrophage phagocytosis, adhesion and migration, thus possibly contributing to atherogenesis. In addition, atorvastatin treatment inhibits CXCR7 induction on macrophages, suggesting a new CXCR7-related mechanism to benefit atherosclerosis treatment independent of lipid-lowering effects of the statin drugs.

In: Medicine Research Summaries. Volume 17
Editors: Zhongwen Liáng and Bibao Zhang
ISBN: 978-1-53612-751-5

Chapter 177

PARTICIPATION OF MICROTUBULES IN INTRACELLULAR CHOLESTEROL TRANSPORT THROUGH CYTOSOLIC LIPID-PROTEIN PARTICLES IN RAT ASTROCYTES[#]

Jin-Ichi Ito[1,•] and Makoto Michikawa[1]
[1]Biochemistry, Graduate School of Medical Sciences,
Nagoya City University, Kawasumi 1, Mizuho-cho, Mizuho-ku, Nagoya, Japan

RESEARCH SUMMARY

Newly synthesized cholesterol is in part translocated from the Endoplasmic Reticulum/Golgi apparatus (ER/Golgi) to the cytosol, followed by incorporation into the cytosolic lipid-protein particles (CLPPs) in rat astrocytes treated with exogenous apolipoprotein A-I (apoA-I). Diameters of the CLPPs are 17 - 18 nm and their densities are 1.09 - 1.16 g/ml, which are similar to those of plasma high-density lipoproteins (HDL), but distributed in the cytoplasm. The cholesterol in the CLPPs is then transported to the plasma membrane for cholesterol release in the CLPP-dependent manner. The CLPPs are cytosolic lipid-protein complexes composed of proteins such as caveolin-1 and cyclophilin A (Cp-A) and lipids such as cholesterol, phosphatidylcholine, and sphingomyelin. Protein kinase Cα (PK-Cα) and tubulins are also included in the CLPPs. A stabilizer of microtubules, paclitaxel (taxol), suppresses not only the apoA-I-mediated intracellular translocation of newly synthesized lipids but also the lipid release from the cells, suggesting the participation of microtubules in intracellular cholesterol transport through CLPP.

Association of CLPP-related lipids and proteins (caveolin-1 and PK-Cα) with the microtubule-like filaments (rMT) prepared in the cytosol fraction of the apoA-I-treated cells is much more greatly increased than in that of control cells without apoA-I treatment. The

---

[#] This chapter was previously published in *Advances in Medicine and Biology. Volume 92,* edited by Leon V. Berhardt, New York: Nova Publishers Inc., 2016.

• Corresponding Author Email: jitoh@med.nagoya-cu.ac.jp.

association of rMT and CLPP-related lipids and proteins is also suppressed by a scaffolding peptide of caveolin-1. These findings imply that the CLPP binds to microtubules through the CLPP-associated caveolin-1. The assemblies of cytosolic caveolin-1 and protein kinase Cα to AffiGel-linked rMT are enhanced more actively in the cytosol of rat astrocytes stimulated with apoA-I than in the cytosol of control cells treated without apoA-I. ApoA-I enhances the phosphorylation of α–tubulin in the PK-C-dependent manner, which induces the dissociation of phosphorylated α–tubulin from caveolin-1. The phosphorylated α–tubulin is no longer associated with caveolin-1. Based on these findings, it is reasonable to assume that apoA-I enhances the association of microtubules with the CLPP containing caveolin-1 and PK-Cα, and that PK-C-dependent phosphorylation of α–tubulin regulates the association and dissociation between microtubules and CLPPs to mediate the microtubules-dependent intracellular cholesterol transport.

In: Medicine Research Summaries. Volume 17
Editors: Zhongwen Liáng and Bibao Zhang
ISBN: 978-1-53612-751-5

Chapter 178

TEETH AND AMELOGENIN IN *XENOPUS*[#]

Hitoshi Ando*
Department of Biophysics, School of Dental Medicine,
Tsurumi University, Tsurumi-ku, Yokohama, Japan

RESEARCH SUMMARY

During various development stages of both *Xenopus laevis* and *X. tropicalis*, numerous small teeth randomly grow on the maxillas, but none on the mandibles. Mature teeth are coated in dental enamel.

Amelogenin mRNA expressing regions and construction of amelogenin gene were examined. Both species of *Xenopus* have two amelogenin mRNAs, and, although one amelogenin gene lies on the sex-determining chromosome XLA2L, their expressions do not vary according to sex.

Amelogenin mRNA expresses only in secreting ameloblasts in *X. tropicalis* tooth germs. Sequence analyses indicate that two types of amelogenin mRNA are alternatively spliced and derived from a single gene in *X. tropicalis*. They are named here as amelogenin mRNA-A and -B. The mRNA-A has a long exon 1, which is much longer than the corresponding exon 1 in other animals. Exon 2 is newly found exon with no corresponding exon in known amelogenins. Exon 2b followed after exon 1 in mRNA-A and mRNA-B starts from exon 2a and 2b. These exons are not confirmed in *X. laevis,* however their existence is easily predicted by a genome browser "Xenbase".

The following five exons of both *Xenopus* may be homologous to each known exon respectively.

The archetype of the amelogenin gene is still unclear because of the relatively low homology of amelogenin sequences among amphibians. *Xenopus* amelogenin may not be the archetype itself, but the newly-discovered exon 2 or elongated exon 1 may transpire to be key in exploring the archetype of the amelogenin gene expected to be found in the ancestor of amphibians.

[#] This chapter was previously published in *Advances in Medicine and Biology. Volume 92,* edited by Leon V. Berhardt, New York: Nova Publishers Inc., 2016.

* Corresponding Author Email: ando-h@tsurumi-u.ac.jp.

In: Medicine Research Summaries. Volume 17 ISBN: 978-1-53612-751-5
Editors: Zhongwen Liáng and Bibao Zhang

Chapter 179

BUILDING COMMUNITY CAPACITY TO IMPROVE POPULATION HEALTH THROUGH INTEGRATING PUBLIC HEALTH AND HEALTH CARE: LESSONS LEARNED FROM THE COMMUNITY HEALTH NEEDS ASSESSMENT CONDUCTED BY NEBRASKA'S RURAL HOSPITALS[#]

Li-Wu Chen*, MHSA, PhD, David Palm, PhD and Kate E. Trout, MPH

Department of Health Services Research and Administration, College of Public Health, University of Nebraska Medical Center, Omaha, Nebraska, US

RESEARCH SUMMARY

The Patient Protection and Affordable Care Act (ACA) contains a provision that requires all nonprofit hospitals to conduct a Community Health Needs Assessment (CHNA) and an Implementation Plan every three years. This chapter provides a comprehensive analysis of the CHNA process, the priorities identified in the CHNA, and the implementation strategies produced by the 31 small nonprofit rural hospitals in Nebraska. Of these 31 hospitals, 30 are classified as critical access hospitals. The majority of the hospitals in the study worked closely with the local health department in their area and this partnership appeared to enhance the quality of the CHNA (e.g., the data analysis, input from the community and the priority setting process). The highest rated priorities among these 31 hospitals were: (1) access to care, (2) obesity, (3) mental health and substance abuse, and (4) cancer. There were also several specific strategies that were recommended to address these issues. Most of these

---

[#] This chapter was previously published in *Capacity Building: Planning, Programs and Prospects*, edited by Diane Brown, New York: Nova Publishers Inc., 2016.

* Corresponding Author Email: liwuchen@unmc.edu.

strategies involved some type of education, increasing or adding new services, developing or implementing a new program, expanding health events or screenings, and expanding staff or providers. The chapter also includes several lessons learned and some key success factors. One of the lessons learned is that it is very important for small hospitals to work closely with their local health department and to align the CHNA with other plans in the area. By involving more partners, it is possible to design interventions that are broader in scope and have a greater collective impact in addressing the complex problems that were identified as the high priorities.

In: Medicine Research Summaries. Volume 17
Editors: Zhongwen Liáng and Bibao Zhang

ISBN: 978-1-53612-751-5

Chapter 180

COLLABORATION OR CONTESTATION? A CRITICAL EVALUATION OF CURRENT CAPACITY BUILDING MECHANISMS IN COMMUNITY-BASED OBESITY PREVENTION PROGRAMMES#

G. Middleton[1,*], A. B. Evans[2], H. Henderson[1] and D. Windard[1]
[1]University of Lincoln, Brayford Campus, Lincoln, Lincolnshire, UK
[2]University of Copenhagen, København, Denmark

RESEARCH SUMMARY

In recent years large community-based obesity prevention programmes have been developed in a number of Western countries in an attempt to reduce the growing epidemic of obesity in children and adults. The construction of community-based programmes revolves around the concept of capacity building. Often described as the ‘invisible work’ in health promotion, capacity building first establishes what structural limitations exist to prevent adoption of healthier lifestyles in communities, with a view to empowering community members to establish healthy behaviours. Typically, programmes attempt to address the main determinants of obesity by deploying an array of interventions at community level. Programmes frequently involve multiple stakeholders; for example, in England, programmes often involve local cross-government departments and networks of organisations acting as partners through a multi-agency approach. The strength of health promotion initiatives relies on formed ‘coalitions’ or partnerships and the subsequent collaboration in the design, delivery and administration of the programme’s multiple components. Advantages of partnership are the pooling of resources, avoiding duplication and potentially understanding the social context more holistically given the engagement of stakeholders’ from different perspectives. Despite best intentions, these large community-based programmes are not without difficulties

This chapter was previously published in *Capacity Building: Planning, Programs and Prospects*, edited by Diane Brown, New York: Nova Publishers Inc., 2016.

* Corresponding Author Email: gmiddleton@lincoln.ac.uk.

and recent literature exposes stakeholder concerns particularly in relation to the development, implementation and evaluation of such programmes (Middleton et al. 2014, Kleij et al. 2015). This includes leadership issues, competing agendas and priorities, the unwieldy nature of large multi-agency networks and the complexities around making a sustained impact. Those involved in the administration of community-based obesity prevention programmes should carefully consider the components which lead to facilitation of efficiency in the capacity building process discussed in this commentary.

In: Medicine Research Summaries. Volume 17
Editors: Zhongwen Liáng and Bibao Zhang
ISBN: 978-1-53612-751-5

Chapter 181

BUILDING CAPACITY TOWARDS HIV PREVENTION IN A LATINO MIGRANT WORKER COMMUNITY IN SOUTH FLORIDA#

Jesús Sánchez*, PhD
Department of Sociobehavioral and Administrative Pharmacy,
College of Pharmacy, Nova Southeastern University,
Fort Lauderdale, FL, US

RESEARCH SUMMARY

Despite an growing array of efficacious interventions tailored to immigrant and migrant populations in the US, there are mounting challenges in developing strategies that prevent and control HIV and other sexually transmitted infections (STIs), and that can be sustained and scaled to meet the needs of those most vulnerable to their impact. Community-based participatory research (CBPR) has received increasing recognition as a public health paradigm that combines epidemiology and behavioral science in order to understand how multiple determinants interact to influence health in a particular community. CBPR requires an equitable partnership between researchers and those directly affected by and knowledgeable of the local circumstances that impact health in a given community. Tangible, lasting health benefits require a balance of rigorous research that respectfully, productively, and equally involves community partners.

In this chapter, we offer our reflections on a CBPR project in partnership with the Latino migrant worker community in South Florida. We first discussed how we forged a partnership (known in the community as Project Salud) between researchers and community members. Next, we present the results and evaluate the efficacy of a community-based intervention to

---

This chapter was previously published in *Capacity Building: Planning, Programs and Prospects*, edited by Diane Brown, New York: Nova Publishers Inc., 2016.

* Corresponding Author: Professor Jesús Sánchez, Ph.D. Associate Professor, Department of Sociobehavioral and Administrative Pharmacy, College of Pharmacy, Nova Southeastern University, 3200 South University Drive, Fort Lauderdale, FL 33328-2018. E-mail: js2769@nova.edu.

reduce risk behaviors and enhance mediators of HIV-preventative behaviors. Finally, we attempt to discuss some of the challenges inherent in CBPR and reflect on the question, "is CBPR a good fit?" We aim for our analysis to contribute a unique perspective to the rich, ongoing discussion about developing community capacity as a means to promote health, ameliorate health disparities, and promote justice in marginalized, vulnerable communities.

In: Medicine Research Summaries. Volume 17
Editors: Zhongwen Liáng and Bibao Zhang
ISBN: 978-1-53612-751-5

Chapter 182

MEASURING COMMUNITY CAPACITIES WITH "KEQ": PSYCHOMETRIC TESTS RESULTS FOR A NEWLY DEVELOPED INSTRUMENT FOR HEALTH PROMOTION PROGRAMS IN GERMANY#

Stefan Nickel*, Waldemar Süß and Alf Trojan
University Medical Center Hamburg, Department of Medical Sociology
Martinistraße, Hamburg, Germany

RESEARCH SUMMARY

Introduction: "KEQ" (Kapazitätsentwicklung im Quartier [Capacity Building in Residential Areas/Neighborhoods]) is the name of a newly developed questionnaire for measuring community capacities considered relevant to health. It is particularly based on the preliminary work of Glenn Laverack and Ronald Labonte who originally differentiated between nine domains of community capacities. KEQ is the first measurement instrument for capacity building in Germany, and can be seen as an intermediate outcome parameter for health promotion programs and activities at the community-level. This research was funded by the Federal Ministry of Education and Research.

Objectives: The general research goal was the development of an instrument for the long-term assessment of health promotion activities in disadvantaged neighborhoods. This chapter will start presenting the neighborhood and health promotion program as the context for developing the instrument. The major section will focus on the psychometric testing of the KEQ instrument according to the classical test theory (objectivity, reliability, and validity). Practicality was analyzed in terms of length of time taken to complete the questionnaire, and number of missing values.

This chapter was previously published in *Capacity Building: Planning, Programs and Prospects*, edited by Diane Brown, New York: Nova Publishers Inc., 2016.

* Corresponding Author Email: nickel@uke.de.

Methods: Surveys were conducted to measure community capacities, each with 40 to 60 stakeholders or change agents, from five socially disadvantaged areas in Hamburg, Germany, at different points in time. The KEQ instrument consists of five domains (participation, local leadership, available resources, networking and cooperation, health care) as a 51 item long-form. (A 31 item short-form is currently under development.) Analyses comprised both descriptive and inference statistics.

Results: Psychometric findings on the basis of N=235 respondents (37% out of 638 in total) permit the application of KEQ in small urban communities (about 3,000 to 20,000 residents). Cronbach's alpha as a coefficient of internal consistency ranged between .82 ("available resources") and .94 ("health care"). The results of the five domains of community capacity and their changes over time can best be depicted in spider diagrams. This form of presentation proved to be highly suitable for feed-back to agents of change in the residential areas involved.

Conclusion: The modular design of the questionnaire allows its flexible use for various assessment goals. Supposedly it is more suitable for measuring quality development than for evidence-producing outcome evaluation. Additional approaches are required to compensate for the possibly one-sided expert perspectives in the KEQ assessments (e.g., "triangulation" or "cross-examination" using groups of residents as informants). Further research is needed to study capacity building in association with final health outcomes.

In: Medicine Research Summaries. Volume 17
Editors: Zhongwen Liáng and Bibao Zhang
ISBN: 978-1-53612-751-5

Chapter 183

BUILDING CAPACITY TO ADAPT TO THE CONSEQUENCES OF DISASTER: LINKING DISASTER RECOVERY AND DISASTER RISK REDUCTION#

Douglas Paton[1], PhD, Li-ju Jang[2], PhD and Melanie Irons[3], PhD

[1]School of Psychological and Clinical Sciences, Charles Darwin University, Darwin, Northern Territory, Australia
[2]Department of Social Work, National Pingtung University of Science and Technology, Pingtung, Taiwan, ROC
[3]School of Psychology, University of Tasmania, Hobart, Tasmania, Australia

RESEARCH SUMMARY

In locations that expose citizens to large scale disasters, a key disaster risk reduction (DRR) goal is developing their adaptive capacity. The atypical nature of disasters make it important to understand how people, individually and collectively, adapt when experiencing disaster. This chapter discusses research on disaster recovery in New Zealand (2011 Christchurch earthquake), Taiwan (1999 Chi Chi earthquake) and Australia (2013 Tasmanian wildfire) and the lessons learnt regarding how personal, family, community and societal factors interact to facilitate adaptation to the consequences of disaster.

Data from the 2011 Christchurch earthquake and 1999 Chi Chi earthquake were obtained as survivors confronted the demands of disaster recovery. By collecting data from the 2013 Tasmanian wildfire using a Facebook page (Tassie Fires – We Can Help) specifically developed to assess response and recovery, the chapter offers rare in situ, real-time insights into adaptive demands and adaptive responses. These analyses are used to provide insights into adaption, and how models and theories of capacity building can be developed from such

This chapter was previously published in *Capacity Building: Planning, Programs and Prospects*, edited by Diane Brown, New York: Nova Publishers Inc., 2016.

experience to inform the planning and design of capacity building programs. By conducting this work in countries that differ extensively in their cultural characteristics (comparing Taiwan and Australia/New Zealand), the chapter affords an opportunity to develop understanding of how cultural similarities and differences inform how capacity is developed, sustained and enacted.

In: Medicine Research Summaries. Volume 17
Editors: Zhongwen Liáng and Bibao Zhang
ISBN: 978-1-53612-751-5

Chapter 184

EFFECTIVE TRAINING TOOLS IN LOCAL AND REGIONAL DEVELOPMENT PLANNING AND MANAGEMENT IN AFRICA*,#

Asfaw Kumssa
United Nations Centre for Regional Development (UNCRD),
Africa Office in Nairobi, Kenya

RESEARCH SUMMARY

Regional development planning is a conscious development strategy designed to bring about change and equity, and to improve the living standards of people by integrating economic, social and environmental policies and programmes in a spatial context. The focus in this chapter is on theoretical issues of training on Local and regional development planning and management, including the trainers, trainees, the subject matter and the training methods. Case example is drawn from a training course by the United Nations Centre Regional Development, Arica Office on Local and Regional Development Planning and Management. The aim is to explore the scope of training and regional approaches, including the choice of relevant modules/subjects, training methods, training materials and challenges of training the critical mass of planners. Particular attention is given to the importance of regionalization of training in Africa.

* The views expressed here are the author's own and not necessarily those of the United Nations.

This chapter was previously published in *Capacity Building: Planning, Programs and Prospects*, edited by Diane Brown, New York: Nova Publishers Inc., 2016.

In: Medicine Research Summaries. Volume 17
Editors: Zhongwen Liáng and Bibao Zhang

ISBN: 978-1-53612-751-5

Chapter 185

THE RELEVANCE OF AMH TO HUMAN REPRODUCTIVE BIOLOGY AND MEDICINE[#]

David B. Seifer[1,2,*], MD, and Reshef Tal[3], MD, PhD
[1]Obstetrics and Gynecology, The Geisel School of Medicine at Dartmouth, Hanover, New Hampshire, US
[2]Division of Reproductive Endocrinology and Infertility, Dartmouth-Hitchcock Medical Center, Lebanon, New Hampshire, US
[3]Division of Reproductive Endocrinology and Infertility, Department of Obstetrics, Gynecology and Reproductive Sciences, Yale University School of Medicine, New Haven, Connecticut, US

RESEARCH SUMMARY

This chapter will provide an overview of AMH as an important hormone in human reproductive biology and medicine. Many of the individual topics mentioned will be further addressed in greater detail in the chapters which follow.

It is our hope that a better understanding of AMH's role in ovarian physiology and human reproduction may expand its growing array of clinical applications and lead to more directed therapeutic options in the future for various reproductive disorders.

[#] This chapter was previously published in *Anti-Müllerian Hormone: Biology, Role in Ovarian Function and Clinical Significance*, edited by David B. Seifer and Reshef Tal, New York: Nova Publishers Inc., 2016.

[*] Corresponding Author: David B. Seifer, Professor of Obstetrics and Gynecology, Director of the Division of Reproductive Endocrinology and Infertility; Email: dseifer@comcast.net.

In: Medicine Research Summaries. Volume 17
Editors: Zhongwen Liáng and Bibao Zhang

ISBN: 978-1-53612-751-5

Chapter 186

BASIC BIOLOGY OF AMH: STRUCTURE, SIGNALING PATHWAYS, AND ROLE IN NORMAL FOLLICULOGENESIS[#]

Jenny A. Visser*
Department of Internal Medicine, Erasmus MC, Rotterdam,
The Netherlands

RESEARCH SUMMARY

Anti-Müllerian hormone (AMH) is a member of the transforming growth factor β superfamily of growth and differentiation factors. Similar to other members of this family, AMH undergoes proteolytic cleavage to generate the bioactive ligand and exerts its effects through a specific type II receptor and potentially three type I receptors, the latter shared by bone morphogenetic proteins. In contrast to other family members, which mostly show a broad expression pattern, the expression of AMH is restricted to the gonads. AMH is best known for inducing Müllerian duct regression during male sex differentiation. However, over the past decade, the specific expression pattern of AMH in small growing follicles of the adult ovary has demanded increasing attention, not in the least as this has implicated a role for serum AMH as a marker for ovarian function. This chapter will summarize our current knowledge of the structure of AMH, and the molecular mechanisms underlying the function of AMH in Müllerian duct regression and gonads. In particular, this chapter will discuss the expression pattern and role of AMH in normal ovarian folliculogenesis.

[#] This chapter was previously published in *Anti-Müllerian Hormone: Biology, Role in Ovarian Function and Clinical Significance*, edited by David B. Seifer and Reshef Tal, New York: Nova Publishers Inc., 2016.
* Corresponding Author Email: j.visser@erasmusmc.nl.

In: Medicine Research Summaries. Volume 17
Editors: Zhongwen Liáng and Bibao Zhang
ISBN: 978-1-53612-751-5

Chapter 187

STUDIES ON ANTI-MÜLLERIAN HORMONE PRODUCTION, ACTION, AND REGULATION IN THE PRIMATE OVARY: INSIGHT INTO HUMAN FOLLICULOGENESIS[#]

Jing Xu[1,*], Mary B. Zelinski[1,2] and Richard L. Stouffer[1,2]
[1]Division of Reproductive and Developmental Sciences,
Oregon National Primate Research Center,
Oregon Health and Science University, Beaverton, Oregon, US
[2]Department of Obstetrics and Gynecology,
Oregon Health and Science University, Portland, Oregon, US

RESEARCH SUMMARY

Although examined over the past decade, our current understanding of anti-Müllerian hormone (AMH) actions in the ovary is primarily based on rodent studies. However, not only are the conclusions from rodent studies inconsistent, but there are apparent species differences in follicular AMH actions according to data from nonhuman primate and human studies. Although the relationship between AMH and clinical outcome in assisted reproduction has been studied extensively, data thus far in humans are almost all correlative. Therefore, studies in nonhuman primates are critical to clearly identify the role of AMH in ovarian physiology due to the similarity of their ovarian structure, function, and regulation to those of women. AMH is produced heterogeneously by primate preantral follicles, with an increased expression during subsequent growth till declining after antrum formation. Actions of AMH appear stage-dependent in the primate ovary in contrast to most rodent data. AMH promotes preantral follicle growth and inhibits antral follicle maturation in primates. The in vitro and in vivo studies conducted in nonhuman primates provide mechanistic data on the

---

[#] This chapter was previously published in *Anti-Müllerian Hormone: Biology, Role in Ovarian Function and Clinical Significance*, edited by David B. Seifer and Reshef Tal, New York: Nova Publishers Inc., 2016.

[*] Corresponding Author Email: xujin@ohsu.edu.

role of AMH, as a paracrine effector, in the primate ovary both qualitatively and quantitatively at the molecular, cellular and systemic levels. New information generated from the nonhuman primate studies for the stage-specific AMH manipulation could portend novel therapeutic approaches to regulate follicular development clinically in women, including those with primary ovarian insufficiency, polycystic ovarian syndrome, and reproductive aging.

In: Medicine Research Summaries. Volume 17
Editors: Zhongwen Liáng and Bibao Zhang
ISBN: 978-1-53612-751-5

Chapter 188

OPTIONS FOR CHOOSING DIFFERENT AMH ASSAYS[#]

Richard Fleming*
Glasgow Centre for Reproductive Medicine
University of Glasgow, UK

RESEARCH SUMMARY

The short history of measuring AMH in human serum or plasma has revealed numerous potential applications in reproductive and paediatric medicine. AMH is a stable metabolite in serum and plasma, but technical practicalities mean that all assays are potentially subject to interference from extraneous factors, and one chapter in the history of AMH measurement is a salutary lesson. Differential abilities of the commercial assays to address particular concentration ranges means that some thought should be given to which assays to deploy in particular circumstances. Both of the automated assays available since the end of 2014 display high degrees of consistency over a wide range of concentrations, and we can look forward to a future with greater precision of assessment. In turn, this should lead to greater consensus about critical concentration criteria.

[#] This chapter was previously published in *Anti-Müllerian Hormone: Biology, Role in Ovarian Function and Clinical Significance*, edited by David B. Seifer and Reshef Tal, New York: Nova Publishers Inc., 2016.

* Corresponding Author: Richard Fleming, Scientific Director, Email: Richard.Fleming@gcrm.co.uk.

In: Medicine Research Summaries. Volume 17
Editors: Zhongwen Liáng and Bibao Zhang

ISBN: 978-1-53612-751-5

Chapter 189

The Value of Normative Data on AMH in Women[#]

Joop S. E. Laven*
Division of Reproductive Medicine, Department OBGYN,
Erasmus MC, Rotterdam, The Netherlands

Research Summary

One of the challenges for the reproductive endocrinologist is to predict whether and how long the ovaries of a woman will function properly. The way to ascertain how long the ovary will function normally is by assessing the number of primordial follicles also referred to as the ovarian reserve. Unfortunately, this ovarian reserve can only be assessed indirectly since primordial follicles are generally metabolically inactive.

Nowadays AMH constitutes the most promising marker to assess ovarian reserve because it is produced by early pre- and antral follicles. AMH levels generally rise during the pre-pubertal and adolescent years and decline in an age dependent manner after the age of 25 years. Moreover, AMH levels are fairly constant throughout the menstrual cycle and are minimally affected by the use of OCPs. A small circadian variation in AMH levels is appreciated. Hence, AMH is good and reliable marker for ovarian ageing.

It seems that apart from inhibiting recruitment of primordial follicles out of the ovarian reserve pool AMH plays an important role in modifying the response of an individual follicle to endogenous FSH. High levels of intrafollicular AMH seem to increase the FSH threshold of individual follicles. Moreover intrafollicular AMH levels seem to be independent of a woman's age and gonadotropin levels since normal levels are recorded during pregnancy. Hence it seems that AMH in particular exerts intra-follicular effects.

Nowadays different assays to measure AMH are on the market. During the last decade some problems arose concerning reproducibility of some assays as well AMH assay-specific

---

This chapter was previously published in *Anti-Müllerian Hormone: Biology, Role in Ovarian Function and Clinical Significance*, edited by David B. Seifer and Reshef Tal, New York: Nova Publishers Inc., 2016.

* Corresponding Author: Joop S. E. Laven, Head of Division of Reproductive Medicine; Email: j.laven@erasmusmc.nl.

preanalytical instability. Comparisons amongst different laboratories indicated that the mean bias for all results was acceptable low, but there was large coefficient of repeatability indicating some inconsistency within and between laboratories. Taking the increasing importance of AMH for the assessment of ovarian reserve into account accurate AMH measurements are required. Moreover, to make results obtained by different assays comparable to each other the need for an international standard is even more urgent than ever. Hence there is an urgent need for reliable assays producing normative data measured against an accepted international standard.

In: Medicine Research Summaries. Volume 17
Editors: Zhongwen Liáng and Bibao Zhang

ISBN: 978-1-53612-751-5

Chapter 190

ANTI-MÜLLERIAN HORMONE AND THE PREDICTION OF AGE AT NATURAL MENOPAUSE#

M. Depmann and F. J. M. Broekmans*
Division of Woman and Baby, Voortplantingsgeneeskunde,
University Medical Center Utrecht, Netherlands

RESEARCH SUMMARY

Menopause occurs within a broad age range varying between 40-60 years. The end of natural fertility is postulated to occur ten years prior to menopause. Recent research has been engaged in providing individual age at natural menopause (ANM) predictions. A precise prediction of ANM can aid in identifying women at risk for future infertility and for diseases associated with timing of menopause. Of the candidate markers for ANM predictions (anti-Müllerian hormone (AMH), the Antral Follicle Count and genetic factors as represented by mother's ANM), AMH is the strongest.

Studies providing data on anti-Müllerian hormone and the prediction of menopause all concluded AMH capable of accurately predicting time to menopause or age at menopause even when added to the prediction made by female age alone, making this marker highly promising for use in the day to day clinical practice. Current limitations in the use of AMH stem from assay variation, from inadequate predictions for the extremes of the menopausal age distribution and broad prediction intervals. Future research should therefore focus on enhancing the precision of individual age at menopause predictions by narrowing the prediction interval and by extending the age range of menopause predictions to incorporate the extreme ages.

This chapter was previously published in *Anti-Müllerian Hormone: Biology, Role in Ovarian Function and Clinical Significance*, edited by David B. Seifer and Reshef Tal, New York: Nova Publishers Inc., 2016.

* Corresponding Author Email: f.broekmans@umcutrecht.nl.

In: Medicine Research Summaries. Volume 17
Editors: Zhongwen Liáng and Bibao Zhang
ISBN: 978-1-53612-751-5

Chapter 191

USING AMH FOR DETERMINING A STRATIFIED GONADOTROPIN DOSING REGIMEN FOR IVF/ICSI AND OPTIMIZING OUTCOMES[#]

Joan-Carles Arce[1,*], MD, PhD, Bjarke M. Klein[2], PhD, and Lars Erichsen[3], PhD

[1]Reproductive Health, Global Clinical R and D, Ferring Pharmaceuticals, Copenhagen, Denmark
[2]Biometrics, Global Clinical R and D, Ferring Pharmaceuticals, Copenhagen, Denmark
[3]Experimental Medicine, Global Clinical R and D, Ferring Pharmaceuticals Ferring Pharmaceuticals, Copenhagen, Denmark

RESEARCH SUMMARY

The use of biomarkers and companion diagnostic approaches should provide valuable tools to aid in the optimization of gonadotropin regimens for better treatment outcomes, improved benefit/risk ratio as well as increased cost-effectiveness. Controlled ovarian stimulation with gonadotropins for IVF/ICSI aims to obtain an adequate number of competent oocytes with the minimum risks for the woman. A large variability in ovarian response across patients given the same dose of gonadotropin is a well-recognized phenomenon. This chapter reviews a strategy for gonadotropin dosing by matching specific patient category characteristics to provide an optimal ovarian response while leading to a reduction of safety risks, fewer cycle transfer cancellations and thereby maximizing the chances for successful treatment outcome. This approach presents a way forward where full information from a diagnostic test (AMH) can be used to begin the journey of truly individualizing and personalizing ovarian stimulation for women undergoing infertility treatment.

[#] This chapter was previously published in *Anti-Müllerian Hormone: Biology, Role in Ovarian Function and Clinical Significance*, edited by David B. Seifer and Reshef Tal, New York: Nova Publishers Inc., 2016.

[*] Corresponding Author Email: joan-carles.arce@ferring.com.

In: Medicine Research Summaries. Volume 17
Editors: Zhongwen Liáng and Bibao Zhang
ISBN: 978-1-53612-751-5

Chapter 192

How AMH Assists Counselling for Fertility Preservation Prior to Treatment for Cancer[#]

C. E. Dunlop and R. A. Anderson*
MRC Centre for Reproductive Health, Queens Medical Research Institute, University of Edinburgh, Edinburgh, Scotland

Research Summary

Due to increasing survival rates from nearly all types of cancer, 'oncofertility' has become an emerging field in clinical medicine. With rising numbers of young girls and women being successfully cured by life-saving, but often gonadotoxic treatments, subsequent reproductive health has become a major quality of life issue, with provision of information on treatment-related fertility issues valued highly by patients. With the development of fertility preservation strategies that can be implemented prior to commencing treatment, such as oocyte, embryo and ovarian cortex cryopreservation, the ability to predict which patients may lose their fertility or more drastically undergo premature ovarian insufficiency (POI) as a result of treatment has become of increasing importance. It is now becoming apparent that AMH levels, measured at the time of cancer diagnosis and prior to beginning treatment, can contribute to prediction of permanent post-treatment amenorrhoea, itself indicating loss of the primordial pool. This would prove extremely valuable in helping clinicians advise patients as to whether fertility preservation is prudent if they wish to have their own family in the future. Fertility preservation strategies continue to develop and improve but not every patient will require them; therefore, in order to assist patients in making informed decisions, an individualised approach is crucial. AMH, measured both pre- and post-treatment is now proving to have great potential as a method of assessing long-term ovarian function in this population of cancer patients. The recent development of prognostic tools utilising pre-

---

[#] This chapter was previously published in *Anti-Müllerian Hormone: Biology, Role in Ovarian Function and Clinical Significance*, edited by David B. Seifer and Reshef Tal, New York: Nova Publishers Inc., 2016.

* Corresponding Author Email: Richard.anderson@ed.ac.uk.

treatment AMH levels and age (with potential refinement with other factors such as BMI) to enhance prediction of the probability of continuing ovarian function and perhaps fertility after treatment is completed is likely to prove valuable in the field of fertility preservation.

In: Medicine Research Summaries. Volume 17
Editors: Zhongwen Liáng and Bibao Zhang

ISBN: 978-1-53612-751-5

Chapter 193

AMH IN DIAGNOSIS AND TREATMENT OF GONADAL TUMORS[#]

Geralyn Lambert-Messerlian[1,*], PhD, FACB, and Rodolfo Rey[2], MD, PhD

[1]Women and Infants Hospital,
Alpert Medical School at Brown University,
Department of Pathology and Laboratory Medicine,
Providence, Rhode Island, US
[2]Centro de Investigaciones Endocrinológicas
"Dr. César Bergadá" (CEDIE), CONICET – FEI – División de Endocrinología,
Hospital de Niños Ricardo Gutiérrez,
Buenos Aires, Argentina

RESEARCH SUMMARY

Tumor marker proteins are an important aid in the diagnosis of gonadal malignancies and are essential for monitoring disease progression in treated patients. Anti-Müllerian hormone (AMH), a member of the transforming growth factor-β family, is synthesized by granulosa cells of the ovary and Sertoli cells of the testis. AMH is useful in the differential diagnosis of sex cord-stromal tumors of the ovary and as a serum marker to monitor disease progression in women after treatment for granulosa cell tumor. AMH is also helpful to identify differentiated types of Sertoli cell tumors by immunocytochemistry. The utility of AMH as a gonadal tumor marker and potential biological roles in oncogenesis are presented in this chapter.

[#] This chapter was previously published in *Anti-Müllerian Hormone: Biology, Role in Ovarian Function and Clinical Significance*, edited by David B. Seifer and Reshef Tal, New York: Nova Publishers Inc., 2016.

[*] Corresponding Author: Director, Women and Infants Hospital, Professor, Alpert Medical School at Brown University; Email: gmesserlian@wihri.org; Phone: 401-453-7793, Fax: 401-276-7882.

In: Medicine Research Summaries. Volume 17
Editors: Zhongwen Liáng and Bibao Zhang
ISBN: 978-1-53612-751-5

Chapter 194

ASSESSMENT OF OVARIAN RESERVE BEFORE AND AFTER GYNECOLOGIC SURGERY[#]

Akira Iwase*
Department of Maternal and Perinatal Medicine,
Nagoya University Hospital, Nagoya, Japan

RESEARCH SUMMARY

Anti-Müllerian hormone (AMH) serum levels have been recently applied to the assessment of ovarian reserve apart from infertility treatments due to the advantages in clinical use, such as intra- and inter-cycle consistency. Surgical interventions for benign gynecologic conditions as well as diseases themselves possibly affect ovarian reserve. Such gynecologic conditions and interventions include endometriosis/endometriomas, benign ovarian tumor, hydrosalpinx, ovarian cystectomy, salpingectomy, and hysterectomy. Most studies demonstrate a decline in serum AMH levels after cystectomy for endometriomas, especially in bilateral cases. It is not conclusive whether electrocoagulation or suturing as a surgical method for hemostasis after cystectomy is preferable for ovarian reserve. The effects of other gynecologic diseases including benign ovarian cysts/tumors and interventions, such as hysterectomy and salpingectomy, on ovarian reserve are controversial. Ovarian reserve is severely decreased following unilateral oophorectomy with/without chemotherapy, in patients with ovarian malignancies who desire future fertility. Serum AMH levels allow quantitative evaluation of ovarian reserve, and should be considered as a marker in determining the indication and selection of operative methods for benign gynecologic conditions. However, there is little available information regarding the correlation between the probabilities of live births and serum AMH levels before and after surgical interventions.

[#] This chapter was previously published in *Anti-Müllerian Hormone: Biology, Role in Ovarian Function and Clinical Significance*, edited by David B. Seifer and Reshef Tal, New York: Nova Publishers Inc., 2016.

[*] Corresponding Author: Akira Iwase, Department of Obstetrics and Gynecology, Nagoya University Graduate School of Medicine, 65 Tsurumai-cho, Showa-ku, Nagoya 466-8550, Japan, Telephone: +81-52-744-2261; Fax: +81-52-744-2268, e-mail: akiwase@med.nagoya-u.ac.jp.

In: Medicine Research Summaries. Volume 17
Editors: Zhongwen Liáng and Bibao Zhang
ISBN: 978-1-53612-751-5

Chapter 195

THE UTILITY OF AMH IN THE DIAGNOSIS AND TREATMENT OF PCOS[#]

A. Dumont*, G. Robin, S. Catteau-Jonard and D. Dewailly
Service de Gynécologie Endocrinienne et de Médecine de la Reproduction,
Hôpital Jeanne de Flandre, CHRU de Lille, France

RESEARCH SUMMARY

Polycystic ovary syndrome (PCOS) is the most common cause of chronic anovulation and hyperandrogenism in young women as it affects 5 to 10% of the world female population. Since 2003, PCOS is mainly defined by the Rotterdam Consensus that considers the antral follicle count (AFC) on ultrasound as one of the diagnostic criteria. With the improvement of ultrasonographic techniques, the number of follicles seen on ultrasound increases every day but remains dependent upon the equipment. Serum AMH (Anti-Müllerian Hormone) has been shown to be synthetized by small antral follicles, which are precisely the ones seen on ultrasound. Serum AMH could therefore be used as a surrogate to the AFC in the diagnosis of PCOS. Serum AMH has also demonstrated its utility in the treatment of infertility, frequently associated with PCOS. It appears to be a predictive factor for ovarian response and also for the laparoscopic ovarian drilling efficacy. However, the lack of an international standard for the serum AMH assay and the difficulty to define thresholds makes it difficult so far to use serum AMH commonly.

[#] This chapter was previously published in *Anti-Müllerian Hormone: Biology, Role in Ovarian Function and Clinical Significance*, edited by David B. Seifer and Reshef Tal, New York: Nova Publishers Inc., 2016.

* Corresponding Author Email: agathe.dumont@hotmail.fr.

In: Medicine Research Summaries. Volume 17
Editors: Zhongwen Liáng and Bibao Zhang
ISBN: 978-1-53612-751-5

Chapter 196

THE ROLE OF AMH IN ENDOMETRIOSIS[#]

Patrizia Carrarelli, Lucia Funghi, Alessandra Gatti, Felice Arcuri* and Felice Petraglia
Università degli Studi di Siena,
Department of Molecular and Developmental Medicine,
Siena, Italy

RESEARCH SUMMARY

Endometriosis is a benign estrogen-dependent gynecologic disorder, characterized by the presence and growth of functional endometrial-like tissue outside the uterus, in which, in addition to immune, environmental and genetic factors, circulating estradiol (E2) contributes to the progression of the disease. AMH acts as a regulator of cell growth in cells and tissues of Müllerian origins, such as endometrium, ovary, cervix and breast; a role for AMH as potential therapeutic factor in tumors originating from these tissues has been proposed. In endometriosis, AMH induces important biological effects on cultured endometrial stromal cells. The high levels reported in ovarian endometrioma (OMA) and deep endometriotic nodules (DIE) indicate a role for AMH in the control of cell proliferation and apoptosis.

[#] This chapter was previously published in *Anti-Müllerian Hormone: Biology, Role in Ovarian Function and Clinical Significance*, edited by David B. Seifer and Reshef Tal, New York: Nova Publishers Inc., 2016.

* Corresponding Author Email: arcuri@unisi.it.

In: Medicine Research Summaries. Volume 17
Editors: Zhongwen Liáng and Bibao Zhang
ISBN: 978-1-53612-751-5

Chapter 197

APPLICATIONS OF AMH IN PEDIATRIC ENDOCRINOLOGY[#]

Analía V. Freire, Romina P. Grinspon and Rodolfo A. Rey*
Centro de Investigaciones Endocrinológicas "Dr. César Bergadá" (CEDIE)
CONICET – FEI – División de Endocrinología, Hospital de Niños Ricardo Gutiérrez,
Buenos Aires, Argentina

RESEARCH SUMMARY

Anti-Müllerian hormone (AMH) is produced by Sertoli cells of the testis at high levels until puberty and by ovarian granulosa cells of primary and small growing follicles until menopausal transition. In children, serum AMH is 20-50-fold higher in boys than in girls. Due to the decrease in adult testicular production, serum AMH is only 2-5-fold higher in adult males than females. AMH is a useful marker to assess ovarian follicular reserve in girls and women in reproductive age. Conditions affecting the pool of small follicles in girls and adolescents, like Turner syndrome, galactosemia or cancer treatment, result in a decrease in circulating AMH. Conversely, serum AMH remains within the normal range in hypogonadal states where the pool of small follicles is not disrupted, like ovarian autoimmunity, FSH resistant ovaries and hypogonadotropic hypogonadism. On the other hand, serum AMH is elevated in conditions presenting with an increased follicular cell mass, like polycystic ovary syndrome or sex-cord stromal tumors. In males, serum AMH is especially useful to assess testicular function during infancy, childhood and puberty. In boys with nonpalpable gonads, AMH detection suggests the existence of intraabdominal testes whereas nondetectable serum AMH is indicative of anorchia. AMH may be low in certain categories of cryptorchid patients, but not in all of them. For instance, Klinefelter boys have normal AMH until mid-puberty. In boys with precocious puberty, AMH is low for age, and recovers normal prepubertal levels when the condition is effectively treated. Serum AMH is low in patients

---

[#] This chapter was previously published in *Anti-Müllerian Hormone: Biology, Role in Ovarian Function and Clinical Significance*, edited by David B. Seifer and Reshef Tal, New York: Nova Publishers Inc., 2016.

* Corresponding Author: rodolforey@cedie.org.ar; Tel. (+54-11) 4963-5931 ext. 133 – Fax: (+54-11) 4963-5930.

with hypogonadotropic hypogonadism but normal in boys with constitutional delay of puberty. Finally, serum AMH determination is helpful in the differential diagnoses of patients with disorders of sex development.

In: Medicine Research Summaries. Volume 17
Editors: Zhongwen Liáng and Bibao Zhang
ISBN: 978-1-53612-751-5

Chapter 198

ANTI-MÜLLERIAN HORMONE AND PREMATURE OVARIAN INSUFFICIENCY#

Laetitia Jacquesson, Anne Bachelot and Philippe Touraine*
Department of Endocrinology and Reproductive Medicine Pitié-Salpêtrière Hospital,
Publique-Hôpitaux de Paris,
Université Pierre et Marie Curie, Paris, France
Center of Rare Gynecologic Diseases,
Center of Rare Growth Hormone Disorders

RESEARCH SUMMARY

Premature ovarian insufficiency (POI) is a disorder affecting approximately 1% of women under 40 years of age. POI encompasses a heterogeneous spectrum of conditions, through two major mechanisms: follicle dysfunction and follicle depletion. POI etiologies include genetic disorder such as Turner syndrome, autoimmune disease, and iatrogenic causes such as surgery, radiotherapy or chemotherapy.

AMH is a dimeric glycoprotein produced by the granulosa cells and acts as an inhibitor of primordial follicles recruitment. Some animal models of premature ovarian failure could help us to understand the possible link between AMH and factors involved in POI.

This chapter was previously published in *Anti-Müllerian Hormone: Biology, Role in Ovarian Function and Clinical Significance*, edited by David B. Seifer and Reshef Tal, New York: Nova Publishers Inc., 2016.

* Corresponding Author: Philippe Touraine, MD, PhD, IE3M, Department of Endocrinology and Reproductive Medicine, Groupe Hospitalier Pitié-Salpêtrière, 47-83, boulevard de l'Hôpital, 75013 Paris, France; Phone: +33 1 42 16 02 54, Fax: +33 1 42 16 02 55, Correspondence e-mail: philippe.touraine@psl.aphp.fr.

In: Medicine Research Summaries. Volume 17
Editors: Zhongwen Liáng and Bibao Zhang
ISBN: 978-1-53612-751-5

Chapter 199

A Critical Evaluation of Whether Circulating Anti-Müllerian Hormone Is a Hormone in Adults, with Special Reference to Its Putative Roles in Men[#]

Ian S. McLennan[1,2*], Yih Harng Chong[1,3], Yui Kawagishi[1] and Michael W. Pankhurst[1]

[1] Department of Anatomy, Otago School of Medical Sciences, Dunedin, New Zealand
[2]Brain Health Research Centre, Dunedin, New Zealand
[3]Department of Medicine, Dunedin School of Medicine,
University of Otago, Dunedin, New Zealand

Research Summary

Anti-Müllerian hormone (AMH) is present in blood but despite its nomenclature has no overt endocrine roles. This chapter reviews the basic endocrinology of AMH, and discusses why its functions might be cryptic. AMH is a member of the TGFβ superfamily that produce context-dependent regulation of development and homeostasis. This large family share a small number of receptors and binding proteins resulting in cellular signalling that emerges from multiple interactions. Consequently, the absence of one ligand typically results in subtle dysregulation, rather than an overt loss of function. AMH has been considered to be an atypical TGFβ, as it uniquely triggers the degeneration of the Müllerian duct. We suggest that AMH displays distinct paracrine and endocrine signalling. Systemic AMH may be a conventional TGFβ superfamily ligand that exerts a gonadal influence to TGFβ signalling in multiple tissues. Circulating AMH is a mixture of the uncleaved prohormone (proAMH) and a non-covalent complex of the N- and C-terminal peptide ($AMH_{N,C}$). ProAMH cannot

This chapter was previously published in *Anti-Müllerian Hormone: Biology, Role in Ovarian Function and Clinical Significance*, edited by David B. Seifer and Reshef Tal, New York: Nova Publishers Inc., 2016.

* Corresponding Author: Ian S. McLennan, Lindo Ferguson Building, Great King Street, PO Box 913, Dunedin 9054, New Zealand. Email: ian.mclennan@otago.ac.nz.

activate AMH receptors, and the AMH-mediated gonadal influence may be modulated by the regulation of its cleavage, both within and outside of the gonads. Ovarian AMH exhibit age-dependent decline, but the age-related changes in testicular secretion are more variable. Elderly men on average have lower levels of AMH than younger men, but with high intrapersonal variation. Some elderly men lack AMH in their circulation. These age-related changes in AMH are only weakly linked to the other Sertoli cell hormone (inhibin B) and the leydig cell hormones. Consequently, elderly men are very diverse in their testicular output. The examination of the traits of men with varying levels of AMH is at an early stage, with initial studies showing multiple associations between AMH and cardiovascular parameters. In conclusion, AMH appears to be a non-classical hormone whose functions have been hidden because it is a component of a complex regulatory system. The importance of AMH and the breadth of its functions are largely unknown.

In: Medicine Research Summaries. Volume 17
Editors: Zhongwen Liáng and Bibao Zhang
ISBN: 978-1-53612-751-5

Chapter 200

SUMMARY OF CURRENT STATE OF AMH UTILISATION IN CLINICAL REPRODUCTIVE MEDICINE[#]

Scott M. Nelson*
Obstetrics and Gynaecology
School of Medicine, University of Glasgow, Scotland

RESEARCH SUMMARY

Personalisation of prognosis and treatment requires accurate phenotyping. AMH provides a critical step towards achieving a precise measure of the functional ovarian reserve and anticipated ovarian response and exhibits superior technical and performance characteristics than any other biomarker including AFC. The actual ovarian response as measured by endocrine parameters or oocyte yield will inevitably be highly variable reflecting differing follicular development patterns and the technical aspects of oocyte retrieval respectively. However, despite these limitations, AMH has now consistently been shown to be useful in prognostication of live birth independent of other amnesic factors and in the stratification of care. That AMH can ensure treatment naïve patients achieve an optimal oocyte yield with a minimal risk of iatrogenic complication is a significant contribution and suggests a future where ovarian stimulation without predetermination of AMH is clinically naïve and potentially negligent.

[#] This chapter was previously published in *Anti-Müllerian Hormone: Biology, Role in Ovarian Function and Clinical Significance*, edited by David B. Seifer and Reshef Tal, New York: Nova Publishers Inc., 2016.

* Corresponding Author: Scott M. Nelson, Muirhead Professor of Obstetrics and Gynaecology, Level 2 New Lister Building, Glasgow Royal Infirmary, University of Glasgow, GLASGOW, G31 2ER, Email: scott.nelson@glasgow.ac.uk.

In: Medicine Research Summaries. Volume 17
Editors: Zhongwen Liáng and Bibao Zhang
ISBN: 978-1-53612-751-5

Chapter 201

RACIAL/ETHNIC DIFFERENCES IN AMH AND POTENTIAL UNDERLYING MECHANISMS[#]

Reshef Tal[1,*], MD, PhD, and David B. Seifer[2,3], MD
[1]Division of Reproductive Endocrinology and Infertility,
Department of Obstetrics, Gynecology and Reproductive Sciences,
Yale University School of Medicine, New Haven, Connecticut, US
[2]Obstetrics and Gynecology, The Geisel School of Medicine
at Dartmouth, Hanover, New Hampshire, US
[3]Division of Reproductive Endocrinology and Infertility,
Dartmouth-Hitchcock Medical Center, Lebanon, New Hampshire, US

RESEARCH SUMMARY

Accumulating evidence suggests that reproductive potential and function may be different across racial and ethnic groups. Racial differences have been demonstrated in pubertal timing, incidence of several gynecologic diseases, infertility, outcomes after assisted reproductive technology (ART) treatment and reproductive aging. Recently, racial differences have also been described in serum anti-Müllerian hormone (AMH), a sensitive biomarker of ovarian reserve, supporting the notion that ovarian reserve differs between racial/ethnic groups.

The existence of such racial/ethnic differences in ovarian reserve, as reflected by AMH, may have important clinical implications for reproductive endocrinologists. However, the mechanisms which may underlie such racial differences in ovarian reserve are unclear. Various genetic factors, and environmental factors such as obesity, smoking and vitamin D deficiency which have been shown to correlate with serum AMH levels and also display significant racial/ethnic variations are discussed in this chapter. Improving our understanding of racial differences in AMH and reproductive aging may lead to better counseling of women

[#] This chapter was previously published in *Anti-Müllerian Hormone: Biology, Role in Ovarian Function and Clinical Significance*, edited by David B. Seifer and Reshef Tal, New York: Nova Publishers Inc., 2016.
[*] Corresponding Author Email: reshef.tal@yale.edu.

regarding their reproductive planning, individualization of infertility treatments and improved outcomes, as well as timely interventions which may prolong reproductive lifespan in these women.

In: Medicine Research Summaries. Volume 17
Editors: Zhongwen Liáng and Bibao Zhang

ISBN: 978-1-53612-751-5

Chapter 202

INFLUENCE OF COMBINED CONTRACEPTIVES ON SERUM AMH[#]

Christopher E. Gibson[1], MD, and Clarisa R. Gracia[2,3,*], MD, MSCE
[1]Division of Pediatric Endocrinology and Diabetes,
Children's Hospital of Philadelphia, Philadelphia, US
[2]Department of Obstetrics/Gynecology,
[3]Division of Reproductive Endocrinology and Infertility,
University of Pennsylvania School of Medicine, Philadelphia, US

RESEARCH SUMMARY

Anti-Müllerian hormone (AMH) levels have become a widely used clinical test in fertility and ovarian reserve evaluations. As the testing used to measure AMH becomes more accurate, the interpretation becomes more important for patients. However, multiple clinical factors and medications can alter AMH and interpretations should be made with caution. This is especially true in women on combined hormonal contraceptive therapy. Although numerous studies have focused on the patterns of AMH during combined contraceptive therapy, the results have been mixed supporting either decreased AMH levels versus no change principally related to limitations in study design. And while most of these studies have shown a decreased antral follicle count (AFC) with a predominance of smaller follicles during combined contraceptive therapy, the connection with AMH is still being explored. There has also been some investigation into the duration of hormonal contraceptive therapy and ethinyl estradiol (EE) dosing, although nothing definitive can be concluded from these studies to date. AMH interpretation during combined hormonal contraceptive therapy is further complicated by specific medical diagnoses, such as polycystic ovarian syndrome or prior cancer history. Therefore, careful emphasis should be placed on both medical history and

[#] This chapter was previously published in *Anti-Müllerian Hormone: Biology, Role in Ovarian Function and Clinical Significance*, edited by David B. Seifer and Reshef Tal, New York: Nova Publishers Inc., 2016.

[*] Corresponding Author Email: cgracia@obgyn.upenn.edu.

hormonal contraceptive use when evaluating AMH levels in women. Moving forward, further studies are needed to help clarify AMH patterns during combined hormonal contraceptive therapy, highlighting the correlation between AMH and hormonal contraceptive duration and dosing as well as prior medical conditions.

In: Medicine Research Summaries. Volume 17
Editors: Zhongwen Liáng and Bibao Zhang
ISBN: 978-1-53612-751-5

Chapter 203

ANTI-MÜLLERIAN HORMONE AND OBESITY[#]

Vicky Moy and Erkan Buyuk*
Department of Obstetrics, Gynecology and Women's Health,
Albert Einstein College of Medicine, Bronx, NY, US

RESEARCH SUMMARY

Obesity continues to be an epidemic in the United States, negatively impacting overall morbidity and mortality, as well as reproductive outcomes. Although the effect of obesity on fertility is likely multi-faceted, obese patients exhibit an altered ovarian follicular environment that impairs steroidogenic action, folliculogenesis and metabolism, and is associated with inflammation, which may contribute to these poor outcomes. Anti-Müllerian hormone (AMH), produced by the granulosa cells of preantral and antral follicles, has been demonstrated to be a useful marker of ovarian reserve; AMH is the earliest marker to change with aging and has minimal inter- and intra-cycle variability. The relation between obesity and serum AMH levels is complex. Age, presence or absence of PCOS, the status of glucose metabolism like insulin resistance states, and potentially race may affect this interaction. The effect of weight loss on serum AMH levels is less clear. It is dependent on the above-mentioned factors, as well as the type of intervention like caloric restriction, physical activity, medical or surgical treatment. Consequently, despite the abundance of publications that study the relationship between obesity and AMH levels, the results are conflicting with lack of a consensus. Elucidation of the mechanisms of the effects of obesity states on serum AMH levels will improve our understanding of these complex interactions, potentially leading to discovery of therapies that may improve reproductive function.

[#] This chapter was previously published in *Anti-Müllerian Hormone: Biology, Role in Ovarian Function and Clinical Significance*, edited by David B. Seifer and Reshef Tal, New York: Nova Publishers Inc., 2016.

* Corresponding Author Email: erbuyuk@yahoo.com.

In: Medicine Research Summaries. Volume 17
Editors: Zhongwen Liáng and Bibao Zhang
ISBN: 978-1-53612-751-5

Chapter 204

ASSOCIATION BETWEEN VITAMIN D AND ANTI-MÜLLERIAN HORMONE[#]

Mohamad Irani[1,*] and Zaher Merhi[2]
[1]Weill Cornell Medical Center, The Ronal O. Perelman and Claudia Cohen Center for Reproductive Medicine, New York, NY, US
[2]NYU School of Medicine, Department of Obstetrics and Gynecology, New York, NY, US

RESEARCH SUMMARY

Vitamin D is a steroid hormone that is mainly synthesized in the skin after exposure to ultraviolet sunlight. 10% of bodily Vitamin D is obtained from diet. Approximately one billion people worldwide have Vitamin D insufficiency/deficiency. Vitamin D receptor is present in many reproductive organs and thus plays an important role in reproduction. This chapter underscores the association between Vitamin D and anti-Müllerian hormone (AMH)- one of the best serum markers of ovarian reserve. Vitamin D induces AMH gene expression in prostate cancer cell line. However, in hen granulosa cells, it decreases AMH mRNA levels and increases FSH sensitivity by upregulating FSH receptor expression. This indicates that Vitamin D might play a role in follicle selection, maturation, and possibly ovulation in the hen. In human cumulus granulosa cells, Vitamin D reduces AMH sensitivity by downregulating AMH receptor gene expression, and possibly facilitating follicular differentiation and maturity. In reproductive-aged women, serum AMH level is positively correlated with serum 25 hydroxy-vitamin D level suggesting that Vitamin D deficiency might be associated with lower ovarian reserve. In Vitamin D-deficient women with PCOS, Vitamin D supplementation decreases the abnormally elevated serum AMH levels. This might represent a mechanism by which Vitamin D improves the ovulatory dysfunction observed in women with PCOS since less AMH indicates higher follicular sensitivity to FSH.

[#] This chapter was previously published in *Anti-Müllerian Hormone: Biology, Role in Ovarian Function and Clinical Significance*, edited by David B. Seifer and Reshef Tal, New York: Nova Publishers Inc., 2016.

[*] Corresponding Author Email: Mohamad.irani@hotmail.com.

Defining the exact role, dose and duration of supplementation, as well as serum cutoff levels of Vitamin D in female reproduction might allow us to use this inexpensive, easily accessible, and relatively safe vitamin as a therapeutic adjunct for ovarian health in reproductive-aged women. Properly designed studies are required to assess the role of Vitamin D in female reproduction particularly in women with diminished ovarian reserve and women with PCOS.

In: Medicine Research Summaries. Volume 17
Editors: Zhongwen Liáng and Bibao Zhang

ISBN: 978-1-53612-751-5

Chapter 205

ANTI-MÜLLERIAN HORMONE (AMH) AND *FMR1* GENOTYPE[#]

A. Shohat-Tal[*] and N. Gleicher
Center for Human Reproduction,
New York, NY, US

RESEARCH SUMMARY

FMR1 (fragile-X mental retardation 1 gene)-associated ovarian dysfunction has historically been linked to carriage of premutation alleles (i.e., 55-200 CGG repeats in the 5'-untranslated region of the gene), though in recent years other forms of ovarian dysfunction, including diminished ovarian reserve, have been associated with carriage of intermediate ($CGG_{n=45\text{-}55}$), low-normal ($CGG_{n<26}$) or high normal ($CGG_{n>35}$) alleles. Molecular studies in mice and *Drosophila* implicate FMR1 protein (FMRP) in folliculogenesis and in inhibition of primordial follicle recruitment, potentially through its role in translational regulation and the miRNA pathway. Anti-müllerian hormone (AMH) is also known to play a role in repressing the primordial to primary follicle transition, suggesting AMH and FMRP may collaborate in regulating the rate of follicular depletion. Clinical studies stratified for age and/or CGG count reveal an association between *FMR1* genotype and AMH levels in infertile women and in fertile women with early ovarian decline. *FMR1* genotype appears to be associated with the dynamics of AMH decline with age. Future longitudinal studies are needed to corroborate these findings and evaluate *FMR1* genotyping as a diagnostic tool to predict diminishing ovarian reserve before the onset of AMH decline, allowing women more informed reproductive planning and evaluation of fertility preservation options.

[#] This chapter was previously published in *Anti-Müllerian Hormone: Biology, Role in Ovarian Function and Clinical Significance*, edited by David B. Seifer and Reshef Tal, New York: Nova Publishers Inc., 2016.

[*] Corresponding Author Email: atal@thechr.com.

In: Medicine Research Summaries. Volume 17
Editors: Zhongwen Liáng and Bibao Zhang
ISBN: 978-1-53612-751-5

Chapter 206

AMH Screening of Ovarian Reserve in the General Population: A Risk-Benefit Analysis[#]

Kelton Tremellen[1,*], MB, BS (Hons), PhD, FRANZCOG, CREI and Neerja Kamal[2], MB, BS, FRANZCOG, MRMed
[1]Gynaecologist and Reproductive Endocrinologist,
Reproductive Medicine, Flinders University,
Bedford Park, SA, Australia
[2]Gynaecologist, Flinders Fertility,
Bedford Park, SA, Australia

Research Summary

AMH based ovarian reserve screening has generally not been supported for two key reasons. Firstly, opponents suggest that since a poor result does not necessarily suggest impaired chances of natural conception in the immediate term, then the test has no value. Secondly, these opponents believe that a poor result may cause anxiety for patients, triggering them to make potentially unwise decisions such as conceiving in an unstable relationship, or undertaking expensive and potentially harmful oocyte cryopreservation procedures. However, in this chapter we will argue that screening of ovarian reserve status does have considerable merit as it prognosticates for IVF related conception, plus identifies diminished ovarian reserve early when symptoms are absent yet the chances of conception are still favourable if plans for starting a family are brought forward. Furthermore, evidence suggests that alternatives to screening such as education of the population about the perils of delaying conception have not been effective in changing reproductive behaviour because women often

---

[#] This chapter was previously published in *Anti-Müllerian Hormone: Biology, Role in Ovarian Function and Clinical Significance*, edited by David B. Seifer and Reshef Tal, New York: Nova Publishers Inc., 2016.

* Corresponding Author: Kelton Tremellen, Consultant Gynaecologist and Reproductive Endocrinologist, Professor of Reproductive Medicine, Flinders University, Bedford Park, South Australia; Email: kelton.tremellen@flinders.edu.au.

overestimate their own personal fertility potential. We contend that AMH based screening of ovarian reserve "personalises" ovarian reserve status, making screening a more effective trigger for changing reproductive behaviour than mere generic advice alone.

However, we do recognise that screening can trigger adverse outcomes and therefore should only be offered to those women who have undergone appropriate pre-screening counselling regarding its merits and potential actions that may arise from adverse results.

In: Medicine Research Summaries. Volume 17
Editors: Zhongwen Liáng and Bibao Zhang

ISBN: 978-1-53612-751-5

Chapter 207

FUTURE RESEARCH AND POTENTIAL THERAPEUTIC APPLICATIONS: AGONISTS AND ANTAGONISTS#

Elodie Adda-Herzog[1,*], Nathalie di Clemente[2,3,4] and Renato Fanchin[1,3,4]

[1]Center of Reproductive Medicine and Biology, Obstetrics and Gynecology Department, Hôpital Antoine Béclère (AP-HP), Paris-Sud University, Orsay, France
[2]Paris Diderot University, Sorbonne Paris Cité, Paris, France
[3]CNRS, UMR 8251, Paris, France
[4]INSERM U1133, Paris, France

RESEARCH SUMMARY

Anti-Müllerian hormone (AMH), a glycoprotein exclusively produced by the granulosa cells of ovarian follicles in the adult female, is not only a putative biomarker of ovarian follicular status but also an important factor in the folliculogenesis process. Manipulating AMH or its specific receptor AMHR-II opens perspectives in controlling both initial follicle recruitment and FSH-dependent, cyclic follicle recruitment. On the one hand, some antibodies directed to AMH could be serviceable to improve follicle recruitment and response of antral follicles to controlled ovarian hyperstimulation. On the other, AMH antagonist administration might be useful in some disorders characterized by follicle excess and arrest as in polycystic ovary syndrome (PCOS). Furthermore, proliferative pathologies such as ovarian malignancies or endometriosis express AMHR-II receptors and, AMH has proven its efficacy in decreasing proliferation of these cells in vitro. Finally, follicular burnout has been described after ovarian toxic agents such as cyclophosphamide or after ovarian graft of cryopreserved tissue. Using

---

This chapter was previously published in *Anti-Müllerian Hormone: Biology, Role in Ovarian Function and Clinical Significance*, edited by David B. Seifer and Reshef Tal, New York: Nova Publishers Inc., 2016.

* Corresponding Author: Elodie Adda-Herzog. Center of Reproductive Medicine and Biology, Obstetrics and gynecology department, Hôpital Antoine Béclère (AP-HP), Paris-Sud University. E-mail: elodie.adda-herzog @abc.aphp.fr.

AMH agonists may prevent this deleterious effect, preserving follicular reserve in these patients. Exploring therapeutically the regulatory role played by AMH in folliculogenesis constitutes a promising research axis for improving ovarian function in infertile patients.